the **health studies** companion

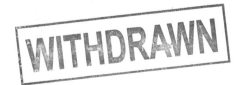

Palgrave Student Companions are a one-stop reference resource that provide essential information for students about the subject – and the course – they've chosen to study.

Friendly and authoritative, **Palgrave Student Companions** support the student throughout their degree. They encourage the reader to think about study skills alongside the subject matter of their course, offer guidance on module and career choices, and act as an invaluable source book and reference that they can return to time and again.

Palgrave Student Companions – your course starts here

Published

The English Language and Linguistics Companion
The English Literature Companion
The Health Studies Companion
The MBA Companion
The Nursing Companion
The Politics Companion
The Psychology Companion
The Social Work Companion

Forthcoming

The Anthropology Companion
The Economics Companion
The History Companion
The Law Companion
The Media Studies Companion
The Sociology Companion
The Theatre, Drama and Performance Companion

Further titles are planned

www.palgravestudentcompanions.com

the **health studies** companion

Sophie Smailes and Clare Street

Your course starts here

palgrave
macmillan

First published 2011 by
PALGRAVE MACMILLAN

Palgrave Macmillan in the UK is an imprint of Macmillan Publishers Limited,
registered in England, company number 785998, of Houndmills, Basingstoke,
Hampshire RG21 6XS.

Palgrave Macmillan in the US is a division of St Martin's Press LLC,
175 Fifth Avenue, New York, NY 10010.

Palgrave Macmillan is the global academic imprint of the above companies
and has companies and representatives throughout the world.

Palgrave® and Macmillan® are registered trademarks in the United States,
the United Kingdom, Europe and other countries

ISBN 978–1–4039–4187–9
ISBN 978–0–230–34552–2 (eBook)
DOI 10.1007/978-0-230-34552-2

This book is printed on paper suitable for recycling and made from fully
managed and sustained forest sources. Logging, pulping and manufacturing
processes are expected to conform to the environmental regulations of the
country of origin.

A catalogue record for this book is available from the British Library.

10 9 8 7 6 5 4 3 2 1
20 19 18 17 16 15 14 13 12 11

contents

acknowledgements   vi

introduction   1

1   studying health: health as a contested concept   9

2   key ideologies   31

3   key terms and concepts   55

4   case studies   124

5   research   185

6   health and social care careers: from the classroom to the workplace   336

glossary   365

references   371

index   401

acknowledgements

Tahira Majothi I would like first to thank Clare and Sophie for suggesting that a careers chapter should be included as part of the Companion, and for allowing me to work on the chapter. Clare and Sophie have both been so supportive of my ideas and provided vital feedback on the overall arc. It's been an innovative approach but, given the vocational nature of the subject matter, an excellent way to contextualise career planning and progress from the classroom to the workplace. I would also like to thank Laura and Julie for agreeing to be interviewed.

Clare Street My thanks go to my colleagues and the students at MMU for their inspiration and support, but also to my friends, parents and particularly my husband Bernard for his sustenance – moral and nutritional.

Sophie Smailes The writing of this book would not have been possible without the support, encouragement and cajolement of my friends; the interest and engagement of my colleagues; the inspiration afforded to me by my students; and the kindly forbearance of my partner. I particularly want to acknowledge the role that my parents' love of the written word and their ever inquiring minds has had in equipping me to embark on this writing journey.

introduction

This text introduces you, the student, to a range of ideas pertaining to the study of health and the field of Health and Social Care Studies, a fairly recent addition to the variety of health-related courses on offer to students at different levels of study. You will notice, for example, that such courses have a range of titles, including 'Health Studies', 'Health and Social Care', 'Health and Social Change', 'Social Change'. For simplification we will refer to this gamut of courses as 'Health Studies'. The term Health Studies can be, on first acquaintance, somewhat of a misnomer – not least because the term 'health' itself is a fluid and contested set of ideas, concepts and experiences. Nevertheless, the experience of health (and illness), the treatment or set of actions taken with regard to health (or illness) and our continuing desire to understand more about what constitutes, affects and fosters health take up a huge proportion of (global) governmental, institutional and individual time, energy and finance and all contribute to our growing interest in 'Health Studies'.

Reflective activity

- Type 'health stories' into an Internet search engine and see just how many news items are listed, and their range.
- What does this suggest to you about the importance of 'health' in our society?

Interest in health is part of our everyday life. Looking at the Reflective Activity below, see if you can recognise practices you might encounter, consume or think about in a single day that could relate to health, and then develop your own list and explore why you engage in these activities:

Reflective activity

What about the following? Do any of these relate to you?
- Brushing your teeth (a habitual daily dental health practice).
- Eating/drinking 'healthily'.
- Prescriptions, vitamins, moisturisers, oils, supplements.
- Visits to the doctor, dentist, hospital, counsellor, reflexologist, masseuse, podiatrist, beautician.
- Visits from the GP, nurse, midwife, healer etc.

- Exercise classes, yoga, pilates, football, meditation, walking.
- Healthy sleep patterns.
- Healthy sex life.
- Spending time with your family and friends.

Add any others you can think of.

Are you influenced by anything in your choices, e.g. choices of food?

Our approach to this text

We have written this text in particular ways, ways that reflect our own 'take' on the study of health (and Health Studies), as well as ways that are designed to get you, the student, fully engaged in the process of learning about 'health'.

First, in terms of your studying 'health' we believe that, at a very fundamental level, it is not the same as studying English or Drama or even Psychology, in that it is an *experience* and *identity* as well as a phenomenon (a 'thing') that can studied. It is as broad and complex as the very notion of 'health' itself and relates to a vast number of professions (and subsections of other professions). Significantly, then, 'health' is more than an interesting subject to study. It is probably the most fundamental concern to individuals and governments (globally, historically) and, in a sense, it is as broad as studying 'life' itself. As daunting as that might sound, it does offer some context to the breadth and diversity of courses on offer.

Second, we acknowledge that all of you reading this text and embarking on the study of health, given that health and illness are imbued within the very fabric of our society, will already have ideas about what health, illness and disease mean, and these ideas are already 'taken-for-granted'. In other words, many of us do not consider that these very assumptions (which we often locate as 'common sense') are underpinned by a set of meanings and values, and have origins that are deeply influential and interwoven within the fabric of our society. Many Health Studies courses may also reflect this stance, being primarily about what we already 'know', i.e. learning about physiological systems, psychosocial approaches to health and how to promote or manage health. Some of those ideas you will find here and you can use this text as a resource to add to your existing knowledge. However, there is more to the study of health (or indeed any academic study) than simply collecting more knowledge. Study at university is also about *challenging* and *expanding* what we already know to *deepen* our knowledge and understanding. It is an (exciting) intellectual journey, which may result in us thinking (and feeling) very differently about health matters at the end of our study from when we started at university. Of course, we may think and feel much the same, but inevitably if we have actively engaged in thinking and learning we will have greater clarity and insight, enabling us to reason out our views and understanding in a far more rigorous and well informed manner.

As a result we would encourage you to think about Health Studies not as a systematic learning of different perspectives related to the field, but rather as an opportunity to unpack the very notion of what an idea of 'health' or **'well-being'** represents, (please note that we will simply refer to the term 'health' throughout this text, as 'well-being' has different meanings). In particular, we will explore some of the 'taken-for-granted' concepts that shape our ideas around health and social care issues and our responses to health and disease (i.e. this is what health is and this is how you promote it).

Reflective activity

Think about how many times you see things to do with health and body image in:

- weekly 'gossip' magazines, newspapers, weekend magazines;
- supermarkets;
- television (how many programmes in one day relate to 'health' issues?).

What advice is being given about 'how to be healthy', and what are the explanations about the causes of our health problems?

Finally, our approach to this text, and indeed our engagement with the area of health studies, is informed by our own interests, concerns and experiences. In this we very much hold with Paul Jewell's (1992) stance that, when reasoning through any ideas or notions, we need to take on board that 'when anyone presents an argument, in fact when anyone communicates or even thinks at all, he/she does from within a world view. This world view is a set of assumptions about the world, along with values, attitudes, standards and so on. Some of these world views are rigid and closed ... other world views are open and flexible, valuing tolerance of other people's positions, though still striving for coherence' (cited in Marshall and Rowland 2006, p. 43).

Who we are

As authors, we share this interest. We have been involved as lecturers and programme leaders of these sorts of courses for many years and it is this very diversity that we enjoy. While our backgrounds differ (one originally from nursing, the other from a more eclectic background of liberal arts and psychotherapy), we have both taken, and still are taking, a long journey in developing our understanding around health and want to share some of this with you. For us, this mostly means looking beyond the narrow confines of 'health as the absence of disease' (more about this in Chapter 1), and delving into the depth and breadth of related (and not so obvious) subjects that help us appreciate and understand the complexity of health and social care issues today. In particular, we recognise that our contemporary thinking does not emerge out of thin air but has a long history of social, cultural, economic, scientific and intellectual development. As a result we have constructed a text that introduces you to some of the ideologies and concepts that influence current thinking. These, themselves, are diverse and at first glance might not seem relevant *at all* to

Health Studies, but bear with us. We make as many links as we are able to show you how different ideas, knowledge, theories and concepts create insights into health (and social care) matters.

Two voices

Our two voices run throughout this text and you may even start to recognise their different 'tones' and 'accents'. Our voices not only reflect our own personal and professional frameworks but are also reflective of particular approaches taken to different sections within the text. Thus, within the research chapter you may find that the 'voice' is one that sounds like a tutor or lecturer concerned with guiding you through, in as engaged a manner as possible, the labyrinthine task of learning about and 'doing' research. On the other hand the 'voice' within Chapters 1, 2 and 3 may 'sound' more formal and academic as we take you through some of the core academic and theoretical debates that underpin health matters. In Chapter 4 you may well find a sense of both these voices and intentions, and this will be evident given both the reflective activities and the complex discourses that we have endeavoured to unpack. Finally, the careers chapter (Chapter 6) once again uses a more student-centred voice for we see this as a fairly practical exercise with which you need to engage.

How we would like you to engage with the text

We ask that you use this text with an open and curious mind. The text will continually remind you that debates and issues around health are constantly shifting, and thus, constantly in need of scrutiny. For a long time in western societies, for example, the study of 'health', 'illness' and disease' has been synonymous with a study of the body and understanding and treating illness and disease. However, you will instinctively know that health and healthy living is more than not being ill. Added to this there will need to be an acknowledgment that the study of heath is also about the study of how *we* live our lives (these sort of questions are often located within **existentialist** debates) and what sanctions and opportunities are legitimate to allow individuals to flourish (be 'healthy') (Seedhouse 1986, 2001, 2004).

We do not ask you to minimise the practical issues such as inter-professional working, mentorship, resources (often lack of) and government priorities in shaping decisions around health. Indeed, as we go to print a new government, with particular priorities and plans for national budgetary cuts within health, is in the midst of putting its manifesto into practice. However, being practical and pragmatic about health does not equate with neglecting intelligent interrogation and debate about health-related matters. You will need to be equipped with deep knowledge and insight, to critically evaluate complex practitioner issues or indeed health matters that affect you as an individual, both personally and professionally.

Reading (suggested and otherwise)

Within several of the chapters you will find recommended reading, labelled as 'Useful Resources'. As with everything within such a hugely diverse field of study this is by no means complete – nor do we imply this to be the case. Our recommendations are based on our own reading, use of material within our own teaching and learning practices, as well as material we have drawn on to write this text. Have a look at the Useful Resources throughout as they give you a fairly clear idea of how we see the role of independent reading – a way of enhancing and developing further your own ideas and interests. Your role as a reader is to start to recognise your own views, have insight into others and then expand on these views in a reasoned and well supported manner. One of the main ways you can do that is to read, read and read.

Reflective activities

You will have already have come across what we have named as a 'Reflective Activity' in the first part of this introduction (see Chapters 5 and 6, for a further discussion of reflection and reflexivity). These exercises are designed to afford you the opportunity to explore a concept further and apply your own experiences and learning to the material we cover in this text. You will find that some of the sections in the text include more of these Reflective Activities than others. This is not to say we don't want you to be reflecting and applying your knowledge throughout, but is instead a pedagogical concern not to influence your interpretations and understandings only through our own interpretations. In other words, our Reflective Activity suggestions say a lot about our own ideas about what might help you to develop as a learner. Given that part of the intention of this text is to equip you with skills to become your own critical reflective learner we would always encourage you to develop strategies of learning that best enhance your development and academic acumen.

How the book is designed to be used

This book can be used in a number of ways. As all parts relate to and feed into each other you can read it from 'beginning to end'. You may, however, find it more likely that you will want to access particular aspects of it that you feel are more relevant to the study you are presently undertaking. Essentially, it is a companion book, whereby relevant sections can be dipped into and consulted as necessary. Though we would encourage you to do some cross-referencing of your own to deepen your understanding, we have at times pointedly cross-referenced to other sections. At other times, we have deliberately not made the links for you as we feel that it is useful for you to make your own connections. You may notice too that there is some repetition of key issues in different sections; this is intentional because, first, we believe that the material within is interlinked and, second, the understanding of concepts can be informed by many ideas and thus take on a slightly different tenor. An example of this is in Chapter 2 where we look at how **social construction** is an approach to understanding health; while in Chapter 5 social construction is positioned as a particular research paradigm. They are clearly associated, informing one another, while at the same time indicating the complexities and indeed applicability of ideas across different disciplines.

The key features of the book are:

> A broad overview of studying health, including concepts of health and contemporary health challenges (Chapter 1).
> An encyclopaedia-like outline of key ideas (ideologies), concepts and terms that provide substance and background to our understanding of contemporary health issues (Chapters 2 and 3).
> Case studies, which explore some diverse, but contemporary, health issues, pulling out knowledge and insights into these subject matters from a range of academic disciplines that inform health and social care (Chapter 4).
> A practically focused chapter on research, which will help you with your own project work and academic study, and will present a critical analysis of different approaches to research (Chapter 5).
> A practical chapter on helping you to plan your future once you have finished your study at college or university (Chapter 6).

Each chapter also includes:

> Frequent cross-referencing, alerting you to the relationship between content in different chapters. This is indicated in the text like this: (see stigma, Chapter x, p. xx).
> Reflective Activities to draw your attention to issues worthy of greater personal consideration.
> A glossary of terms in the form of brief explanations (terms in the glossary are presented in the text in **bold**).
> Further reading, both within the text and at the end of various sections to identify texts, or other sources, that explore relevant issues in greater depth – see the 'Useful Resources' boxes.

Chapter-by-chapter summary

Chapter 1 Studying health: health as a contested notion

In this chapter, we start by taking you through an exploration of what is meant by health in order to construct some mental picture of the contentious nature of the study of health. No attempt is made here to settle the debate about the nature of health because concepts of health are contingent upon time, place, social priorities and values (Naidoo and Wills 1994, 2000), but the chapter draws attention to the fact that various conceptualisations of health are *preferred* in a particular temporal and social context. These preferred concepts of health emerge from contemporary epistemologies (i.e. how theories and social issues at a particular time shape ideas about health) and all versions are essentially **social constructions**. This exploration includes a brief overview of related terms and contemporary health/health policy issues. From this, a much more eclectic and critical awareness of the identity of 'health' and therefore what constitutes and contributes to 'Health Studies' should emerge and inform your understanding and readings of later sections too. We also provide a brief guide to some key principles regarding studying and learning.

Chapter 2 Key ideologies: shaping the way we think

Usually, texts on Health Studies or those contributing to the study of health take a single discipline focus (such as biology, biomedicine, sociology, psychology) and introduce the student to the relevance of these disciplines to health. Instead, in this chapter we have chosen to look at some core ideologies and theories, which inform discourse around the study of health. They are provided alphabetically for your ease of reference. The content within this section includes an overview of the particular ideology or theory and outlines how it has informed or contributed to our understanding of health matters. The content is *not* exhaustive, and we acknowledge that your tutors may notice some exclusions and inclusions that do not reflect all the issues and content that might be explored in your particular courses, but our choices have been informed by over ten years' experience of teaching health studies. They include ideologies and theories that help to explain and clarify the origins of some of the contentious and polemic debate that exists around health.

Chapter 3 Key terms and concepts: informing ideas and actions

In this chapter, we turn our attention to some of the key terms, issues and academic disciplines that have been influential in the sphere of health studies. This chapter essentially acts as a reference point for a quick reading on key subject matters. The items are also listed alphabetically.

Chapter 4 Case studies

In order to see how these different domains affect the construction, treatment, policy-making and (global) experience of health, we introduce some contemporary health examples in this chapter. The aim here is to work across the domains by exploring a small number of health issues in detail, ones that illustrate the complexity of knowledge construction and how this can affect treatment, decision-making, policy-making and ultimately the experience of health and illness. This will allow you to see just how many perspectives there can be on one particular health topic. These case studies, in particular, will extend your understanding of how health matters are constructed and managed and illustrate the contentious and controversial nature of knowledge. The case studies focus on obesity, artificial reproductive technologies (e.g. IVF), HIV and AIDS, and dementia.

Chapter 5 Research

This chapter introduces you to the field of health research and focuses on a selection of research designs relevant to health studies. The chapter begins with a discussion about the purpose of research and related philosophical issues (some of which you may have encountered already, such as **epistemology** and **ontology**, as well as methodology, ethics, **evidence-based practice** etc.). Different approaches and methods used in research are then outlined and examples of the different methodological approaches are given. Throughout this chapter research articles, from a wide variety of journals available to us through our library licensing agreements with publishers, are used to illustrate and unpack some of the applications of research. The examples used all relate to HIV/AIDS, obesity, dementia and ART. The overall intention of this chapter is for you to actually reflect on your own engagement with research, providing you with practical activities to enhance your learning as well as encouraging you to reflect on how research, in its many forms, can enhance and inform our understandings of complex ideas. It is therefore designed to be 'student-centred' – that is, deliberately written to equip you with some of the skills needed to embark on your own research.

Chapter 6 Career pathways: from the classroom to the workplace

Chapter 6 is written by Tahira Majothi, a careers consultant. The focus of this chapter is on starting to put your short- and long-term career planning into action. It is a very practical chapter that aims to identify the skills and competencies necessary to help you prepare for the transition to work, which can be gained through academic studies, placements and work experience (paid or unpaid). An exploration of the opportunities within the health and social care fields that may be available to you is also included.

1 studying health: health as a contested concept

This chapter explores:

> different concepts of health;
> a broad overview of public health and health promotion in contemporary health policy;
> the importance of establishing a clear definition of health to underpin work to promote health;
> implications for studying and learning around health.

Introduction

It is a widely accepted understanding that 'health' is value-laden and shaped by context, politics and power. No 'sense' can be made of the study of 'health' without acknowledging that various epistemologies also shape notions of 'health'. **Epistemology** (see also Chapter 5, pp. 223–4) refers to the production and promotion of *knowledge* about a certain phenomenon. The idea of epistemology has become very important in academic research in recent years, as people have started to question where our knowledge of certain things comes from and how they become popular or 'taken-for-granted'. In this chapter, the 'taken-for-granted' concept under question is 'health'. This may seem a strange idea, as most of us think that health is something you have, or don't have, and that there are certain, definite things that contribute to, or detract from, health. In thinking this, we are automatically seeing health as a tangible 'thing' that exists without change, has always existed (in the same form) and will remain the same forever (we would call this an **ontological** position on health – relating to the nature of existence). However, this is not the case, as there are many different conceptualisations of what is meant by 'health'.

Reflective activity

- Think about your own experiences. In one week, are there times when you feel more 'healthy' than others?
  - Does this depend on whether you have an illness or disease?
  - Does it depend on how you feel 'in yourself' or how you feel physically?
- At times when you have felt 'healthy' have you acknowledged this feeling? Or did you only know you were healthy when you felt less healthy?

Concepts of health

No attempt will be made to settle any debate about the nature of health because concepts of health are contingent upon time, place, social priorities and values (Naidoo and Wills 1994, 2000), but it is important to recognise that various conceptualisations of health are *preferred* in a particular temporal and social context as well as emerging from contemporary epistemologies (i.e. how theories and social issues at a particular time shape ideas about health). Additionally, all versions are essentially social constructions. For example, the theory of health that remained influential and underpinned action to tackle disease until the rise of the bacteriological age from the 1860s (Pasteur, 1822–95; Villermin, 1827–92; Koch, 1843–1910; and Ehrlich, 1854–1915; see Webster 1994) was the miasma theory. According to this theory, disease, death and pestilence emerged from bad smells – vapours from rotting vegetables or rotting bodies, marshy places or polluted rivers. Close contact with any of the above was believed to result in disease (Davey and Seale 1994). Typically in the newly industrialised cities of the early nineteenth century such as Manchester and Liverpool, there were plenty of 'bad smells' emerging from, among other things, untreated sewage and unregulated commercial processes, e.g. slaughter houses in residential areas, and these were blamed for diseases such as cholera, which became epidemic in the 1830s. Edwin Chadwick (1800–90) became convinced that disease caused poverty and that unsanitary conditions and squalor were ultimately to blame for early deaths (expertly and graphically illustrated in his *Report on the Sanitary Conditions of the Labouring Population of Great Britain 1842*). The solution thus became simple – remove the bad smells! Poverty could not be eliminated (without massive social, economic and political upheaval), but the unsanitary conditions could be improved.

> The primary and most important measures, and at the same time the most practicable, and within the recognised province of administration, are drainage, and the removal of all refuse from habitations, streets and roads, and the improvement of the supplies of water. (Porter 1997, p. 411)

What this example illustrates is how epistemology – the nature, sources and limits of knowledge – shapes responses to events and the solutions and actions that emerge. Belief in 'bad smells' (the miasma theory of health) logically results in action to remove the bad smells. We know now, of course, that the smells emerged from putrefaction caused by bacteria and so forth, and that these are the real culprits of disease, but this knowledge came only with advances in science.

Useful resource

If you want to look at some of Chadwick's findings presented in the report go to: http://www.spartacus.schoolnet.co.uk/PHchadwick.htm

Moreover, an undisputed 'truth' regarding health is not possible, as concepts of health embody 'beyond-the-facts' value judgements (Seedhouse 2001), which serve a purpose within a given society:

> conflict and competition between accounts of health reflects disputes that are basically epistemological in origin – they revolve around differences of view about what counts as 'reliable' or 'true' knowledge. (Wright and Treacher 1982, cited by Beattie 1993, p. 261)

Beyond-the-facts judgements

In our current climate of **evidence-based practice**, it is easy to believe that all decisions are solely evidence-based. This is clearly not the case, as demonstrated by Seedhouse (1997a, 2004). Values shape what is considered a 'problem', e.g. a health problem. Hence, sports-related injuries and deaths are tolerated, while smoking is unanimously vilified (Seedhouse 1997a, 2004). This is not necessarily a 'wrong' choice. It is an inevitable outcome of *decision-making*. However, what does need to be acknowledged is that decisions can *never* be based on 'facts' alone. For example, decisions concerning whether or not women should be given the right to vote are not influenced by '**facts**' alone, nor indeed can ideas about what constitutes a 'person' simply be considered a 'factual' matter. John Locke (1632–1704), for example, stated that the notion of what constitutes a 'person' was a forensic (legal) term. It is up to society to decide what constitutes a 'person', as *facts* do not exist to solve the problem or prove who is, or is not, a 'person'. Fundamentally, judgements about a matter have to be made and 'categories' created that represent current thinking on a matter. What is important is that the decisions can be justified in some way and moral reasoning can support this process.

Seedhouse (2004) asserts that it is important to develop a position between the two extremes of 'values-first' (relativism) or 'evidence-first' (which presupposes evidence exists in a vacuum). Evidence is in fact interpreted in some way or other and it *is* possible to have better or worse interpretations of facts, e.g. interpretations that do more good than harm. In fact, both 'facts' and 'values' about a matter exist. The example given by Seedhouse (2004) is that it is plain 'fact' that some people in the UK and USA live in luxury while others live on the streets. Where values come in is in the *interpretation* of whether this is a 'good' thing or not, whether it was luck, skill or talent that produced these results, and whether it is acceptable to have such extremes in a society. These sorts of decisions can only be made on a 'beyond-the-facts' basis.

Another example provided by Seedhouse (2004) relates to alcohol use. Epidemiological studies have demonstrated that heavy drinking (somewhere in the region of 50 plus units of alcohol consumed a week) is detrimental to health (a fact). Whether someone who drinks heavily leads a 'bad' life, however, is *not* a matter of 'fact'. It depends on how one thinks a life ought to be lived: 'the causation of the disease is a matter of evidence or even fact, the interpretation of the behaviour that caused the disease depends upon what the interpreter values – that is, it depends upon her prejudice' (Seedhouse 2004, p. 89). In the matter of health, evidence and values can never entirely be separated: 'the evidence is not mute – but it never entirely speaks for itself' (Seedhouse 2004, p. 89). Using the example of excessive consumption of alcohol to demonstrate how evidence *and* values play a separate part in decisions about whether something is 'good' or not may not be immediately obvious. This stems from axiomatic assumptions that often emerge in discussion around health promotion and 'healthy lifestyles', i.e. that what constitutes 'being healthy' is the absence of disease. Death and disease are seen as bad things in themselves (Seedhouse 1997a, 2004) and as the excessive consumption of alcohol is known to cause death and disease, it is automatically a *bad* thing too. Thus the notion of health is often conflated with the idea of what constitutes a 'good life' (Seedhouse 1997a, 2004).

Health as the 'good life'

The term 'good life' is essentially linked to the word '**well-being**'. Broadly speaking the term 'well-being' is intrinsically connected to ideas about what constitutes human happiness and what sort of life is good to lead (Walsh 1995). This implies a connection between what is morally good (which in itself embodies values – what is the 'right' thing to do) and what sort of life most people will find enjoyable and comfortable. 'Well-being' is more likely to refer to the latter than the former although both components are seen to be relevant features – Aristotle, for example, believed that a morally good life was essential to human flourishing (Walsh 1995). 'Well-being' is thus a highly complex notion and embodies aspirations concerning 'what sort of life one wants to lead'.

Thus while an 'early' death *might* be avoided by only consuming alcohol in moderation, an **abstemious** lifestyle may mean that other ways of achieving fulfilment and potential are curtailed (the 'good life') and hence 'well-being' is limited. Ernest Hemingway's 'hard-living' lifestyle, for example, was full of rich experiences and opportunities and creative fulfilment. It is, therefore, in part a matter of opinion that the best way to live a life is to be prudent in all matters.

Another example might help to clarify this relationship between evidence/ fact and values in matters of health. Asceticism is a doctrine in which the enjoyment of bodily pleasures, comfort and ease is denied as they tie an individual to the 'illusory' world of matter and away from the contemplation of 'higher' things (Dent 1995a). St Simeon Stylites (*c*.390–459), for example, who lived on top of a pillar, represents an extreme example of an ascetic lifestyle. Asceticism formed part of the philosophy of St Augustine (founder of Western Christianity) and for St Augustine sexual abstinence and virginity were highly commended (although he did commend marriage to others). While a lifestyle of such denial would undoubtedly curtail the current rise in sexually transmitted infections (STIs) – for example, visits to GUM clinics have doubled over the decade 1990–2000 (DoH 2001) – it is unlikely that the values in the twenty-first century would support the extremes of ascetic behaviour: it is no longer seen to constitute the 'good life'. So what is seen to constitute the 'good life' is *not* simply derived from evidence and facts, but also from social values.

According to Seedhouse (2004), values prevalent in society will shape what is deemed necessary and possible to do (e.g. in the name of health), and contrary values will self-evidently be deemed wrong and be rejected as the foundation for action in a matter. These 'values' include political/ideological values, and, for example, while evidence concerning the existence and impact of inequalities in wealth and health has existed for many years (e.g. the Black Report in the late 1970s), past governments rejected recommendations for state intervention as they did not fit with their political and ideological values (those embodied by liberal individualism, see p. 44). Beyond-the-facts judgements shaped social policy throughout the 1980s – and they continue to do so.

Theories of health

In order to illustrate this further we will now spend some time considering various *theories* of health. Some of the basic premises and principles, along with a brief critique, of each of these will be presented. While any grouping of theories of health is artificial (and different authors may group theories differently), they enable the reader to gain a clear impression of the many and varied ways in which the notion of 'health' or 'being healthy' is conceived.

We start with the concept of health that can be broadly categorised as the *bio-medical, Western/scientific* view of health, as it is the concept of health that dominates current thinking and health and health promotion policy in the UK (Naidoo and Wills 2000; Earle 2007).

The biomedical, Western/scientific theory of health

This view of health underpins many of the features of modern health care and medicine and the basic premises are associated with scientific and medical thinking. It has been described as having several key features:

> It is *biomedical*, whereby health is seen to equate to the 'normal' functioning of the *biological* aspects of the human body. It is assumed that this 'perfect' functioning is the normal state of being.

> It is *reductionist*, in that the 'normal'/healthy function of the body can be assessed by examining the body at a molecular/chemical level. Bits of the body can be treated as separate entities. Illness equates to some form of malfunction that is measurable (Cedar 2008).

> Finally, a *mechanistic* metaphor is applied. In other words, the healthy functioning of the body/person is analogous to that of a well functioning machine and some internal process causes disease, e.g. degeneration through ageing or system failure, or an external process such as attack by germs.

According to Seedhouse (1986, 2001) this medical, Westernised theory view equates health to a commodity (see commodification, p. 71). Health is something that can be 'lost' but also 're-supplied'. The restoration of health is akin to the buying and selling of produce. Medical treatment aims to restore functioning or health to body systems and once functioning is restored health returns. It can be re-supplied thorough the provision of drugs or via technologically based interventions such as surgery. Treatment and care take place in 'specialised' settings and separate from 'everyday' life, with little active involvement of the 'patient'.

Health and disease are opposites: health equates with the absence of disease.

Critique of the Western/scientific concept of health

While the biomedical, Western/scientific view of health underpins much of the work done for health in industrialised Western nations, it is also widely criticised. This theory equates health with the absence of disease, thus implying that as someone becomes more diseased they will automatically become less healthy. Health and disease are seen as opposite ends of a continuum. This, however, seems too simplistic, and while it *might* be the case, it is not always so. For example, I may have a cold, but am on my dream holiday and so am feeling happy and contented, and am enjoying life. To consider myself as not being healthy *simply* because I have a virus in my system seems far too unsophisticated. As noted above, there are many ways in which human beings think of the notion 'health', and physical perfection is only part of this.

This is one of the key limitations of the biomedical Western/scientific view of health, as it connotes health with the *physical* integrity and functioning of a person. Many people instinctively feel this is too narrow a way of thinking about health as we frequently recognise the importance of *social* and *psychological* states in the attainment, and subjective assessment, of health. In practice, too, many health care professionals do not confine themselves to this restrictive view of health (i.e. simply physical matters) when practising their medicine or health care (Seedhouse 2001).

This emphasis on health as being a biological affair can also lead to the separation of 'health' – its attainment and restoration – from everyday life and the social and economic environment people inhabit. For example, people usually consult medical 'experts' or are treated in hospitals when they are poorly and they are prescribed medical regimes even when their 'illness' may clearly have social and psychological roots, as with depression.

Ivan Illich (1976) adds to this critique in his claim that 'The medical establishment has become a major threat to health' (his opening lines in *Limits to Medicine*), and uses the word **iatrogenesis** to describe problems relating to health that stem from the Western/scientific concept of health and the resulting prominent role of medical physicians. He particularly comments on professional control and considers the over-medicalisation of life as an obstacle to autonomy because of the dependence it fosters on 'expert medical systems'. He believes medicine created three types of iatrogenesis:

> *Clinical*. Where the medical intervention/action itself causes damage or ill-health (for example, drug therapies that cause unpleasant, unwanted and sometimes life threatening side effects).
> *Social*. When policies reinforce the role and function of industrial, and other, organisational systems that cause ill-health (e.g. pollution generated by industry that damages environments and harsh and dangerous working practices that cause ill-health, injury and death).
> *Cultural and symbolic*. when medically sponsored behaviour restricts and undermines the competence of people to care for themselves and each other or manage their own suffering (e.g. the tendency to call in counsellors and social workers whenever there has been some sort of disaster).

Salutogenic health

The medical model can be termed a pathogenic conceptualisation of health and concentrates on disease and the prevention of disease (Jones 2000). It works within the illusion of attaining perfect health, whereas the normal state of health for humans is one of imperfection (Dubos 1959; Antonovsky 1987, 1993: cited in Jones 2000). Instead Antonovsky (1987, 1993) proposes a *salutogenic* concept of health, which emphasises that 'most people are neither diseased nor healthy but somewhere along a 'health-ease' continuum' (Jones 2000, p. 31), and what is of interest is to explore factors that help people remain healthy (Earle 2007; Watt 2007). From his work with survivors of concentration camps, Antonovsky identified three principle ingredients that are 'health promoting'. These are comprehensibility (the ability to understand the 'dynamics' of living), manageability (the ability to cope with life demands) and meaningfulness (that effort and actions to meet life challenges are worthwhile) (Antonovsky 1987). This equates, for example, to experiences in the workplace where an individual feels that her work is meaningful, but not over-stressful, and that she is able to operate as an autonomous, participatory individual (Jones 2000). What is crucial from the salutogenic perspective is not only the internal resources of individuals, but the environment within which they live and the opportunities for relationships, and support, it affords. This sort of dialogue gives value to the development of broader concepts of health, which attempt to move away from the focus on disease and pathology.

Health as an ideal state

There are several concepts of health that broadly fit into this category (Seedhouse 2001). The most famous embodiment of this way of picturing health is the World Health Organisation (WHO) definition, first presented in 1946:

> Health is a state of complete physical, mental and social well-being and not merely the absence of disease and infirmity.

This definition of health points to broader aspects of health. Things other than the physical functioning of the body are acknowledged as being important aspects of *being healthy*.

Other such concepts refer to *health as personal strength or ability*. This way of thinking about *health* and *being healthy* comes out of the work of people such as Sacks (1973) and Williams (1983) (see Boxes 1.1 and 1.2). You may well have seen some of Sacks's work depicted in the film *Awakenings*. This is based on Sacks's real life experiences working with people suffering from **encephalitis lethargica** and their treatment with the so-called miracle drug **L-dopa** (**laevo-dihydroxyphenylalanine**).

Box 1.1 'Awakenings'

Oliver Sacks is a physician and psychiatrist who in the late 1970s worked at Mount Carmel hospital, New York, with patients suffering from the extremely debilitating condition of encephalitis lethargia (a sort of 'sleeping sickness'). This was a viral disease that swept Europe and America in the first two decades of the twentieth century. People who were struck down with this illness presented with a multitude of symptoms from delirium to Parkinsonian symptoms. More than a third of the victims died. For many of those who did not die, their recovery was characterised by progressive states of illness. The worst of these were people left in a sort of 'waking coma', a state of motionless, speechless, consciousness.

It is from Sacks's experiences of working with this group of people that he started to formulate his ideas of being a *healthy* human being. He saw an abundance of dignity and 'spirit' in the people caught under the spell of encephalitis lethargica. Something that transcended the body and made him feel that these people were 'healthy' and robust *despite* being severely physically restricted. He recalls conversations with one of his patients in the week before he died:

> We had several talks in those final days, the tone of which was set by Mr O. 'Don't give me any guff', he said. 'I *know* the score. Bob's down to skin and bone. He's *ready* to go'. In his last few days he joked with the nurses, and asked the Rabbi to read him a psalm. A few hours before his death he said: 'I was going to kill myself, in '22 … I'm glad I didn't … it's been a good game, encephalitis and all. (Sacks 1973, p. 80)

Of another patient he writes:

> all in all, Miss H has done well – amazingly so, considering the existence she has led. Against all odds, Miss H has always managed to be a real *person* and to face reality without denial or madness. She draws strength unfathomable to me, a health which is deeper than the depth of her illness. (Sacks 1973, p. 115)

Box 1.2 Williams (1983)

Williams's (1983) ideas came out of his work with elderly Aberdonians. In his study Williams noted that people talked about health in terms of *strength*. Health was sometimes equated with being not being ill or diseased, but he found that people felt that health could exist even when people had a serious illness. People were considered healthy if they 'had the power to "come through" or "come up"' (Williams 1983; cited in Seedhouse 2001, p. 51) and he reports accounts describing people with severe physical diseases (in one instance, gangrene of the leg) as 'being healthy', because of the strength they exhibited to survive this trauma. Williams concluded that health is far more complex than the absence of disease, but is a positive state of 'activity and moral effort' (Williams 1983; cited in Seedhouse 2001, p. 51).

The work of both Sacks and Williams fits under the humanist banner: that of free-thinking, rationality and the view that we as humans have the ability to shape our lives.

From this perspective, the presence of disease, illness and suffering per se does not mean that a person does not have health. Instead, disease, illness and suffering are seen as potential obstacles to the achievement of health. The work of Sacks and Williams led them to conclude that *health* was an unquantifiable resilience or ability to be positive and adapt to life circumstances – not just about the absence of disease, as with the biomedical, Western/scientific concept of health. Health does not simply equate to 'normal' biological functioning or the absence of disease, as they concluded that the people they met could be considered healthy *despite* (in some cases) alarming levels of sickness and disease. Thus, as with the WHO definition of health, being healthy is considered in holistic, and not simply physical, terms.

Another similar way of conceiving health is that it relates to the *ability to adapt*. Significant authors who present ideas of being healthy as equating to the ability to adapt are Dubos (1987), Illich (1976) and Mansfield (1977). To Dubos, Illich and Mansfield the essence of health is human beings' ability to adapt to the environment within which they live and to face the challenges that arise in their everyday lives. Illich (1976, p. 273), for example, sees health as being to do with autonomy:

> Health designates a process of adaptation. It is not the result of instinct, but of an autonomous yet culturally shaped reaction to socially created reality. It designates the ability to adapt to changing environments, to growing up and to aging, to healing when damaged, to suffering, and to the peaceful expectation of death.

Self-awareness, self-discipline and inner resources are needed for health:

health is seen as a 'task', a process of adaptation. What is key to health is that a person is *autonomous enough* to adapt. Autonomy is necessary for health.

Thus for Dubos (1987), Illich (1976) and Mansfield (1977), freedom of the human spirit is the essence of health and health is not an absolute and specific state of being. The capacity to explore and face dangers and challenges is an essential aspect of human life and to define one way of life, e.g. living the sort of lifestyle that is currently considered 'healthy' (taking regular exercise, drinking alcohol in moderation, not smoking, having a healthy diet etc.), as *the* way of being healthy is tantamount to dictatorship.

There are recognised strengths and weaknesses in all of these concepts of health. David Seedhouse (1986, 2001) offers an insightful and comprehensive critique of many of these theories as either unrealistic and idealistic (WHO/ideal state theories), too vague (inner strength/ability to adapt) or too narrow and prescriptive (biomedical, Western/scientific).

The need for a broader theory of health

The other theories of health, noted above, do redress some of the limitations of the Western/scientific concept of health, because they explicitly or implicitly recognise the importance of the social and psychological dimensions of health. Some (e.g. ability to adapt) also acknowledge that health is not a 'perfect' state. However, they are often vague or idealistic and therefore fail to provide a useful theory of health (Seedhouse 1986, 2001).

It is David Seedhouse's (1986, 2001) contention that a concept of health is needed that acknowledges many of these facets of health (physical, social, psychological and spiritual), as it provides a more concrete basis from which to develop work to promote health and does not prescribe only one way of life as being healthy, and we will deal with this concept in some depth. Seedhouse (1986, 2001) asserts that a concept of health must account for the complex and different (real and envisaged) dimensions of 'health' because what constitutes being healthy may differ significantly, person to person. A particular form or 'state' cannot typify being healthy. He amply illustrates this in the following quote taken from the first edition of his book *Health: The Foundations for Achievement* (1986).

> The idea that health is a specific, definable, fully describable state to which everyone can aspire equally is nonsense. It is as meaningless as the idea that there can be a perfect person. What would such a being look like? Individuals are occasionally described as perfect by people whose faculties of reason are temporarily clouded by romantic mists. A 'Mr' or 'Mrs Right' sometimes rides into a person's life. They are not, of course, everyone's choice of candidate for a perfect human being. The issue of health is similar. People are different – they have different ages, abilities, intelligences, disabilities, environments, ambitions, stresses, jobs and so on. (Seedhouse 1986, p. 56)

In other words, there is no such thing as *one type* of 'perfect person' that would be considered suitable for everyone and represent their ideal partner. Similarly, there is no such thing as *one type* of life/ lifestyle that is considered suitable for 'health', and represents 'being healthy' to *all* individuals.

Thus, Seedhouse (1986,2001) presents a different theory of health – health as the *foundations for achievement*. Seedhouse's basic premise is that: 'A person's health is equivalent to the state of the set of conditions which fulfill or enable her to work to fulfill her realistic chosen and biological potentials' (Seedhouse 2001, p. 103). The extent to which a person can function successfully (i.e. the extent to which a person is autonomous) is roughly the extent of his or her health. These potentials are influenced by internal physical problems (what diseases or disabilities they may have), internal mental problems, external pathogens (the circumstances they live and work in, for example) and external impacts such as accidents, but for someone's potential to be achieved certain foundations are essential (Seedhouse 2001). Seedhouse (1986, 2001) identified five foundations as follows:

Foundation one
For good health, we all have basic needs of food, drink, shelter, warmth and purpose in life (the specific constituents of this will differ person-to-person, place to place and so forth).

Foundation two
People also need access to the widest possible information about all factors, which have an influence on a person's life (the nature and type of information will differ according to circumstances etc.).

Foundation three
This foundation draws attention to the vital importance of education to enable people to fulfil their potential. Essentially, it is important to have the knowledge, skills and confidence to assimilate information. Literacy and numeracy are a basic necessary but people also need to understand information and how it applies to them and be able to make *reasoned* and *informed decisions* regarding actions they may take.

Foundation four
This refers to the importance of *community*. Individuals are never totally isolated from other people and the external world – being part of a community is essential to good health (although the 'community' may come in many different forms). In addition, people should not strive to fulfil personal potentials, which undermine basic foundations of others. People must be aware of implications of any actions and the basic duties which follow from living in community/society, i.e. how actions, behaviours and choices impact on others.

Foundation five
This represents things such as medical services and support, social services and improved facilities for disabled people. This relates to *whatever* is

needed when a particular life problem becomes bad enough to impede a person's attainment of their potential. The need for these 'special' services may be permanent (such as continuing support for special needs) or temporary (such as life-saving, life-sustaining medical/healthcare). (Adapted from Seedhouse 2001)

What is noted is that foundation five is not necessary for *all* individuals, *all* of the time, and specifically highlights that medical, health and social care and welfare are not central to good health. Instead they provide specific benefits for people in accordance with specific needs. Good health is as much dependent on the other foundations as it is on foundation five, and work to promote health, in theory, can encompass this breadth.

The importance of defining health

The meanings and values accorded to health underpin 'health promotion'. Establishing an understanding of what is meant by health is therefore an essential prerequisite prior to any action being taken to 'promote' health, and helps to resolve the lack of clarification that exists around the term 'health promotion' (Naidoo and Wills 2000). Work to promote health *must* be based on some comprehension of what health is, as the meanings accorded to this concept shape what type of activity and intervention is deemed necessary.

For example, if the biomedical, Western/scientific theory of health, outlined above, is taken as the basis for work to promote health, the general emphasis will be on *disease prevention* – usually by encouraging people to adopt *healthy lifestyles* – and medically/healthcare orientated action (because being healthy/health is equated with the absence of disease). Action on a broader scale, e.g. against material and structural inequalities that influence health, *may* be seen as important but only in so far as tackling these sorts of inequalities reduces the incidence and prevalence of disease (i.e. prevents disease).

In contrast, if the foundations theory of health is used as the basis for work to promote health, attention is directed towards the need to ensure that *all* foundations are as solid as they can be and this might not be related to traditional disease matters or healthcare provision at all. For example, as people generally need shelter to be as healthy as they can be (not just physically healthy), providing shelter for a homeless person becomes a legitimate concern *in itself*. It contributes to health on a *foundational* level, not primarily because they are more likely to get ill if they sleep rough but because they can then start to do *other things* with their life (if they choose) – which are arguably more important goals for living than simply the 'goal' of avoiding illness/disease. The value of this broad approach to health is clearly articulated by Barbara Stilwell, who writes in the foreword of the second edition of *Health: The Foundations for Achievement* (Seedhouse 2001):

> I was ... working ... as a nurse practitioner in a shelter for single homeless men. ... Most medical visitors to the hostel spent a long time talking to

the men about stopping smoking. The men clearly thought these visitors were crazy: imagine worrying about smoking when your 'home' is the size of a single bed and locker, with all the privacy and amenities you might expect. ... I welcomed being able to think about health as the foundations for achievement – where I could have a legitimate concern with the basic needs of food and drink, shelter, warmth and a purpose in life ... and still be a nurse practitioner. (Stilwell, p. vii in Seedhouse 2001)

If the 'foundations for health' concept is used to underpin work for health, it can be *much* broader and less prescriptive in nature. It provides the flexibility for meeting people's varying, actual and everyday needs as the focus is not simply on physical (social and psychological) aspects of people's lives that are linked with disease (mortality and morbidity) alone. It also encapsulates the value of the broader health agenda recognised in reports such as the Black Report (1980) and the Lalonde Report (1974), for example, via the importance of ensuring that foundation one is as solid as it can be.

This brings us to an exploration of the themes and policies that currently underpin work to promote health and provides additional insight into how concepts of health shape priorities and perspectives therein.

Health promotion, public health and recent health policy

Many attempts have been made to establish a theoretical basis for health promotion (Cross 2010) but according to Seedhouse (1997a, 2004) these remain essentially flawed. The meanings accorded to this term are as complex as those pertaining to health, and discussion in various key texts (Naidoo and Wills 2000; Douglas et al. 2007; Earle et al. 2007) tends to concentrate on the development and progression of 'health promotion', rather than providing detailed definitions. Some useful texts have been identified under the useful resources at the end of this chapter if you want to explore this in greater depth, but the pertinent points are addressed here.

The origins of health promotion itself are recognised in public health. Public health has a long history, but in more modern times was shaped by the social and industrial upheaval of the nineteenth century and the actions taken to manage the high rates of morbidity and mortality experienced, particularly, in the new industrialised towns of the nation. The initial manifestations of public health could be considered wide-ranging, involving engineering and social solutions (sanitation and regulation of working hours and so forth) as well as broadly medical, and this is reflected in this classical definition of public health:

Public health is the science and art of preventing disease, prolonging life and promoting physical health and efficiency through organized community efforts for the sanitation of the environment, the control of community infections, the education of the individual in the principles of personal hygiene, the organisation of medical and nursing services for the early diagnosis and preventive treatment of disease, the development of social machinery which will ensure to every individual in the community a standard of living adequate for the maintenance of health. (Winslow 1920, cited by Baggott 2000, p. 1)

However, as Jones and Pickstone (2008) comment, until the late 1970s and early 1980s public health (which by then was referred to as community medicine) became increasingly associated with epidemiology (see p. 194) and medicine, with health education as an associated discipline. This narrow focus on medically inspired intervention and 'education about health and hygiene' (health education) (Earle 2007) was gradually eroded by the emergence of a more critical **discourse** within the Lalonde Report (*A New Perspective on the Health of Canadians* 1974) and writings of people such as McKeown and Lowe (1974), along with the publication of *The Black Report* in the 1980s. This shifted awareness towards a re-engagement of public health with the broader social and economic agenda and recognised the important of 'making healthier choices, easier choices' (Earle 2007). In other words, the social, economic and policy environment should be 'health promoting' and address the root causes of poor health. This shift was termed the 'New Public Health' era and reference to health promotion became more commonplace (Earle 2007).

In terms of actions and interventions, the new public health/health promotion remained a 'very broad church' (Baggott 2000, p. 1), one that, in theory, could encapsulate a huge array of interventions and actions (Baggott 2000). This diversity itself creates confusion, and although reference is made to socio-economic and environmental matters in public health/health promotion and health policy documents and texts, there is a tendency for work to largely focus on individually orientated interventions around health education and lifestyle change, particularly among health professionals such as nurses (Cross 2010).

The root of this problem, according to Naidoo and Wills (2000, p. 71), lies in the fact that there is 'no agreed consensus on what health promotion is or what health promoters do when they try to promote health ... The term health promotion is used in a number of ways, often without clarification of meaning'. This lack of clarification and mix of meanings is noticeable in several policy documents (see Box 1.3).

Box 1.3 suggests that the undeclared vision regarding public health/health promotion is one associated with disease prevention, and is therefore based on the biomedical, Western/scientific concepts of health and reflects what Seedhouse (1997a, 2004) asserts: that health is essentially a complex, contested and poorly understood concept. Hence, a 'default position' is *health as the absence of disease.*

the health studies companion

Box 1.3 Reference to Specific Terms: Health Promotion and Public Health in Recent Public Health/Health Policy Documents.

Saving Lives – Our Healthier Nation (DoH 1999a)

No specific definition is provided in this document and while reference is made to service interventions and the importance of not simply focusing on the individual, the key content does reflect individual action, behaviour change and disease prevention. For example,

> We want to move beyond the old arguments and tired debates which have characterised so much consideration of public health issues, including those who say that nothing can be done to improve the health of the poorest, and those who say that individuals are solely to blame for their own ill-health.

> ... develop mental health promotion strategies in schools, workplaces and prisons which enhance social support and coping strategies and which tackle bullying.

> ... development of more comprehensive sex and relationships education, more coherent health promotion messages and more effective service interventions ... number of public health promotion campaigns for young people which aim to increase their understanding of sexually transmitted infections and how to prevent them.

> Ten Tips for Better Health: 1 Don't smoke. If you can, stop. If you can't, cut down. 2 Follow a balanced diet with plenty of fruit and vegetables. 3 Keep physically active. 4 Manage stress by, for example, talking things through and making time to relax. 5 If you drink alcohol, do so in moderation. 6 Cover up in the sun, and protect children from sunburn. 7 Practise safer sex. 8 Take up cancer screening opportunities. 9 Be safe on the roads: follow the Highway Code. 10 Learn the First Aid ABC – airways, breathing, circulation. (DoH 1999 – from the introduction)

Wanless Report: *Securing Good Health for the Whole Population – Final Report* (Wanless 2004)

Out of the reports looked at, this is the only one that provides a specific definition, and other references to public health/health promotion made in the document at least infer a strong relationship between disease prevention, lifestyle and health.

The definition of public health for this review has been drawn very widely; essentially it considers public health to be:

> the science and art of preventing disease, prolonging life and promoting health through the organised efforts and informed choices of society,

organisations, public and private, communities and individuals. (Wanless 2004, p. 3)

Smoking … in England … very important; it and obesity remain the most important lifestyle determinants of future health. (Wanless 2004 p. 6)

… creating a 'fully engaged' population through individualised health promotion and disease prevention (Wanless 2004, p. 9; this is the only mention of Health Promotion)

Choosing Health – Making Healthier Choices Easier (DoH 2004a)

No specific definition of public health or health promotion can be found in the Choosing Health (DoH 2004) document. Reference is made to health promotion as a process of information dissemination and awareness-raising. For example:

An Action Diabetes bus is already taking testing and health promotion services out to schools, temples, mosques, businesses and community centres. There are also videos and magazines now being produced and trained voluntary health counsellors will work within local communities to provide advice to those most at risk on how to obtain information on diabetes and improving health (DoH 2004, p. 24)

… we will equip all frontline staff to recognise the opportunities for health promotion and improvement, and use skills in health psychology to help people change their lifestyles (DoH 2004, p. 124)

… The NHS and its partner organisations, including local government, will benefit from this stronger evidence base both as to what works within the field of public health, inequalities and ill-health prevention and on the case for investment upstream. (DoH 2004, p. 190)

Darzi Report (DoH 2008a)

The general reference here is to strengthening programme and service interventions. Targets mentioned relate to diseases, states of health or risk factors and include: obesity, drugs, smoking, sexual health and mental health.

The Child and Young People's Health Strategy due in the autumn will seek to build on the new Child Health Promotion Programme that sees highly skilled health visitors and school nurses supporting families on health and parenting from pregnancy onwards. It will also bring with it a further focus on improving services for adolescents (DoH 2008a, p. 34)

Reference is made to 'the importance of extending services in the community, and the benefits to general wellbeing and to physical from stronger mental health promotion' (p. 18). No reference is made to public health except in the context of job titles and functions.

Work to promote health

Since the 1970s, the shifting pattern of mortality and morbidity (from infectious diseases to chronic conditions such as cancer and heart disease), the growing number of elderly and the changing social and cultural landscape have reshaped healthcare priorities, with an increasing emphasis in recent health (and social) care policy documents on prevention (health promotion) work and consumer choice (DoH 2004a, 2008a). Moreover, aetiological explanations of these diseases have increasingly been couched in terms of individual behaviour rather than environmental factors – 'many of the current major problems in prevention are related less to man's outside environment than to his own personal behaviour' (DHSS 1976, p. 17) – and this emphasis continues. For instance, Lord Darzi's report (DoH 2008a, p. 3), highlighted the role of the NHS in keeping people healthy rather then treating disease: 'the NHS has a responsibility to promote good health as well as tackle disease ... to improve the prevention of ill-health'.

Consequently, the priorities set for healthcare now revolve around our biggest killers – heart disease, cancer, strokes – or other factors that cause morbidity within the community (and are in theory preventable), such as HIV/AIDS (sexual health), obesity, drug use and mental health (DoH 1992, 1999a, 2004a, 2008a), and consumerism and choice within health care (DoH 2004a, 2008a). In the *Choosing Health – Making Healthy Choices Easier* document (DoH 2004a), for example, the following principles are outlined:

> At the start of the twenty-first century England needs a new approach to health of the public, reflecting the rapid and radical transformation of English society in the latter half of the twentieth century, responding to the needs and wishes of its citizens as individuals and harnessing the new opportunities open to it. ... The opportunities are now opening up rapidly for everyone to make their own individual informed healthy choices which together will sustain and drive further the improvement in the health of the people of England. (DoH 2004a, pp. 2, 18)

There are limitations to these approaches, and the emphasis placed in recent policy documents on disease prevention, lifestyle change and individual choices and a critique of these is dealt with in relevant sections of Chapter 2, 3 and 5 (see individualism, autonomy, free will, consumerism and behaviour change, for instance). However, to briefly comment at this point, what this focus does reflect is that the term 'health' (and therefore work to promote health) 'is a largely socially determined category predicated upon the particular characteristics and dynamics of the society under investigation' (Kelman 1988, p. 23). In other words, health priorities are selected, along with the means of addressing these health priorities (*inter alia*, prevention, public health and health promotion), according to the dominant values, needs, evidence and practical considerations within twentieth- and twenty-first-century societies, and this is still primarily focused on 'health as the absence of disease'.

Studying health

It is unpacking these influences and understanding key socio-cultural, ideo-logical and theoretical concepts that will help you in your 'study' of health. We will not rehearse details of studying and learning, or study skills, here, as there are some excellent texts on the market (see recommendations below) and the careers chapter (Chapter 6) also explores some practical reflective activities such as using a SWOT analysis, but we do want to mention, here, some key issues about academic study.

In essence, academic study involves building up your knowledge of evidence, ideas and theories around a subject matter (in this case health), but, more significantly, developing your understanding and ability to critique these ideas. What will become evident is that studying and learning is not a passive process that merely involves the absorption of information because, as we have already demonstrated in this chapter, ideas ('information') about health, for example, are far from straightforward. Some ideas are also more robust than others, either because of their evidential or philosophical foundations, or because they provide more acceptable, and practical, ways forward.

What should also become obvious as you study and learn is that you, as an individual, will have preferences regarding ideas and evidence. Some ideas and evidence you will accept more enthusiastically than others, using them to inform your analysis and actions, as they will fit more readily with your values or reflect your experiences. However, your challenge, as a student, is to retain an open mind and critically reflect upon, analyse and evaluate *all* ideas and evidence. Remember, actions and evidence within contemporary society are shaped by complex and competing demands and you should aim to develop a deep understanding of these matters in the study of health and social care.

Critical analysis

Critical analysis, critical evaluation or critical reflection essentially involve asking the question '*why?*', asking for *reasons* for doing something, or coming to informed judgements about the quality of evidence or opinion before believing what you are told. As Bowell and Kemp (2010, p. 3) note, 'Every day we are bombarded with messages … telling us what to do or not to do, what to believe or not believe; … to vote for Mrs Bloggs; practice safe sex; … don't use drugs … euthanasia is murder; … capitalism is just … etc.', and it is important for us to use our critical faculties to make sense of all these admonishments. Feldman and Marks (2005) add that without the skills of critical analysis, we have no means of distinguishing between different views on a subject and separating fact or sound argument from sophistry or opinion: 'All opinions are not equal. Some are a great deal more robust, sophisticated and well supported in logic and argument than others' (Douglas Adams, quoted in Feldman and Marks 2005, p. 4). What we should be seeking is a sound *justification* for accepting an argument or advice or taking a particular course of action, rather than propaganda, good marketing and other forms of persuasion (Bowell and Kemp 2010).

Reflective activity: as seen on TV!

How many 'health' products or activities can you list. Here are some of mine:

Benecol™
Olay sun cream™
Weetabix™
'You are what you eat' TV
Fitness club membership
Climbing stairs

- What evidence or justification is used in association with the product, programme or health advice?
- Do you believe what they are telling you? Is that evidence or justification sound or open to question?

Feldman and Marks (2005) suggest a broad hierarchy of opinion we can trust, with scientific and epidemiological evidence reproduced in peer-reviewed journals at the top, and propaganda (press statements and interviews) and folk-lore at the bottom, but they acknowledge that even experts *interpret* facts and this is shaped by ideology and values. Some of these concerns emerge when we scrutinise issues in the case studies in Chapter 5.

In essence, the point of critical thinking is to 'liberate yourself from accepting what others try to persuade you of without knowing whether you actually have good reason to be persuaded' (Bowell and Kemp 2010, p. 5). Bowell and Kemp add that while it might seem much easier just to 'go with the flow', and not think too deeply, this can often lead to inappropriate or bad decisions and action, on your behalf or by others (who accept poor argument and advice). It can lead to feelings of bewilderment over the different, and often conflicting, pieces of information sent our way, or indeed feelings of being duped when the promised benefits of an action do not come to fruition (if we have done what we have been told to do to, for example, to avoid disease but we still get ill).

To avoid these limitations and poor outcomes, you need to actively engage in your own learning. As Walton (2006) asserts, critical argument and critical thinking require a certain attitude, one that accepts that it is important to work through a problem or make thoughtful decisions. Critical thinking involves active learning, such as reading around a subject matter, thinking about the associated issues and gaining knowledge that helps you to interpret or understand different points of view and argument.

Knowledge helps us to get to the truth of a matter (Bowell and Kemp 2010). We have knowledge if what we think (and believe) is supported by sound evidence and therefore what we claim is justified. It is difficult to judge exactly what constitutes sound, or 'enough', evidence to be confident in our knowledge about something, but it is certainly easier to detect flawed or incomplete knowledge when we explore a matter in depth and from different perspectives and become wary of generalised declarations. An example of this sort of sloppy knowledge is referred to by Bowell and Kemp (2010) in the context of arguments that immigrants and asylum seekers have luxurious lifestyles. Frequently, one or two (alleged) examples are cited (often from newspapers) that paint a picture of wealth and security so powerfully that those who do not stop to question 'Is this true?', 'Does this relate to *all* immigrants and asylum seekers?' become subject to what Seedhouse (2004, p. 88) refers to as 'blinkered prejudice'. In other words, something other than reason and sound knowledge is in operation (Bowell and Kemp 2010) and while Seedhouse (2004) argues that values (prejudices) always shape our views, these should be attained and supported through critical evaluation and reflection and should always be open to scrutiny.

Developing your skills of critical thinking and improving your knowledge around health and social care issues will not necessarily mean that all argument is resolved and agreement is reached, but it will help to clarify the different perspectives called into play and the foundations of the views and ideas held by yourself and others (Walton 2006). As Bowell and Kemp (2010, p. 6) declare, critical thinking is also extremely empowering: 'those in power sometimes fear the effects of those who can think critically about moral, social, economic and political issues. The ability to think critically … is essential if one is to function properly in one's role as a citizen.'

This is why we have included information and discussion on many different theories, concepts, ideologies and examples within this text, as they provide you with foundational knowledge but also broader insights into the complex matters of health. You will need to put your point of view and argument over in your college and university work, and once you are in employment, to assert the necessity of a particular course of action or demonstrate the validity of a particular issue to reach an informed understanding of the issues under scrutiny.

How much reading is enough, and does it all need to be really up-to-date?

This is a very good question, and one that is not easy to answer. You do need to read around a subject matter and should explore enough material so that you are confident that the issues and ideas have been explored thoroughly. For example, if your seventh piece of literature (journal article, book, book chapter) includes the same, or similar, arguments and evidence as all the others, then you have probably got a good grounding in the topic. This is *not to say* that one text that says something different is not relevant to the subject. It might in fact be most important, as the content is offering an alternative perspective on the topic under scrutiny.

You also do not have to restrict yourself only to recent texts. It depends on the nature and purpose of the topic you are studying. For example, philosophical traditions from over 300 years ago are still relevant as they inform our ethical understanding today. Immanuel Kant's (1724–1804) work is an example of this, as is Enlightenment thinking, which you will read about later in this text. However, if you are exploring health policy, you do really need to look at the latest documents too. While the principles may be very similar across various policies (as you can see from the sections above), the detail will be different, and if you are exploring contemporary health and social care issues, they should be just that, i.e. contemporary. On that note you will notice within this text that some of the policy documents we refer to here may date from 2008 or 2009 and this is because a more recent version has not been produced and because of the inevitable time lag between writing and publishing. Nevertheless, the information will be pertinent and should spur you into seeing if there is anything more up-to-date too, and your tutors will be able to help with this.

Not putting opinion … only what others say?

The tradition in academic study is that you write in the 'third person' (unless otherwise instructed) and you should avoid making ill-informed statements e.g. 'I think …'. Argument, based on opinion, with little or no knowledge to support the claims made does not constitute critical analysis or critical thinking. Similarly, simply stating a disagreement, e.g. 'I do not agree, I think this course is too long', without evidence or argument does not constitute critical analysis either, but is merely an unsupported **proposition**. However, this does not mean that you should simply, robotically, synopsise other people's ideas or quote their words directly. Rather, you should always be using your critical thinking skills, and be making informed judgements and assessments about what you are reading. You should present your work in a manner that clearly demonstrates *your* current thinking; thinking that is supported by the evidence and arguments of others. So your 'opinion' is always in an essay, in so far as you are the one selecting the materials to demonstrate your insights into the debates surrounding the matter under scrutiny, but this should be presented in a balanced and evidenced manner.

Conclusion

Studying health is complex and challenging and requires developing knowledge but also critical thinking skills. Exploring concepts of health illustrates this dynamic and also the importance of basing ideas and actions on clear, reasoned, constructs. As Hamlin (1995, p. 1030) notes, 'Shouldn't medical folk be expected to be able to talk about what health is and what we are called on to do to foster it?', and it is with this in mind that the next two chapters introduce some key ideologies and terms and concepts that shape contemporary thinking and knowledge around health.

Key points to consider include:

> Many different ideas shape our thinking around health and work to promote health.

> These ideas are shaped by values and are controversial and contested.

> Critical thinking and developing our knowledge and critical understanding are vital to be able to navigate our way around the complex world of contemporary health and social care issues.

Useful resources

On health and health promotion

Earle, S., Lloyd, C. E., Sidell, M. and Spurr, S. (eds) (2007) *Theory and Research in Promoting Health*. London: Sage Publications in association with the Open University. This book will provide you with an overview of the historical development of health promotion and principles and practices of work to promote health.

Porter, R. (1997) *The Greatest Benefit to Mankind*. London: Fontana Press. This book provides the reader with an excellent journey through the history of medicine and includes a chapter on public health (public medicine).

Seedhouse, D. (1986, 2001) *Health: The Foundations for Achievement*. Chichester: John Wiley and Sons. This is essential reading for a well considered, critical analysis of health and work to promote health.

Seedhouse, D. (1997a, 2004) *Health Promotion: Philosophy, Prejudice and Practice*. Chichester: John Wiley and Sons. This provides a coherent analysis of the pitfalls and limitations of many traditional approaches to work to promote health and presents an alternative way of perceiving work to promote health that maintains its ethical as well as practical integrity.

On health policy

Baggott, R. (2007) *Understanding Health Policy*. Bristol: Policy Press.

Ham, C. (2004) *Health Policy in Britain: The Politics and Organisation of the National Health Service*, 5th edn. Basingstoke: Macmillan.

On study skills

Cotterell, S. (2008) *The Study Skills Handbook*, 3rd edn. Basingstoke: Palgrave Macmillan. A very user-friendly text with lots of exercises and practical examples.

Race, P. (1999) *How to Get a Good Degree. Making the Most of Your Time at University*. Buckingham: Open University Press.

On critical thinking

Bowell, T. and Kemp, G. (2010) *Critical Thinking. A Concise Guide*, 3rd edn. London: Routledge. This book presents an excellent and accessible overview of critical thinking and critical argument. Exercises (and answers) are provided too.

Walton, D. (2006) *Fundamentals of Critical Argumentation*. Cambridge: Cambridge University Press. Another excellent text introducing critical argument that is easy to read with some interesting examples.

2 key ideologies

2.1 INTRODUCTION

This chapter explores:

> different ideologies that directly, or indirectly shape ideas around health;
> where appropriate, the implications for health (and social care) that emerge from the particular ideology.

This chapter explores key ideologies and theories that shape contemporary attitudes and beliefs, particularly in relation to how we perceive and act upon matters around health. Ideology refers to an organised system of beliefs, values and ideas, which form the basis of a social, economic or political philosophy and which shape the way individuals or a group (e.g. a social class group) act and understand the world. It was a term introduced by the French philosopher Destutt de Tracy to refer to the 'science of ideas', through which de Tracy asserted that the 'biases and prejudices' which underpin our thinking will be revealed. The word fell into disuse but was revived through the writings of **Karl Marx**. Ideologies themselves are social creations (Bell 1999). 'Classification is a matter of human interest and convenience ... general words stand for "nominal essences", mental abstract ideas which we ourselves construct' (Woolhouse 1995, p. 495), and ideologies are products of a particular social, cultural and economic history and context. For instance, the notion of individual freedom emerges as an ideology within liberal capitalist societies and the operation of the **free market** economy.

They are not true representations of reality and the ideas and values that a particular ideology represents are not necessarily shared by all. You may recognise this from disagreements that emerge in your discussions in class, and this demonstrates how ideologies shape our interpretations, understandings, actions and decision-making within society, such as health policy decision-making.

Understanding the nature and content of various contemporary ideologies is therefore central to recognising the contested territory of decision-making within health, healthcare and work to promote health, and this in itself helps to form the foundations of effective critical analysis of such matters.

The key features of each ideology are described, followed by a discussion of how this perspective contributes to shaping, and resolving, the debates and dilemmas that emerge within contemporary health and healthcare practice. This is brief, by the very nature of this text, but provides you with a broad outline of the ideology or theory. It was difficult to make decisions about which ideologies to include and inevitably choices and inclusions are imperfect. What we have chosen to present are some key '**grand narratives**' and critiques, and alternatives to these grand narratives that have influenced directly, or indirectly, our thinking and understanding around health, the shape of contemporary health policy and issues regarded as pertinent to health. In practice the presentation of this section is alphabetical, and not exhaustive, and in no way implies a hierarchical value attributed to the concepts.

This latter point is important because this content is here to serve a purpose for you as a student. The intention is that you can 'dip into' ideas that help you in your analysis of the issues you come across in your study on your course.

We cross-reference to other ideologies or indeed key concepts in Chapter 3 as appropriate.

2.2 KEY IDEOLOGIES AND THEORIES SHAPING THE WAY WE THINK

Capitalism

Capitalism is included because it reflects the social and economic structures of most contemporary Western societies and is increasingly a dominant force across the world.

What is capitalism?

Most Western societies have economic systems based, to a greater or lesser extent, on capitalism. Capitalism describes an economic system rooted in the production of commodities and the accumulation of profit, operating within a free-market (Wood 1995; Pampel 2000; Bilton et al. 2002). During the late eighteenth and nineteenth centuries capitalism, combined with new industrial inventions, provided the means for rapid growth in factory-based production, fuelling the Industrial Revolution, of which Britain was the pioneer. The origins of capitalism lie in the work of Adam Smith (1723–90) (see, for example, *The Wealth of Nations* 1776), championing a general **laissez-faire** philosophy of governance, which contributed to the shift from protectionist mercantile policy to those that embraced free trade and competition. Fundamental to laissez-faire philosophy is the principle of minimal state intervention, stimulating individual innovation unfettered by unnecessary regulation, and based on the assumption that free markets, competition and self-interest produce economic efficiency and national wealth (Pampel 2000) (see also liberal individualism, p. 44).

The relationship between capitalism and health: the benefits of capitalism?

During the Industrial Revolution the loosening of regulation under laissez-faire capitalism undoubtedly brought benefits, particularly to consumers (Mathias 1969). It enabled the production of goods and basic commodities at prices that many more in the population could afford (Myers 2007). Industrial capitalism also brought about overall improvements in material conditions, a rise in health (represented by declining mortality) (Hart 1985; Handy 1998; Myers 2007), more individual freedom, the ability to strive for personal achievement and greater mobility and privacy (Myers 2007) (see individualism, p. 92).

The relationship between capitalism and health: the negative impact of capitalism on health

The fragmentation of community and kinship networks is regarded as an inevitable outcome of capitalism (Pampel 2000), as capitalism requires a mobile workforce, and the importance of 'production' supersedes other social goals (Daykin and Jones 2008), with cultural images and ideas developing to serve the economy, not people's psychological and social realities (Eckersley 2006; cited in Carlisle et al. 2008). Myers (2007, p. 43) asserts that a 'socially toxic individualism' emerges from capitalism, which contributes to undermining the development, *inter alia*, of collective, national, policies for health (Stampar 2008), with medicine and health work increasingly becoming a marketable commodity (Hart 1985; Scott-Jones 2002; French 2007; Carlisle et al. 2008) (see commodification, p. 71).

While the extreme forms of worker exploitation, observed in Britain in the nineteenth century with child labour and work-days of 12 hours or more, have largely disappeared (in the UK at least), modern methods of organising work have become dehumanising and potentially health-damaging, through the monotonous and mechanised nature of some forms of industrial processes (White 2009). The potential for 'boom and bust' economic cycles threatens employment and economic security (a very real threat with the 2008–9 credit crunch in Western capitalist economies), although, as Hart (1985) comments, this does not have to be an *inevitable* consequence of capitalism, as states can elect to provide welfare and support to protect against the worst

vagaries of market forces. Doyal and Pennell (1979) and Navarro (1976) also comment on the role of capitalism in encouraging the consumption of 'unhealthy' goods such as cigarettes, processed foods and use of the car, and the health-harms of industrial processes themselves (e.g. accidents, occupational disease).

Conclusion

As a dominant social, economic and political force, capitalism has shaped health in several ways through its influence on socio-economic conditions and the commodification of many aspects of life. In order to constructively, critically analyse health in the twenty-first century at least a basic understanding and awareness of these factors that contribute to, and detract from, social, community and individual experiences of health is essential.

Communitarianism

Communitarianism is included because it has been an important sub-theme in modern government policy in the UK (for example, tackling social exclusion and strengthening communities).

What is communitarianism?

Authors such as Sandel (1982), Walzer (1983), MacIntyre (1985) and Shiell and Hawe (1996) argue that people cannot be regarded simply as individuals immune from social circumstances and the lives we inhabit. Language, ethnicity, heritage and environment all shape our identities and the decisions and choices we make. These ideas, also embodied within communitarianism, recognise the value of the social in human relationships and propound the importance of recognising *collective* needs and responsibilities above individual aspirations (Calder 2003).

The notion of rights and responsibility is core to the dialogue of communitarianism (Etzioni 1993; Calder 2003), debating the flaws of what is sometimes termed the 'me-ist' society (the growth of assertion of individual rights and freedom of choice) (Etizioni 1993) (see individualism, p. 92, and free will, p. 80). Choice is often asserted as a key mechanism for improving services, facilities and experiences but Etzioni (1993) asserts that it is facile to assume that individual rights or individual choice are sacrosanct and will solve problems such as bad schools. Choice, for example, is much more likely to lead to, and consolidate, ghettoisation, as those with the opportunity for choice (e.g. money and access to other resources) are able to live in better-resourced areas, send their children to fee-paying schools and so forth. Rights too are often in practice the pursuit of individual aspirations (Etzioni 1993). This seriously undermines the principles of rights, as they cannot be divorced from the social context, including a consideration of the rights of others (the community), legal determinants and the resources available (Etzioni 1993). Warnock (1998) points out that it is nonsensical to assert a right, for example, to a blood transfusion when no blood is available. The assertion of this right becomes meaningless without the resources to make fulfilment of the right possible.

Essentially communitarianism requires the establishment and practice of shared values, which operate in the interests of community members per se, not merely individuals, fostering social bonds. Communitarianism is about making environments good for all and represents ideas close to the heart of recent governments, such as that of New Labour (1997–2010) (Calder 2003).

How is communitarianism developed?
The existence and development of trust between citizens and the dominant hegemony (those with dominant political, economic and social control) within society is vital to establishing more communitarian societies. Trust itself is established

through reciprocity, mutuality, the creation and support of social bonds, better community representation and equity as a foundation to decision-making (Mooney 2005; Mooney and Houston 2008), and through the operation of institutions such as health care (Travassos 2008). Open and frequent dialogue over issues that affect both individuals and communities is essential in identifying and establishing a new consensus, as illustrated by the campaigning over smoking and smoking in public over the years (Etzioni 1993; Hoedemaekers and Dekkers 2003).

Establishing communitarian – shared values – inevitably involves an element of self-policing (Etzioni 1993). The relationship between the state and its citizens shifts. For example, the direct role of the state in people's lives, particularly with regard to legislative control, becomes reduced. Communities become much more like constitutional democracies. The state, however, retains a strong role to support communities affected by the vagaries of capitalist market forces, which lead, for example, to industrial closures and unemployment.

Establishing communitarian values depends on developing a middle-way between abdicating individual responsibility (blaming all problems on society or government) and ignoring the barriers (social, economic and environmental) and prejudices that do shapes opportunities and aspirations (Etizioni 1993). Informed debate about options for action is essential and rules, boundaries and other controls must be established to ensure that options in one area do not precipitate a general decay of freedoms elsewhere (Etzioni 1993).

Improving communities requires improvements in local facilities and services and in education and training to support the development of community members, as well as admonishments to responsibility and punishments for transgressions of community/societal rules (National Crime Prevention Council 1995).

Criticisms of communitarianism

Etizioni (1993) notes that the values of communitarianism are criticised as being based on both fuzzy and rather rosy concepts of what constitutes a community (Calder 2003) and for the potential of curbing individual freedoms. Particular versions of 'community' could become reified (Calder 2003), and enforcing and asserting community values over individual freedoms may culminate in sanctions, stigmatising and alienating members of society who are cast as deviating from these shared values (Etzioni 1993; Roberts and Reich 2002) (see stigma, p. 118). Paradoxically communitarian aspirations could lead to more central control of communities, e.g. a zero tolerance policy (Calder 2003).

For communitarian values to flourish, the responsibility for monitoring and managing social behaviour inevitably becomes a more community/individual duty. This focus is at odds with the increasing individualism observed within society. Etzioni (1993) notes, for example, that citizens in the USA want trial by jury but do not themselves wish to be jurors, and wish to pay less in tax and have greater individual freedom, while placing greater and greater responsibilities onto government. Simultaneously, under the guise of individual choice, we also witness increasing decentralisation of the provision of services such as accessible and affordable childcare and perhaps, ironically, communitarian impulses are frequently played out through individual behaviour, such as not dropping litter and volunteer work. Myers (2007) notes too that broad societal aspirations and expectations do not necessarily support or sustain a more communitarian orientation.

Communitarianism and health

The health benefits of supportive communities are increasingly recognised (Scheff 1990; Calder 2003; Kagan 2006; White 2009). Lomas (1998, p. 1181) asserts that:

We ignore what our everyday experience tells us, i.e. the way we organise our society, the extent to which we encourage interaction among the citizenry and the degree to which we trust and associate with each other in caring communities is probably the most important determinant of our health.

Supportive communities also contribute to improving children's welfare and achievements, and reducing crime and deviance within society (National Crime Prevention Council 1995; Voydanoff 2001) and according to Mooney (2005), Gilson (2003) and Mooney and Houston (2008), more community, collectivist, orientated societies reflect a particular perspective on **morality** and **justice** in a society. For example, a more communitarian society would be one in which healthcare is regarded as a community good, not merely an individual good, and a society based on greater trust can facilitate and promote access to healthcare among disadvantaged and marginalised members of society (Travassos 2008).

Conclusion

Communitarian principles are reflected in various guises and in many discussions around contemporary health and social care issues. Fulfilling a communitarian agenda, though, would require considerable shifts in social priorities and the current focus on individualism.

Democracy

Democracy has been chosen for the same reasons as capitalism.

The origin of the word democracy is from the Greek, referring to the rule of the *demos*, i.e. the citizenry or people make decisions about matters that affect all members of the city-state (Bullock 1999). Both Plato and Aristotle included in this only the 'best' citizens (*aristos* – Greek for 'best', as in aristocracy) and were highly critical about the rule of the 'mob' (Ncayiyana 2004).

Democratic principles essentially recognise the importance of the individual (Bullock 1999) and refer to the notion of 'government by the people'. It is generally considered to be the best form of government (Hardin 1995). Essentially its principle foundation is 'one person, one vote', therefore reputedly exemplifying government by the people, through the right to vote on policy via a mandate to the elected party. It is worth noting that those who have had the right to vote have until recent times been a narrow range of the population, with women, for instance, only being given equal voting rights to men in 1928 in the UK.

Democracy is considered to create positive outcomes for its population in the form of welfare, autonomy, equality and agreement, though the extent and nature of any of these in reality are open to dispute (Hardin 1995). For example, welfare provision is not necessarily as egalitarian in practice as in principle and participation cannot be the only mechanism for attaining autonomy (as active participation and deliberation within populations counted in the millions are impracticable) (Hardin 1995). Nevertheless, the principles of democracy endorse the extension of certain rights to all citizens: freedom of speech, freedom from persecution, freedom of assembly (e.g. to join trade unions), equal rights under the law, freedom of movement, freedom of religion and education (Bullock 1999).

Reflective activity

Look up the proportion of people who voted in the 2010 UK election (try http://www.ukpolitical.info/Turnout45.htm).

- Do you think this should be improved?
- What are the disadvantages of people not voting?

Other more recognisable characteristics of a democracy are that of free voting in elections (held at regular intervals, with the potential to change the constituents of the governing party or parties), freedom for candidates to campaign against the government, freedom for elected governments to create legislative and fiscal policy and raise taxes, and the right for our representatives to vote on such matters. Finally, there is freedom to criticise, discuss, argue and dispute such policies without fear of retribution.

In reality few, if any, modern democracies would claim to be as egalitarian as this principle presumes and a more accurate description of modern societies such as the UK would be to describe them as 'representative democracies' (Bullock 1999). In other words, we vote for a Member of Parliament (MP) as the intermediary between us as individual citizens and the policy-makers (government).

Criticisms of democracy

Hardin (1995) notes that one of the limitations of democracy lies with the difficulty in translating individual choices and preferences to collective decision-making, and the problematic nature of participation when a population (its constituent individuals) is ill-informed about matters of state and the needs of whole populations: 'Self interest leads to public ignorance' (Hardin 1995, p. 183). Bullock (1999) adds to these criticisms and notes that democracies in practice do not create the necessary conditions for active participation and often operate to the lowest common denominator, with prevarication in terms of decision-making. Bullock (1999) also comments on the rise of bureaucracy associated with democracies, which diminishes opportunities for effective participation. Despite these flaws, there are increasing calls for greater democracy at all levels of decision-making, particularly within local government and other organisations such as trade unions.

Democracy and health

'A country's political structure affects virtually every aspect of society, including health' (Ruger 2005, p. 299). Various commentators (Reich 1994; Franco et al. 2004) note that democracies demonstrate better health performance, as judged by various indicators such as maternal and infant mortality, and longevity, than states operating under other political regimes. Ruger (2005) points out that it is unclear what particular mechanism(s) within democratic countries contribute to the relative health advantages observed, but one aspect may be the effect of greater political and social participation: for example, the opportunity to vote. In non-democratic countries the needs of the poor may ignored (as they have no veto), and it may be in the interests of those vested with power to maintain ignorance and not invest in health, education and economic security, as this stifles population advocacy (Ruger 2005; Bowell and Kemp 2010). Non-democratic countries may provide few opportunities for their citizens to avoid health hazards, through non-provision of resources and services, or the lack of a chance for public participation and social choice. Lack of freedom, particularly lack of freedom of speech between groups and within the media, may also obscure problems that exist within a society. Ruger (2005) suggests that lack of transparency and information contributed to the devastating famine in China in the late 1950s and early 1960s. Neither the reality of the situation nor the failings of government policy were disclosed to the population en masse, enabling the government to act with impunity.

Democratic practice alone, though, will not eliminate disparate health experiences, as what also seem to matter *within* countries are experiences of poverty and equality, particularly income distribution. More egalitarian distribution of wealth,

rather than the overall wealth of a country, is linked to better overall health outcomes (Wilkinson 1996; Franco et al. 2004; Ncayiyana 2004) and this varies even in democratic countries (see capitalism, p. 32, and inequalities, p. 95).

Democracies do have the potential for participation to blossom and this can be particularly valuable, both in general and within the health sphere: 'a commitment to improving public participation practices can reap dividends for both service delivery and democratic decision-making' (Andersson et al. n.d., p. 5), and is strongly advocated in recent health policy (DoH 2004a).

Conclusion

Overall, what can be concluded is that 'how the way a society organises and conducts itself affects the health of its members' (Martyn 2004, p. 1424). A society based on a democratic social system is not without its flaws and full equality of power and representation appears elusive. However, within democratic societies, participation and equality are made possible, with certain rights being asserted for all citizens, and perhaps the best conclusion that can be drawn about democracy is embodied in Winston Churchill's witticism that 'democracy is the worst form of government, other than all the other forms we know' (Hardin 1995).

The Enlightenment

The Enlightenment has been chosen because it represents a time of profound changes in thinking and scientific and medical discovery which has helped shape the nature of society today.

Useful resource

Sir Isaac Newton (1642–1727) was a significant figure of influence to the Enlightenment. On 14 May 2010, to celebrate 350 years of the Royal Society, ↘

pieces of wood from the apple tree that inspired Sir Isaac Newton's theory of gravity were launched into space on the NASA shuttle *Atlantis*, representing the monumental progress and contribution of scientific experimentation and discovery inspired by the Enlightenment. Go to: http://news.bbc.co.uk/1hi/8671627.stm for more about the story.

The Enlightenment was a period in the history of Western nations when significant shifts in thinking took place (Bilton et al. 2002). The Enlightenment spawned modernity (see p. 46) (Chisick 2008) and was itself influenced by the work of Francis Bacon (1561–1626), who advocated the use of the scientific method, and René Descartes (1596–1650), who promoted **rationalism** (Jones 2008). In essence the Enlightenment saw the expansion of knowledge, the application of reason and the development and growth of the scientific method. It was considered that society would steadily improve, informed by rational thought, science and personal freedom. People (and thinking) were released from the constraints of religious myth and aristocratic power, opening up the possibility for people to live in societies in which social institutions could improve life and create greater happiness (Pampel 2000). There was a huge growth in confidence in the power of reason to solve societal problems. The key attributes of Enlightenment thinking were that intellectual enquiry was core to progressing humanity and happiness, and that iniquities, inequalities, social injustice, superstition and so forth must be challenged. Enlightenment thinking, for instance, was used to inform anti-slavery enquiry, such as that led by William Wilberforce (1759–1833) – although it was also used to argue *for* slavery (Open University Learning Space n.d.).

The acquisition of knowledge was fundamental to Enlightenment thinking.

At the heart of the Enlightenment in France, for example, was the *Encyclopédie* complied by Diderot (1713–84) and D'Alembert (1717–83), one of the first encyclopaedias, which included contributions from Voltaire (1694–1778), Rousseau (1712–78) and other contemporary thinkers of the eighteenth century. It included a total of 72,000 articles. The *Encyclopédie* was banned in 1759, which suggests concern about the effect of ideas and knowledge on the status quo. One of the guiding principles behind the Enlightenment was that knowledge should have substantive foundations, rather than simply being based on authority, convention, tradition or prejudice. Instead knowledge was acquired through evidence gathered via the senses (observation and experimentation), i.e. empirically. Medicine made great strides through the Enlightenment period and the benefits, for instance, of surgery and inoculation (such as inoculation against smallpox, which was banned by the Church) demonstrated the valuable contribution to society of scientific and rational thought. The confidence in the power of scientific and rational thought extended to the ability to identify moral absolutes and universal standards, such as what constitutes 'right' from 'wrong'. Moral debates increasingly focused on increasing individual and social well-being rather than adhering to religious doctrine (see modernism, p. 46).

Alongside this emphasis on knowledge and rational thought, perhaps contrarily, grew an interest in the sublime qualities of nature, with writers such as Rousseau (1712–78) (also associated with **romanticism**) arguing that humanity should return to the laws of nature, and expressing an interest in the emotional responses and unique identity of persons. These shifts in thinking contributed to the rise of individualism (see p. 92), the hedonism of the eighteenth and early nineteenth centuries and the recognition that feelings as well as reason were important.

Criticism of Enlightenment thinking

The egalitarian and progressive ideas that emerged from the Enlightenment thinking were still limited by social prejudice. The 'mob' or 'masses' were still regarded as dangerous and educated, wealthy men remained at the centre of power. Women were excluded from power, or contributing to debates around social and political change (Open University Learning Space n.d.), although influential women did emerge during this period, such as Mary Wollstonecraft (1759–97), who was an early proponent of the rights of women (see feminism, p. 43), Jane Austen (1775–1817), the novelist, and Mme de Staël (1766–1817), the author.

The focus on knowledge and rationality and the faith invested in this as enabling access to *the* truth, the ideal society and the perfectability of humankind has also been criticised (Sutcliffe 2008). Sutcliffe highlights the perspectives of individuals such as Bayle (1647–1706), who argued that the Enlightenment quest for *all* encompassing intellectual/philosophical systems was simply an alternative form of dogma (to that of religious dogma). Instead, Bayle asserted that it was essential to avoid certainty. Postmodernist thought, eventually emerged to contest the certainty of the claims of Enlightenment thinking (see postmodernism, p. 47).

Enlightenment and health

The ideologies of different epochs inform contemporary thinking, either directly or as a reaction against the preceding dogmas, and the thinking that emerged prior to, and during, the Enlightenment continues to be a powerful discourse that influences contemporary thinking. For example, the gradual acceptance of women's rights, and the importance of discovery via experimentation and science rather than religious or imperial dictate, were established by Enlightenment thinking. 'Reason ... would create a better future; science and technology, as Francis Bacon had taught, would enhance man's control over nature, and social progress, prosperity and the conquest of disease would follow' (Porter 1997, p. 245).

Enlightenment thinkers declared aspirations to use medical advances to improve longevity and usher in the end of disease and illness, and medical and scientific discovery emerging from the Enlightenment still informs healthcare practice today. For example, measurements such as monitoring the pulse were advocated in the early eighteenth century when Sir John Floyer (1649–1734) recommended using a watch with a special second hand when checking the pulse (Porter 1997). The mechanistic explanations of disease also emerged during this time and anatomical and physiological investigation became established. Some of these investigations were inventive and not always pleasant. For example, much experimentation involved vivisection, spawning an anti-vivisection movement (Samuel Johnson, 1709–84, thought vivisection abhorrent) and self-experimentation. For example, Spallanzani (1729–99) swallowed and regurgitated linen bags to test the effects of saliva (Porter 1997).

Useful resource

Moore, W. (2005) *The Knife Man: Blood, Body-Snatching and the Birth of Modern Surgery*. London: Bantam Books. This is an interesting read about the life and times of John Hunter and his contemporaries. John Hunter was a key figure in the Enlightenment and is credited as being the founder of modern surgery. The anatomical ↘

and pathological specimens of John and his brother, William, form the foundation of the collection in the Hunterian Museum in London. The museum is located inside the Royal College of Surgeons. For more information about the museum go to http://www.rcseng.ac.uk/museums/

Conclusion

Overall, the Enlightenment established experimentation as a legitimate method of discovery, and saw developments in the understanding and classification of disease, including pathology and therapeutics. It built on older traditions (such as 'smallpox' parties among the peasantry of Turkey and folk-lore medicaments), but also colonised traditional areas of care, such as midwifery, and the role and function of religion by offering scientific and medical solace rather than religious guidance at the end of life. As Porter (1997, p. 302) puts it, 'Science and medicine were challenging religion as meanings of existence. ... The Enlightenment ... sped the medicalization of life and death ... gaining cultural authority.' Arguably this is still true today given the continuing dominance of the biomedical, Western/scientific concept of health, discussed in Chapter 1, and does have negative and positive consequences too (see commodification, p. 71).

Useful resource

For a comprehensive overview of the Enlightenment see http://openlearn.open.ac.uk/course/view.php?id=2090. Access to this initially is as a guest log-in but you can register for free. The information here is comprehensive and interesting.

Environmentalism

Environmentalism has been chosen because it represents ideas that are increasingly shaping our modern world: for example, green issues and concerns over carbon emissions.

Environmentalism is a political and ethical movement that focuses on improving the natural environment through economic, social and political change. Founded on interest in humankind's relationship with the natural environment, concerns have emerged about various harms and damage being done to various aspects of the environment. There are broadly two perspectives within environmentalism, anthropocentric and biocentric environmentalism. Anthropocentric environmentalism is primarily concerned with the impact of environmental degradation on human society rather than a concern for the environment, or other living creatures, per se. Biocentric environmentalism is broader, asserting that we have a duty and moral obligation to the environment and planet itself (Elliot 2008).

Concern about the environment filtered into human consciousness in recent times through the work of authors such as Rachel Carson, James Lovelock and Edward Goldsmith and colleagues. Carson published her book *Silent Spring* in 1962, and documented the impact, among other things, of pesticides on living creatures. Attention was drawn, for example, to the effects of DDT (dichlorodiphenyltrichloroethane). DDT was a commonly used and highly effective pesticide against diseases such as malaria and typhoid but was also implicated in the aetiology of cancers and disruption of genetic material. DDT was noted to accumulate in fatty tissues and was linked to observed problems experienced by birds of prey (the laying of thin shelled eggs, which cracked during incubation). The use of DDT was banned in the USA in 1972. According to James Lovelock's, Gaia theory (Gaia being the Greek earth goddess), the Earth is a finely tuned, self-regulating system, and Edward Goldsmith and colleagues (*Blueprint for Survival* 1972), drew attention to current and future damage to the Earth's ecosystem through human activity. In 1985 a hole was identified in the ozone layer over Antarctica, linked to the use of chlorofluorocarbons (CFCs, found in aerosols and refrigerators), and the Chernobyl disaster in 1986 drew attention to the fragility of the environment, along with more recent episodes of flooding, heat waves, cyclones and forest fires (Denney 2005). Attention has also increasingly focused on concerns over energy consumption and global warming (Lomborg 2001; Denney 2005; McKibben 2006). All of these events have galvanised attention to the impact of environmental degradation on people's state of health and quality of life (Elliot 2008).

Impact of environmentalism

Whatever the specific focus, the impact of environmental concerns can be seen on national and international politics. This is partly in terms of domestic politics and the rise of political parties such as the Green Party (the first Green Party MP was elected in the 2010 general election), along with grass-roots environmental activity asserting the rights, for instance, of indigenous people over logging companies (Elliot 2008), but also in the shape of international treaties and legislative proposals. The phasing out of DDT and other organic pesticides (organic because they contain carbon) was approved at the Stockholm Convention on Persistent Organic Pollutants (POPs) in 2000, and the United Nations Conference on Environment and Development held in Rio de Janeiro in 1992 (known as the Earth Summit) focused specifically on environmental issues and sustainable development. Significant documents emerged from this conference, including Agenda 21, the Rio Declaration on Environment and Development and the United Nations Framework Convention on Climate Change (which spawned the Kyoto Protocol's enforceable target reductions in emissions in 1997). The Kyoto agreement specifically set

targets for a reduction in the production of greenhouse gases between 2008 and 2012 by 5.2 per cent (Denney 2005).

Useful resource

For more information on the Earth Summit look on http://www.un.org/geninfo/bp/enviro.html

Increasingly, therefore, the matter of the environment shapes and features in our everyday lives, with McKibben (2006) calling for a general curtailment of consumption and increase in sustainable use of resources, and a fundamental shift in our 'consumption mindset'. These shifts influence people's health and quality of life (Elliot 2008), but also their behaviours and opportunities (see capitalism, p. 32). Consider, for instance, the recycling of waste products (plastics, glass, paper and so forth) that many do on a weekly, if not daily, basis, and the potential impact of local and national policy to control the use of energy and emissions of greenhouse gases. The latter is seen, at least in part, as spurring action towards congestion charges in cities such as London and Greater Manchester (put to the vote in Greater Manchester in December 2008, and resoundingly rejected) and you may even observe TV adverts urging you to 'know your carbon footprint' (see 'Act on CO_2': http://www.un.org/geninfo/bp/enviro.html).

Criticisms of mainstream environmentalism

While the environmental lobby is likely to remain an influential actor in the development of economic and energy policy over the next decades, this impact is far from uncontroversial. Lomborg (2001, 2007), for instance, while accepting that climate change is occurring and that human activity contributes to this change, argues that the extent of climate change is often exaggerated and the solutions embodied in the **Kyoto Agreement** are unlikely to be cost effective. Instead he suggests that human society should work towards developing strategies and systems that enable us to cope with changes more effectively, rather than trying to stop global warming. This argument is partly based on the expense and difficulty of actions to reduce carbon emissions, which inconvenience and inhibit individuals and states (for no certain gain), but also because this detracts us from spending money on actions and interventions that we *know* will save lives, now, such as tackling malaria and ensuring access to clean water (Lomborg 2001, 2007).

O'Neill (2007) takes his criticism of environmentalism even further, locating environmental dialogue with that of religious doctrine. He points to how the 'End of Days', flood, famine and catastrophe claims of environmentalists resonate with biblical accounts of the demise of mankind and the positioning of 'anti-environmentalists' as heretics and 'deniers' (O'Neill 2006). Environmentalism has become an unquestioning, unquestionable, doctrine (O'Neill 2006). O'Neill (2007) further equates the calls of the environmentalist with the preaching of priests and other religious leaders, with the only difference between the two doctrines being the origins of salvation, one residing in Mother Earth, the other in heaven. This connection between moral decay and capitalist consumption has been a powerful argument for decades and, according to Furedi (2007), has been captured and utilised by the environmental lobby, with its call for prudence and restraint of human activity:

The 'science' of global warming has been transformed into a moral denunciation of human activity, to a point where the term 'human impact' is instantly identified with destructive and irresponsible behaviour.
(Furedi 2007, p. 4)

Environmentalism and health

Despite these criticisms of the environmentalist lobby, concern over the health impact of environmental change, and global warming in particular, is becoming an increasing force in contemporary political and health debate. Shircore (2009), for example, asserts that climate instability is one of the greatest threats to the long-term health of populations. It is recognised too, that the impact of global warming is likely to fall, disproportionately, on the poorest and most vulnerable members of the world's community, those who, ironically, contribute least to the causes of climate change (Committee on Environmental Health 2007; Patz et al. 2007). Children are regarded as being especially vulnerable from a variety of consequences of global warming, including risk of injury and death due to extreme weather conditions, increase in climate-sensitive infectious disease, air pollution, leading to increased problems associated with respiratory disease (D'Amato and Cecchi 2008), and heat-related diseases as well as the effect of disruption to crop yield, disruption and contamination of water supply and consequent impact on social stability (Committee on Environmental Health 2007; Bernardi 2008; Patz et al. 2008; Shea et al. 2008). Other environmental events such serious flooding exacerbated by deforestation cause serious harm and injury as well as economic disruption, and malaria could increase if climates become warmer and more humid (Patz et al. 2007).

Within Western nations, Bloomberg and Aggarwala (2008) argue, action to reduce the impact of climate change, through reducing carbon emissions, could have a positive impact on health. Reductions in carbon emissions will decrease the prevalence, for instance, not only of respiratory disease but also of obesity and associated chronic disease through reduction in the use of cars and the promotion of cycling and walking (see also Case Study 1 in Chapter 4).

Conclusion

Environmentalism draws our attention to the contested notion of debates with the public sphere and how evidence and argument can be used in a variety of ways. It is likely that the consensus around environmentalism and global warming will gradually shift and will remain an important consideration for human health too.

Feminism

Feminism is included because it is a social and political ideology and movement that has had a profound impact on modern Western society. It continues to be a source of debate regarding the role and health of women in societies across the world.

There is a huge amount that can be written about feminism and this section provides only the broadest outline of its key components. In essence, feminism encompasses a range of ideas, all of which focus in one way or another on the rights of women, equal political rights, economic liberation, equal pay and opportunities and sexual freedom. The origins of feminist thinking are diverse and date at least from medieval times but gained momentum with the eighteenth-century Enlightenment (see p. 37), which, among other things, encapsulated shifts in thinking around the rights of man (woman). For example, Mary Wollstonecraft (1759–97), the mother of Mary Shelley (who was the wife of the poet Percy Shelley, and author of *Frankenstein*), wrote *A Vindication of the Rights of Women* in 1792. During this and subsequent decades, concern grew over the legal rights of women in marriage, education and employment. The suffrage movement of the latter part of the nineteenth century and early part of the

twentieth century was an active political manifestation of this trend (Swingewood 1999), although achieving even the modest goal of the right to vote took a significant number of years, not being granted until 1918, to women over the age of 30, providing they, or their husband, qualified under certain property rules. It took a further ten years for these rights to equal those of men (eligible to vote at the age of 21). Further radicalisation in feminist politics took place in the 1960s and 1970s, linked with other social and political protest (for example, for black rights in the USA) and eventually many strands of feminism emerged: for example, women's emancipation, women's liberation, the women's movement, social feminism and radical feminism (from the 1970s onwards) (Grimshaw 1999).

> ### Reflective activity: women's images on TV adverts
>
> - Over the next week or so, make a note of how women are portrayed in advertisements on TV.
> - What is the subject matter of the advert?
> - Are the women pictured in domestic settings or work settings?
> - If they are pictured in work settings, what sort of job are they depicted doing?
> - Overall, what have you observed as the most dominant media representation of women?

Whatever the particular focus, the common strand within feminist discourse is exploring the origins and nature of equality and difference (Grimshaw 1999) and the invisibility of women's roles and female perspectives within society (Maynard 1999).

Feminist study increasingly scrutinised the nature of male and female identity, challenging fixed notions of gender based on biological characteristics, in favour of ones acknowledging the patriarchal oppression of women (Grimshaw 1999) and social construction of masculine/feminine roles (Butler 1990; Maynard 1999), including the trivialising nature of female imagery in the public forum, e.g. media images based on sexual attractiveness or domestic competence (Tuchman et al. 1978).

Feminism and health

White (2009) highlights how the socialisation of male and female roles and the contribution of **patriarchal** gender stereotyping around women and motherhood contribute significantly to women's experiences of health and illness, including the medicalisation of women's health, particularly around the reproductive life cycle (see Case Study 2 on artificial reproductive techniques in Chapter 4). As a consequence, among other things the feminist movement from the 1970s onwards responded by encouraging women to take control of their own health and bodies, focusing on self-health, women health clinics and so forth (See for instance, Phillips and Rakusen's *Our Bodies, Ourselves* originally published in the 1970s). However, gender issues in health remain important, particularly in relation to women-only services and the importance of female practitioners being actively involved in service delivery such as cervical and breast screening.

Conclusion

Feminism as a social and political movement has enabled women to become increasingly empowered members of society. Women now have far greater opportunities for education, employment, financial security and legal and social rights, but inequalities remain and feminist discourse will continue to provide valuable insights into the experiences of women.

Liberal individualism

This is included because it represents a dominant ideology underpinning many Western nations' economies and social and political systems. It strongly shapes attitudes and policies associated with health.

Liberal individualism represents a particular theoretical and political ideology, which emerged in eighteenth- and nineteenth-century philosophical thinking. Its distinguishing features are the rights (civil and political) it ascribes to individuals (Kymlicka 1995). Liberty, equality of opportunity and personal freedom – freedom of speech, conscience, association, occupation and sexuality (Kymlicka 1995) – are central tenants of liberalist thinking. Key liberalist philosophers are John Locke (1632–1704), Immanuel Kant (1724–1804), John Stuart Mill (1806–73) and John Rawls (1921–2002). John Locke asserted that the state should have minimal involvement in the lives of individuals (see individualism, p. 92). The role of the state was essentially to enable individual freedom, and limit actions to the protection of property rights and personal liberty (Roberts and Reich 2002). Immanuel Kant argued that individuals should be treated with respect (as ends in themselves) and seen as having the capacity to develop and make life plans. It is still the dominant ideology in much of the world (Kymlicka 1995). Liberalism is strongly associated with capitalism and the rise of the **free market** (Kymlicka 1995) (see democracy, p. 35, and capitalism, p. 32).

A core commitment within liberalism is *liberty*, and essentially there are two versions of this concept. Each version of liberty has implications for what is determined to be the proper role of the state in terms of policy development and government involvement in the actions and options of its citizens. Negative liberty emphasises a minimal role for the state, with individuals free to pursue activities without interference (including risk-taking), providing other are not harmed (actions within the law) (Baggott 2000). All values are given equal credence (Kymlicka

1995). Freedom is considered to be the absence of restraint (Mills 1993). Positive liberty suggests a more active role for the state. Positive liberty is linked to a person's capacity to act to realise their life goals, and the state must act to enable these. Certain preventable risks, especially if not voluntarily chosen, should be controlled, in so far as they disable the optimising of freedoms for individuals. Barriers, for instance, could legitimately be placed in the way of individual action that may be deleterious to health, such as control of drugs.

> A State which does not act in certain ways to minimise certain preventable risk, especially if they are not voluntarily assumed and often even if they are to some degree, is actually choosing not to optimise the sum total of freedoms experienced by its subject population.
> (Mills and Saward 1993, p. 165)

It was recognised, over time, that unfettered individual action, and free-market activity through corporate capitalism (negative liberty), contributed to large-scale inequalities, generating acute inequalities in distribution of property as well as other social and economic resources, and thereby disabling choice and opportunities for many citizens. Policies and resources applied by government (e.g. through legal and fiscal measures) are required too (Roberts and Reich 2002).

Liberalism and health

The ideologies of liberal individualism remain core to issues pertinent to current debates around health, particularly the emphasis of liberalism on individuals' freedom of choice and rejection of state interference (Baggott 2000). Consider, for instance, the introduction of the smoking ban in England in July 2007. Some will argue that this infringes personal freedom of choice to smoke, while the general consensus it that it is necessary to protect people from the harms associated with passive smoking. Amartya Sen (cited by Roberts and Reich 2002) would argue that the state should limit itself to facilitating choice (via education), rather than prescribing choice (via policy control), but should, for example, provide healthcare, as this is needed as one of the resources to enable choice. Liberal individualists are particularly critical of any expansion of the state into the regulation of health matters for individual citizens (Baggott 2000). Part of this criticism emerges because the state exaggerates particular risks (reflecting vested interests in controlling certain activities), which can lead to what Strabanek (1994) called 'healthism'. Healthism refers to the state-directed, population-based, promotion of health. Nazi Germany reflects an extreme version of this, with the state population purged to improve the 'national stock' (Strabanek 1994; Baggott 2000). Liberal individualists are particularly critical of the creation of medical, state, bureaucracies, which dictate and prescribe certain modes of behaviour to individuals (Strabanek 1994; Baggott 2000).

Problems with liberal individualism

The extent of acceptable state involvement in enabling or prescribing choice (e.g. where it is permissible to smoke) remains a central and controversial component of contemporary political policy debate. In particular, Kymlicka (1995) questions the reality of choice within society if either the extremes of liberalist thinking are applied (which create inequalities) or state sanctions over particular behaviour (which limit and prescribe action) are put in place, because 'freedom of choice is only meaningful if individuals have an adequate range of options to choose from – that is, if diverse life-styles and customs exist in society' (Kymlicka 1995, p. 484).

Conclusion

Liberal individualism remains a powerful influence on health and social policy and related matters within contemporary society. In the context of health and social care, the challenge remains to establish the necessary and appropriate balance between freedom and control, as well as determining which values, choices and actions are more appropriate than others (Kymlicka 1995).

Modernism/modernity

The next few entries – modernism, postmodernism, poststructuralism and social constructivism – have been included because they constitute important social theories that have fed into discourse and ideas in the Western world.

Modernism refers to a 'meta-narrative' (an overarching commentary on human society) that prescribes clear, defined and indisputable certainties about the nature of the world and reality, i.e. an **ontological** reality. It created an intellectual climate that asserted the possibility of infallible progress and human and social improvement through the objective endeavours of science and rationality (originating with the Enlightenment (see p. 37) (Fox 1998; Francis 2000; Bilton et al. 2002). From such enquiry it was considered possible to understand and identify how the world worked, and, through structured interventions (including controlling nature), to improve circumstances for humanity, creating a 'ideal' society (Holborn 1999). The decline of religion and absolute monarchy changed the nature and structure of society and social order, gradually creating a more individualistic society (Pampel 2000). While it was acknowledged that individualism enabled industrialisation and the modernisation of society, early sociologists such as Comte and Durkheim observed that it also created an unstable social order. Modernist thought developed out of quests to explore how society might function as effectively, orderly and morally as possible (Pampel 2000). The modernist

era is associated with many significant social, economic, structural, scientific and industrial changes and new ideas such as democracy, liberalism, citizenship, nationalism, socialism and conservatism (Bilton et al. 2002).

Criticism of modernism
Modernist ideas are now largely viewed with some scepticism and indeed alarm. Assertions about the nature of an 'ideal' society contributed to the creation of an intellectual climate whereby persecution was made possible: for example, within the Nazi state in Germany in the 1930s and 1940s. Furthermore, modernist ideas rely on the unquestioning acceptance of rules of behaviour imposed by the state (Cameron 2004), something that is at odds with the increasing recognition of diversity within and across nation states (Bilton et al. 2002).

Modernism and health
As indicated in other sections, much of our thinking around health is shaped by values and ideas of what constitutes health, what factors influence health (social, economic, individual) and what is called on to 'foster' or promote health. Changes associated with modernism certainly altered the conditions and context of human activities and structures of society through industrialisation, urbanisation, rationalisation, the rise of the nation state and shifts in public and private spheres, contributing to structural, social and economic inequalities that impact on health (Bilton et al. 2002; White 2009). Tonnies (1855–1936) argued that urbanisation fractured traditional kinship relationships and the nature of support provided to and by individuals, creating what Simmel (1858–1918) described as a network of impersonal relationships, the impact of which has been increasingly criticised,

by Etizioni (1993), for example (see communitarianism, p. 33). Modernity is associated with the rise of consumerism (see p. 73) and bureaucracies (Weber 1864–1920). Bureaucracies in particular changed the nature of relationships between individuals and organisations, becoming more impersonal and bound by duties and responsibilities, with the power base residing within the organisational structure rather than individuals (Bilton et al. 2002). Bureaucracies also represent the increasing power of the nation state through rules, regulations, laws and surveillance of its citizens.

Reflective activity

Think about the bureaucratic structures you come across (e.g. at college, university, when you apply for a job).

- What are the positive aspects of how these systems work?
- What are the negative aspects of how these systems work?

In particular the growth in scientific and technical aspects of life and solutions to problems has contributed to the creation of an environment in which individuals increasingly rely on experts. This is observed in the context of health and health care, with access to care and treatment primarily being through professionals (doctors, nurses, professions allied to medicine, such as physiotherapists). Science and technology has also contributed to growing expectations regarding what is possible, for instance, in terms of treatment and cure of disease (Le Fanu 1999; Bilton et al. 2002). For example, Clarke (1998) highlights the modernist quest from the early twentieth century to the 1960s for meta-solutions, almost industrial mass production and 'control over' health, in this case with reference to reproductive matters.

Conclusion

Many of us will be able to recognise the impact of modernist thinking on everyday life, e.g. in terms of the rules and regulations we are subject to, and modernist patterns do contribute to the development of social order. However, as noted, there are significant flaws in this idealised way of thinking and attempts to construct an ordered society. Acknowledging these limitations has contributed, according to Lyotard (1984), Bauman (1989) and Bilton et al. (2002), to societies now more accurately being described as entering a postmodernist era (from the 1970s onwards) as a reaction against the extremes of modernist thinking.

Postmodernism
See the modernism entry.

Postmodernist thinking takes a very different perspective to modernism. As implied by the name, it suggests that modernism is no longer relevant. Postmodernism disputes modernist claims of certainty and the potential for ideal societies. Postmodernists argue that the social world is fluid and fragmented and even scientific discovery cannot be accepted unquestioningly. No objective criteria can be used to determine if one theory, one idea, one perspective is *better* than another. To Postmodernists, 'truth' itself becomes a nonsensical concept (Warnock 1998). Instead, the diversity of the world (values, cultures, social systems) needs to be acknowledged and captured within any deliberations or social commentary. The value and importance of theory is judged, from a postmodernist perspective, not as though it were a 'truth' but simply for its practical value and utility, and consequently postmodernists are suspicious of grand narratives, which are overarching explanations of how things are, how society is structured, how society works, such as **Marxism** (Taylor 1999a). 'Postmodernism reminds us that there is no one right way of thinking about human societies' (Taylor 1999a, pp. 16–17).

Foucault (1926–84), influenced by Nietzsche (1844–1900), argued that throughout history there had existed a series of different 'knowledges' or 'archaeologies' (Warnock 1998), which far from being 'objective' treatise on the truth, were merely descriptions designed to assert power and oppress others (for example, criminals and criminality, sexual deviance and sexual deviants, madness and the insane) (see stigma, p. 118). Values and beliefs were in fact masquerading as objective 'fact' and 'truth', and it is no longer possible to determine a 'correct' point of view. According to Dunning (1993, p. 132), 'the profusion of alternative modes of thinking and consciousness, derived from other cultures, ... prompts informed viewers to question the completeness, if not the veracity, of any world view that can be fully depicted from a single view point'. In other words, it is considered that any interpretation is possible and equally valid as any other (Warnock 1998).

Criticisms of postmodernism

One key criticism of postmodernism is its consequential impact on the rise of relativism (see p. 113). If no 'truths' can be determined, it becomes impossible to position any value or belief as good or bad, acceptable or unacceptable, right or wrong, or to discriminate between competing perspectives or courses of action. For example, one set of cultural values may judge women to be inferior to men, and this is given equal status to other values, which promote egalitarianism and equality. This is clearly an untenable position and does not reflect how societies actually work (Seedhouse 1997a, 2004). Moreover, postmodernist discourse is itself contradictory – 'to be consistent, the belief that all beliefs and practices should be thought of as being of equal value must be just as biased as any other' (Seedhouse 2004, pp. 84–5) – and while postmodernism is critical of grand narratives, it is, in effect, one itself, albeit one with greater diversity.

Postmodernism and health

The central tenant of postmodernist thought, that no one value or perspective is 'better' than another, has significant implications for work for health in several ways. At a fundamental level the postmodernist perspective maintains that the values upon which work for health (treatment, care or prevention) are founded are not fixed and cannot represent an indisputable idea of what constitutes health itself. Diversity and difference are at the very root of postmodernist discourse, acknowledging the concomitant nature of values and beliefs about health: 'the only incontrovertible knowledge any person has its their autobiography' (Cameron 2004, p. 9). Consequently, a disputed territory of what constitutes the most effective, most appropriate approaches to health and social care, treatment and prevention emerges. The 'one-model fits all' approach becomes unsustainable, indeed inappropriate, from the postmodernist perspective.

Reflective activity: different values and choices around health

A good example of the different opinions, arguments and actions related to health is embodied in arguments around female circumcision (sometimes called female genital mutilation). For interesting arguments about this see a series of articles in the journal *Health Care Analysis*, vol. 6, no. 1, March 1998 and reflect on these.

- On a less controversial matter, just consider the range of views on what people consider to be a 'healthy diet' (from veganism to meat-eating, French cuisine to Chinese food).

It becomes equally unsustainable, therefore, to make any recommendations about health-related behaviour lest they be considered as imposing specific, often 'white middle-class', values on others (Warnock 1998; Cribb 2002): 'the state (or its policies or agents) should have regard to the basic conditions for well-being but should in no way promote "well-being" according to any particular conception' (Cribb 2002, p. 271). In practice an understanding of this diversity and critique of a naive acceptance of the dominant **hegemony** around health and healthy lifestyles, 'to … manipulate, judge and moralise about lifestyle … exposing the connections between empowering people and exercising power over them' (Cribb 2002, p. 273), helps to explain why many matters to do with health and social care remain controversial. Different people, groups, communities and societies present different descriptions and make different choices around health matters.

Conclusion

Postmodernist thinking paves the way for diversity and acceptance of other ideas and perspectives. However, in terms of work for health, this diversity renders specific policy dictates untenable and work to promote health meaningless, as the ability to assert and justify any particular course of action, health advice or information or policy option is unsustainable (Warnock 1998; Cribb 2002; Seedhouse 2004). A middle ground between the postmodernist perspective (that all values are equal) and the modernist perspective (that of certainty and indisputable truths) is needed. In reality too, both *indisputable facts* and values, which are open to debate, contribute to our decision-making (Seedhouse 2004). It is a fact, for example, that the more cigarettes someone smokes the more likely they are to develop lung cancer. To assert, though, that smoking cigarettes is unreservedly bad reflects particular values about choices and lifestyle, rather than being a 'matter of fact'

(Seedhouse 2004). What postmodernist thinking helps to establish is that decisions and policies need to remain open to debate.

Poststructuralism and social constructivism
See the modernism entry.

Poststructuralism
Poststructuralism is akin to postmodernism (see above) in not being a unified philosophy, and in evoking a rejection of **grand narratives** and structuralist descriptions of society (which attempts to identify and describe overarching themes and structures of a society). Both poststructuralism and social constructivism question the objective nature of reality and set out to explore the construction of ideas, concepts, power, language and knowledge. Poststructuralism, for example, sees the processes of social functioning as being about difference and the subjectivity of experience. The term '**discourse**' is associated with poststructuralism. Discourse refers to a 'framework of meaning' representing the language used to construct particular meanings in a given context: for example, the nature of childcare, the nature of what constitutes health and so forth.

The French philosopher Michel Foucault (1926–84), early on considered a postmodernist, later a poststructuralist commentator, asserted that there were no absolutes to explain the human condition, or that it was possible to study humans objectively (Lye 2004): 'The Poststructuralist view holds that persons are culturally and discursively created in interaction as situated, symbolic beings. The common term for a person so conceived is a "subject".' Within the poststructuralist perspective there is no mechanism for assessing the relative validity or importance of different perspectives or discourses (Francis 2000). Subjects, i.e. people, are created by cultural meanings and practices (economically, socially,

2

occupationally and so forth) and therefore have multiple identities (Lye 2004). No one objective reality exists, but reality is shaped by language and ideologies and what we take for granted about the world is mediated through selection and control of ideas, information, knowledge and so forth.

Another influence of poststructuralism is in the use and interpretation of language. For Derrida (1930–2004), the French philosopher and grammatologist, everyday language is not neutral but embodies cultural assumptions and presuppositions (Lechte 1994). Hence 'texts' (taken to mean anything from books to pictures) could be interpreted in multiple ways. Language signifies meaning but the interpretation of meaning is filtered through an individual's own experiences. For a rather simple example, take the letters F R U I T, which signify the word 'fruit'. This word creates a certain mental image, but one that may vary considerably between individuals. The sender (who says the word) may have apples, pears and bananas in mind. The receiver (who hears the word) instead may have grapes, paw-paw and prickly pear in mind (influenced by a recent viewing of the Walt Disney film *The Jungle Book*). Derrida's idea came to prominence in the 1960s and 1970s when many cultural and social institutions were being challenged. People latched onto the idea of challenging the 'Western canon' and elitism, and embraced the freedom of interpretation posited by Derrida, Foucault and other poststructuralists.

Social constructivism

Social constructivists are anti-realists, and for them the material world does not exist, only concepts and various socially and culturally embedded discourses (Parker 1992). 'For the constructivist, our stories about the world cause that world to come into being' (Philippson 2001, p. 11), and as Ogden (2002) puts it the discourse 'constructs' the object. The object has no independent existence. For example, 'a discourse that describes sex as biological is considered to actually construct sex as being biological' (Ogden 2002, p. 11). Ogden goes on to suggest that 'fact' and 'truth' are problematic, they are constructed from social processes, social relations and social interactions. So, for example, physical illness and the experience of illness are social products (Taylor 1999b; Ogden 2002).

Reflective activity: the social construction of reality

For some further philosophical exploration of this matter (i.e. that 'reality' is a subjective social construct, rather than objective 'fact') type the following sentence into a search engine: 'If a tree falls in the forest and no one is there, does it still make a sound?'

- What do you think about this statement?
- Look at the comments on and discussion of the question. You will find both scientific (objective) and psychological (subjective) explanations – very illuminating!

Criticism of poststructuralism and social constructivism

These perspectives are criticised for presenting an egocentric 'anti-realistic' view of reality and poststructuralists and social constructivists are considered to be relativists (Taylor 1999b) (see p. 113). Warnock (1998) warns that a quest to explore, challenge and analyse should not be conflated into relativism. Taken to its logical conclusion, these assertions imply that it is not possible to come to a definitive meaning, understanding or reading on any matter (or of any text). This, Maynard (1994) suggests, renders social research pointless, and if this 'interpretive' perspective were literal, the lack of shared meaning would make communication and the use of language both impossible and meaningless. Belsey

(2002) notes that the meaning of language is *not* totally at our disposal. Meanings are largely predetermined and we absorb the explicit meanings and values inherent within a particular culture, which help us to depict our world and the characteristics therein. Without some 'agreed' (albeit often invisible) criteria and convention of meaning we would be unable to interact with each other or make judgements, distinctions and choices between different options and objects and courses of action. Hence, contrary to Ogden's (2002) claim that we are now 'intra-active' beings (we construct the world by the way we think about the world), our experiences are actually shaped by 'interactions' (Philippson 2001).

Poststructuralism and social constructivism and health

Taylor (1999b) describes how the development of medicine in the nineteenth century reflected significant changes and 'constructions' in the way health and medicine presented itself:

> most doctors in the eighteenth century had taken a more holistic approach, seeing disease in very general terms as symptoms of some disturbance with the whole *person*, the observation, dissection and systematic classification of patients gave rise to a new form of clinical medicine where diseases were located in specific parts of the human *anatomy*, such as the heart or the liver. For the social constructivists, this development was not the result of some progressive enlightenment, where the truth about the body was 'revealed' through clinical examination, but simply a different way of constructing or 'reading' the body ... as Armstrong, one of the leading social constructionists, puts it: 'the fact that the body became legible does not imply that some invariant biological reality was finally revealed to medical inquiry. The body was only legible in that there existed

the new clinical techniques a language by which it could be read' (1983, p. 2). (Taylor 1999b, p. 272–3)

Therefore, poststructuralists and social constructivists are only interested in discussions of health and biological matters in so far as they provide insight into culturally situated 'discourses' about the nature of health and illness in contemporary society; they do not provide comment on the *reality* of a matter. What this approach negates, though, is the actual impact of particular 'constructions' on health (Taylor 1999b). These 'constructions' themselves do have a reality as they have a real impact on how we approach the management, treatment and prevention of disease and the promotion of health. This is reflected, for instance, in the growing emphasis on lifestyle behaviour and choices and disease prevention (Taylor 1999b; Fitzpatrick 2001; DoH 2004a, 2008a).

The insights presented to us by the poststructural and social constructivist perspectives reflect the complex nature of humans and human society, acknowledging that humans are both physical *and* psychological entities, 'with ... physical rules ... (I can't walk through walls), but ... psychological processes which can't be reduced to physics (e.g. commitment and choice)' (Philippson 2001, p.5). It is certainly true that the way we describe, and therefore experience, certain illnesses, conditions or diseases has changed over time. What is now called post traumatic stress disorder (and treated medically and psychologically) was once labelled 'shell-shock' and prior to that simply cowardice (and 'treated' by a firing squad)! Moreover, as Phillips (2004) points out, our perceptions of issues are not always as factual and objective as they might seem. This can include the exclusion of knowledge that does not fit the prevailing view, thereby shifting the balance of 'knowledge' and over-representing particular outcomes. This can lead to incorrect decision-making, as published information, for instance, does not reflect the totality of knowledge in society (Cochrane Collaboration 2002).

These insights do not, however, deny the existence of the object (disease, illness or condition) itself but reflect changes in our understanding, diagnosis and experiences. As Taylor (1999b, p. 274) points out 'The fact that knowledge is culturally constructed need not rule out objective knowledge'. The generation of data and knowledge is to evaluate theories and help choose between them. Eliminating one or other body of knowledge (biological or social-cultural) seems an inadequate strategy to enable us to understand the richness and complexity of human societies and seek improvements in lives, conditions and circumstances (Taylor 1999b).

Conclusion

The themes embodied within poststructuralist and constructivist thinking are subject to the same criticisms as those levelled at postmodernism. However, despite these limitations, poststructuralism and social constructivism provide us with some interesting insights into the complex nature of modern, diverse, societies. Poststructuralism and social constructivism alert us to the need to identify, and understand, subjective experiences and interpretations of social-cultural life, and acknowledge the importance of exploring alternative explanations and perspectives, and of applying informed, critical analysis at all times when considering health and social care issues.

Socialism

Socialism has been included because its principles still underpin calls for socio-economic structural reform to create greater equality in society and in particular as an alternative system of social organisation to that driven by **laissez-faire** capitalism.

Socialism refers to a variety of socio-economic theories that broadly focus on what are considered to be fundamental flaws within the capitalist system and advocate another system for ameliorating the core problems within society. The ideas linked with socialism are not new, having emerged, for example, in works such as Plato's *Republic*, but the specific term emerged in the nineteenth century, linked with social critics such as Robert Owen (1771–1858) and Charles Fourier (1772–1837). Socialism also formed part of **Karl Marx**'s (1818–83) theory, known as **Marxism**. These critics, Owen, Fourier et al., were commenting on the terrible social and economic injustices observed during the development of the early capitalist societies of the Industrial Revolution. These injustices were in relation to vast disparities of wealth and income, power and opportunities within society and excessive individualism (see p. 92), competition and materialism, and socialism typifies a sense of outrage over exploitation and oppression of those within the lower socio-economic groups within society (Haslett 1995) (see capitalism, p. 32). More contemporary commentary on inequalities in health – notably publications such as the Black Report (1980), the Acheson Report (DoH 1998) and Marmot et al. (2010) – arguably stem from socialist-type concerns over what are deemed to be unacceptable inequalities in modern society. Socialism would broadly consider that a good society would emerge if selfish ends were constrained: for example, not pursuing profit or advantage at the expense of others, i.e. not treating people as 'a means to an end', but instead treating people equally, as 'ends in themselves' (Seedhouse 1997b).

Core socialist principles are the redistribution of wealth and abolition of private property. Socialist constructed government systems would feature the state ownership of the 'means of production' (industry and other institutions of wealth production), control over economic investment (potentially including centralised control over economic planning and investment), more equal distribution of income and wealth and the democratic election of government officials. The mechanisms by which these principles might be put into practice are varied. For example, should redistribution of wealth be 'according to need', 'according to effort' or simply 'equally distributed'?

Reflective activity: redistribution of wealth

What benefits and problems do you think there might be with the three potential systems for redistributing wealth?

- According to need.
- According to effort.
- Equally distributed.

Criticism of socialism

There are wide-ranging criticisms of socialism. Generally, socialist planning systems, such as that in the former USSR, are criticised for stifling entrepreneurial endeavour, and for being oppressive to their citizens (sometimes exerting excessive control through imprisonment and capital punishment).

Reflective activity

- For an overview of Barack Obama's healthcare reforms in America watch http://www.youtube.com/watch?v=RagbVl29JiQ
- What is the central purpose of his reforms?

In terms of health, frequently, strong ideologically driven criticisms of socialism emerge too. Ausman (2003, p. 89), writing about the American healthcare system, claims that 'Our elected representatives have created a socialized system of healthcare that has been operating for years and is an excellent example of the failure of socialism. … Everyone is forced to bear the costs of care for those who practice poor health habits. This is also socialism.' Ausman's comments illustrate that collectivist approaches to care are strongly resisted by those likely to have a more liberal-individualist (see p. 44) stance and these claims about healthcare have more recently emerged over the US President Barack Obama's proposed health reforms in 2010.

Socialism and health (care)

Socialism is inherently sceptical of focusing on individuals as the source of agency within society, as it is deemed impossible for sole enterprise to overcome the complex and powerful determinants of health (Baggott 2000). Instead, state intervention is required to improve social, material and structural conditions that produce circumstances conducive to good health (Baggott 2000). **Public health** with its long history of state intervention (for example, improved sanitation in the nineteenth century, the Clean Air Act 1956) has a socialist (collectivist) flavour (Baggott 2000), and would be deemed essential to any strategy to promote population health and ameliorate the consequences of socio-economic disparities generated by capitalism (Navarro 1976; Allsop 1990; Baggott 2000). Equity is a key principle that drives health policy and practice from a socialist perspective. The basic constituents of a more socialist healthcare system would be central funding, equal opportunity irrespective of ability to pay and funding according to workload (but not market driven). According to Paton (1997) a more equitable health service equates with a more equitable society and contributes to fulfilling a redistributive principle via taxation (especially of the wealthy) to provide a service for all (Powell 1997). International evidence suggests too that privately financed healthcare is more expensive and less efficient than a more 'socialised' system (see rationing, p. 85).

Conclusion

Overall, socialist-orientated state interventions are deemed to produce more individual freedom for all in the long run (Baggott 2000) as they provide the means for overcoming obstacles to fulfilling the potential of individuals and thereby of society's citizens as a whole. A truly socialist perspective would put prevention in the public policy arena too, as all policy would in effect be health policy to create better conditions for living (Powell 1997).

2.3 CONCLUDING COMMENT

What these ideologies contribute to our insights about health-related matters is to demonstrate the importance of engaging with different and multiple ideas, insights and interpretations when attempting to understand the complexity of human and social issues. Some of these ideologies draw our attention to the socially and culturally constructed nature of knowledge. Concepts of health, for example, are socially constructed (as discussed in Chapter 1), as are our ideas about what is important in the realms of options and actions around health and social care work. However, a more careful reading of these matters does highlight that ideas, policy, doctrine and strategy *are* based on substantive principles and contemporary thinking does not emerge from a vacuum but is informed by the themes embodied in the ideas explored in this chapter. For instance, the shifts in thinking associated with the Enlightenment (see p. 37) still influence our emphasis on rational thinking and empirical experimentation, over belief, faith and superstition. These different ideas and debates can therefore be used when constructing your own insights and arguments and help to inform your ideas about contemporary health and social care debates and are essential to improve your skills of critical analysis in your study of health.

Key points to consider include:

> Different ideologies and theories create very different understandings of issues and health matters.

> Ideology and theory strongly influence ideas, options and actions in contemporary society.

> All ideologies and theories have strengths and weaknesses but understanding this can help to shape your own conceptualisation of health and social care needs, diversity and intervention.

3 key terms and concepts

3.1 INTRODUCTION

This chapter explores:

> key terms, concepts and theories critically, identifying their impact on health and healthcare;
> a range of issues that inform, and emerge from, contemporary discourse in health studies;
> the value of conceiving of health matters from a particular perspective.

The purpose of this chapter is to introduce you to some terms, concepts and theories that shape health and social care interventions. It includes some applied philosophical concepts such as *individualism, rights* and *responsibilities,* some reference to social trends such as *globalisation* and *consumerism* and terms that you are likely to come across in Health Studies such as *chaos theory, behaviour change* and *empowerment.* As we have already stressed, all these ideas and theories shape our approaches in the field of health and healthcare, and increasing your knowledge about these matters will provide you with greater insight into some contemporary dilemmas. To facilitate this we critique the core components of the term or concept under scrutiny and make reference to the associated health implications.

The entries in this chapter are presented in alphabetical order, so you can dip into each entry to gather some basic knowledge to help you with your studies. You will notice, too, that there is some repetition of themes and ideas under different terms, and this illustrates the interconnectedness of matters to do with health.

3.2 KEY TERMS AND CONCEPTS: INFORMING IDEAS AND ACTIONS

Autonomy

Autonomy is from the Greek for self-rule (*auto* – self, *nomos* – law). Autonomy refers to an individual's capacity to choose freely for himself and be able to direct his own life. The concept of autonomy emerges through the philosophising of Enlightenment thinkers (see Chapter 2, p. 37). John Stuart Mill

(1806–73), a nineteenth-century philosopher, in his work *On Liberty* asserted that autonomy was the central feature of being a person and that this was implicitly linked with happiness. John Stuart Mill argued that each person is the best judge of their own happiness and that the autonomous pursuit of goals is itself a major source of happiness. However, autonomy is restricted by law, social tradition, the autonomy of others and the circumstances of a person's life (age, class, financial position, ambitions and personality etc). 'All of our decisions should take account of the needs of … shared relationships, not just our own wants and desires' (Barratt and Sipos 2005, pp. 3–4). Personal autonomy depends on the physical wherewithal to carry out chosen tasks, having knowledge and understanding of options, an ability to select appropriate goals and suitable environmental circumstances. Waller (2005) asserts that autonomy is good for you. Choices promote physical and psychological well-being, whereas loss of control creates helplessness. Autonomy is also identified as an important component in several concepts of health (Illich 1976, Seedhouse 1986, 2001), which are discussed in greater detail in Chapter 1. Autonomy is closely linked to concepts of free will (see p. 80).

Autonomy and health

There are two aspects of autonomy that are relevant to any health-related activity designed to improve or maintain health status. These are *respecting autonomy* and *creating autonomy*.

Respecting autonomy refers to a respect for the rights of individuals and the right for them to determine their own lives. Harris (1985, p. 80) asserts that this is *the* most important principle: 'Since it is my life, its value to me consists precisely in doing with it what I choose.' This has implications for any work for health. It means that we *must* respect the choices people make whether or not we agree with them, even if this might lead someone to harm. There are times when we might override this: for example, if the decision is based on biased or incomplete information. Another reason, Seedhouse (1988) and Barratt and Sipos (2005) would suggest, for not respecting someone's autonomy is if it would harm one or more other people: for instance, if someone had consumed too much alcohol but still intended to drive. On occasions these limits are also embodied in law, as with drink-driving. However, Seedhouse (1988, 1998a, 2009) and Cribb and Duncan (2002) suggest it is of primary importance to respect autonomy unless there are defensible grounds upon which autonomy should be overridden. This principle is deeply embedded in Western philosophical tradition since the Enlightenment. John Locke (1632–1704) wrote: 'No man can be forced to be healthful, whether he will or no' (cited by Feldman and Marks 2005, p. 8).

Creating autonomy, on the other hand, refers to any work aimed at enabling an individual and improving their capacity to do things and achieve life goals. It is particularly relevant to health work as the focus is, usually, on individuals who have some form of disabling problem, a dysfunction or difficulty that blocks or inhibits normal functioning, ability and achievement. According to Seedhouse (1988, 2009), health work must always be about creating autonomy and must aim to enable people to flourish as much as possible. Creating autonomy is dependent on providing the tools to enable free-thinking, informed choice. It can include activities such as providing information to someone about their medication (including side-effects) and offering a particular treatment such as surgery to improve the functioning of (part of) the body, or it can be about creating opportunities per se. Work for health may sometimes focus initially on creating autonomy rather than respecting autonomy (an individual's specific choice) in order to create greater autonomy at a later stage, and at times requires active engagement from health professionals. Autonomy may not be created by simply allowing people to make their own choices (a **laissez-faire** approach), as individuals may have insufficient knowledge, skill or understanding to make a fully informed, autonomous choice (Seedhouse 2009). Creating autonomy, too, may require the imposition of something that, at least initially, is unpopular or undesired: for example, compelling children to go to school. This may not be their choice at the time but will ultimately improve their options and choices later in life. This is what Beauchamp and Childress (1994) identify as facilitating freedom from personal limitations that ultimately prevent meaningful choices.

3

One of the challenges for health work and health workers is navigating the balance between creating and respecting autonomy. As Barratt and Sipos (2005, p. 1) note, autonomy within healthcare 'involves independence, self-reliance, and the patient's right to make decisions about his or her life, including decisions about the treatments he or she wishes to receive'. Thus, as mentioned earlier, the central imperative for work for health (care, treatment or health promotion) is that of creating autonomy. However, there comes a point at which the decision to *stop* the pursuance of further action to improve someone else's health has to be made. This is particularly the case if the person concerned is not in agreement with further action and is content with their current state (Seedhouse 2009). This is what Seedhouse (2009) refers to as the 'autonomy flip', where *respecting* autonomy takes precedence over *creating* autonomy in health work.

Both Barratt and Sipos (2005) and Seedhouse (2009) warn that such decisions should not be taken lightly, as an emphasis on self-determinism (i.e. autonomy) and freedom (non-intervention) could leave people without appropriate care or treatment.

> Neither is it an implication of a commitment to respect autonomy that whatever a person wishes should be provided. It does not follow that because a patient wants ampules of heroin on prescription a doctor has a duty to oblige. But what is implied is that once choice is possible, once the human faculty of reason is present, then the doctor should not positively prevent this choice unless respecting the wish would cause harm to others,

or seriously undermine the subject's welfare and the subject does not recognise this. (Seedhouse 2009, p. 159)

However, unfettered paternalism ought to be avoided, as it should be recognised that 'human freedom even extends to the ability to make poor choices' (Barratt and Sipos 2005, p. 2). Berofsky (2003), using the example of an individual who chooses to temporarily deny themselves access to food to enable medical aid to be delivered to a remote region of the world, argues that the exercise of autonomy can specifically lead to action detrimental to an individual, but that this remains an autonomous choice.

Conclusion

Autonomy is central to key concepts of health such as the *foundations concept of health* (Seedhouse 1986, 2001). Much activity within health and social care is aimed at creating and maintaining autonomy. Respecting autonomy is also a vital consideration and can present significant challenges for health and social care practitioners, but autonomy should always be recognised as a core human attribute.

Behaviour change

Personal behaviour has long been associated with health and disease, particularly in more recent times, following the ground-breaking discovery of the link between smoking (a personal behaviour) and lung cancer. This spurred increasing interest in the possibility of reducing mortality and morbidity through other lifestyle changes such as dietary change and increased physical activity (Fitzpatrick 2001). As Le Fanu (1999, pp. 47–8) puts it, 'the preventability of lung cancer was enormously influential in promoting the notion that cancers and the other common causes of death might also be preventable by similar "lifestyle" changes'. Consequently, behaviour change is a major component of contemporary public health strategies to promote health and prevent disease (Stroebe and Stroebe 1995; Conner and Norman 1996; National Institute for Health and Clinical Excellence (NICE) 2007; Thirlaway and Upton 2009). At the heart of the Wanless report (Wanless 2004) for instance, is a call for a 'fully engaged' public as a route to improved health through changes in behaviour and associated social, economic and environmental context (which enable healthier choices) and the Darzi Report (DoH 2008a) re-emphasises the role of the NHS in keeping people healthy rather than simply treating illness and disease.

The lifestyles and behaviours that contribute to the construction and production of health and disease are referred to as the 'Holy Four' by McQueen (1987, cited by Irvine 2010). These are smoking, alcohol 'misuse', poor nutrition and low levels of exercise, with sexual activity added later following the advent of HIV and AIDS (Crossley 2000; Fitzpatrick 2001; Irvine 2010; see also Chapter 4, Case study 3) .

Apart from the evidential base – the limitations of which are discussed later – one of the main reasons why behaviour change and healthy lifestyles form a core strand of contemporary health strategy is that they reflect core Western ideological and ethical values around autonomy (see p. 55) and free will (see p. 80). Western philosophical thinking places significant value on individual self-determination (Dougherty 1993; Seedhouse 1997a; Warnock 1998), choice and responsibility. A core feature that distinguishes human beings from other life forms is that we have the cognitive ability to make choices and it is generally accepted that our behaviours are *not* determined in a pre-programmed and predictable way like other things in nature, e.g. as the law of gravity 'makes' a leaf fall from a branch (Warnock 1998; Seedhouse 2009). The French philosopher Jean-Paul Sartre (1905–80), for example, observed that individuals have a fundamental capacity for choice and personal responsibility. Sartre acknowledges that frequently this is obscured by social convention and, consequently, individuals often act in what he called *bad faith*; in other words, acting according to roles and rules. Bad faith refers to people claiming 'that they had no choice but to do X'. However, this is because people allow themselves to be constrained by social rules and convention, although these social rules and conventions are social constructs. They are not fixed or pre-determined (Seedhouse 2009). Essentially, 'bad faith is the failure to realise that any role has originally been a matter of choice, and that it remains a matter of choice whether we continue to perform it or not ... no matter what the rules, there is always choice' (Seedhouse 2009, p. 105). Sartre's work reinforces the claim that as human beings we do indeed have the capacity for choice, although it must also be acknowledged that choice, options and capacity are not limitless (Seedhouse 2009).

Nevertheless, it is important to acknowledge here that we are not merely passive 'victims' of our circumstances and if we deny this fact not only are we acting in bad faith, but we also deny human dignity and can encourage passivity and lack of effort (Dougherty 1993). Mary Warnock (1998) also suggests that if we treat people as though they have no choice and will always behave in the future as they have behaved in the past, we objectify and dehumanise them. Denying the existence of free will thus prevents us from fulfilling our full potential and taking responsibility for our behaviour. Embracing free will and choice generates the capacity to act appropriately and ethically too. Hence, being able to make a choice about how we live is a fundamental human attribute and underpins assertions around behaviour change, i.e. that we can 'choose' to behave differently.

Relying on behaviour change as a mechanism for health improvement is politically attractive too. It is acknowledged in a NICE report (2007, p. 6) that behaviour change is, at least in part, a focus of action on health because 'people's behaviour – as individuals and collectively – may be easier to change' than genetic or socio-economic or environmental conditions, as it does not need great social investment. Instead, the responsibility for health is placed with the individuals themselves (Baric 1995) and very much fits with the contemporary focus on the **ontology** of the individual (Baric 1995; Bennett et al. 1995; Leichter 1997; Seedhouse 1997a, 2004; Fitzpatrick 2001; Ogden 2002; White 2002; Denney 2005) and the delivery of health care systems whereby the health care delivery package is established and regulated by the individual relationship between health care professionals and 'patients' (White 2002; Bambra et al. 2007). The particular lifestyle package and way we behave also represents behaviours approved of by society. Conforming to these behaviours denotes social position, status and image and, according to Leichter (1997), represents the value systems of the dominant **hegemony** (ideologies, values of those in power) (see also individualism, p. 92).

Changing behaviour: models of behaviour change

Reflective activity

- Consider a behaviour you enjoy (whether it is 'good' for you or 'bad' for you). You might consider watching TV, drinking tea, coffee or soft drinks, going to the gym, listening to music, texting your friends etc.
- How easy do you think it would be to change this behaviour?
- What would help you change this behaviour?

There are a plethora of behaviour change models that inform practice, and the main features of the most dominant models are mentioned here. These are the Health Belief Model (HBM), the Theory of Reasoned Action (TRA) and the Transtheoretical Model of Health Behaviour (Stages of Change). Self-Efficacy, a key component of the HBM and theory that informs programmes such as the Expert Patient Programme (EPP) is also discussed in this section.

The HBM (Rosenstock 1974; Becker 1974; Kirscht 1974; Janz and Becker 1984; cited by Janz et al. 2002) grew out of attempts to understand what contributed to people's engagement with prevention initiatives, such as health screening, and has been widely used to explain the adoption and maintenance of health behaviours. Early evidence suggested that the two key elements underpinning action were an individual's perceptions of seriousness of a particular disease and their personal susceptibility (Janz et al. 2002). Of importance here is the recognition that these are perceptions rather than objective calculations of risk, and action is also shaped by perceptions of benefits to be gained from a particular course of action and the perceived (and actual) barriers to action (or the cost incurred by a given choice), all of which are informally constructed by the individual (Janz et al. 2002). All of these domains are influenced by socio-psychological, demographic, structural factors and cues to action are recognised as an important component within this model (Family Health International 2004). Cues to action include a poster campaign (e.g. encouraging the use of the stairs rather than the lift), being sent an invitation letter to attend for a screening test or experiencing a physical symptom of a disease. Self-efficacy is also recognised as an important psychological state that stimulates and enables action, and is discussed in greater detail later.

Empirical evidence of the value of the HBM in shaping prevention campaigns indicates that perceived barriers and perceptions of susceptibility are more influential in shaping choices than perception of seriousness (Janz et al. 2002; Family Health International 2004). The influence of perceptions of benefits to be gained through behaviour change is less clear-cut given the contingent nature of the outcome, i.e. the benefits cannot be guaranteed (Thirlaway and Upton 2009).

The Theory of Reasoned Action (TRA) and Theory of Planned Behaviour (TPB) (Ajzen and Fishbein 1980; cited by Family Health International 2004; Montaño and Kasprzyk 2002) link beliefs and attitudes to behaviour, suggesting that behaviour change is ultimately the result of change in beliefs. In other words, people perform behaviour if they think they should and two things influence this perception: first, attitudes towards the behaviour, i.e. personal belief in the good or bad attributes of the behaviour; second, perceptions of the social pressure to perform the behaviour (normative belief), which strongly influence decision-making around behavioural choices. The TPB developed from the TRA and differs only in its inclusion of perceptions of behavioural control, e.g. perceived self-efficacy or time constraints (Thirlaway and Upton 2009). The TRA and TBA are based on the assumption that human beings are rational and make decisions following considerations of options. Furthermore, it is contended that intentions shape action, i.e. that the most important determinant of behaviour is *behavioural intent* (Montaño and Kasprzyk 2002).

Studies have shown that subjective elements strongly influence intentions (not just external factors). Thirlaway and Upton (2009), for instance, note that perceptions of behavioural control seem to be a vital component in the prediction of choices and actions, along with perceived and actual social norms. However, it is acknowledged that an intention to do something may be thwarted by actual barriers to action, e.g. environmental conditions (Montaño and Kasprzyk 2002). Finally, it is increasingly being recognised that the relationship between behaviours, intentions and action is a two-way dynamic, with behaviour shaping attitudes as well as intentions driving choices. This makes the relationship between the two difficult to predict without insight into past behaviours (Thirlaway and Upton 2009) or accounting for all the behavioural dynamics that shape actions (Montaño and Kasprzyk 2002).

The Transtheoretical Model of Change (Stages of Change) (Prochaska and DiClemente 1986; Prochaska et al. 2002) was initially developed in the context of addictive behaviours, has been applied, for example, to alcoholism

3

treatment and smoking cessation and initially emerged from empirical research exploring how people managed to quit smoking (Prochaska et al. 2002). It is based on the notion that change is not a linear, predictive, process. Instead, it is a journey, during which people succeed in their quest to change by using different processes at different times, or 'stages'. Six stages of change have been identified: *pre-contemplation, contemplation, preparation, action, maintenance* and *termination*. An individual needs to pass through a series of stages before they have established the 'new' behaviour.

Each stage typifies certain characteristics. At the *pre-contemplation* stage, the individual will often be termed 'hard-to-reach' as they have no interest or motivation to change, possibly having tried and failed to change in the past, and will frequently avoid any reference to the behaviour, e.g. smoking. The *contemplation* stage represents a shift in this pattern of thinking during which an individual might consider the possibility of change and be acutely aware of the pros and cons of such action. This stage usually represents an intention to change within the next six months, but individuals may procrastinate for a considerable period of time (Prochaska et al. 2002). *Preparation* is the stage at which an individual is ready for action, often having done some ground-work such as joining a gym, consulting a self-help book or seeking another form of guidance. Individuals at this stage are very receptive to action-orientated activity such as joining a weight-loss or smoking cessation group. *Action* is the stage at which people make deliberate changes, and is considered 'action' in terms of attaining some risk reduction such as quitting smoking. *Maintenance* then emerges as an ongoing stage (lasting from six months to five years), whereby an individual is less actively engaging in behaviour change strategies but is attempting not to return to old habits. The setting of (realistic) goals is a central feature of the process of change. Relapse is seen as a natural and normal part of the process of change too. A lot can be learnt by an individual when they 'relapse' about the triggers and stress points that sabotage intentions. This can then feed back into the 'action' or 'maintenance' stage.

Prochaska et al. (2002) note that the percentage of individuals who start to smoke again is 43 per cent at one year, only declining to 7 per cent after five years of abstinence. During both the *action* and *maintenance* stages, relapse of behavioural intent remains a possibility. It is only at the *termination* stage, when an individual is no longer likely to return to the behavioural habit as a coping strategy, that an individual can be considered to have changed their behaviour. Prochaska et al. (2002) acknowledge that it is rare that individuals are completely temptation free, with fewer than 20 per cent of smokers or alcoholics, for example, achieving this state.

Ultimately, it is recognised that people will only change when they are ready to do so and it is argued that at the pre-contemplation stage a smoker, for instance, will not be aware that his or her behaviour is a problem and will therefore have no intention of stopping. They are in effect 'happy' smokers (Conner and Norman 1996). The balance of pros and cons needs to alter, to promote a shift in behavioural intent. Of particular importance is an increasing recognition of the benefits (pros) of change supplemented by a continuing, decreasing, negative (cons) to returning to old habits (Prochaska et al. 2002). A re-evaluation of the pros and cons of behaviour change can be stimulated by several actions including awareness raising activities (feedback, confrontations and media campaigns), self-re-evaluation, such as considering oneself as an active individual (e.g. identifying with healthy role models), and helping relationships, such as buddy systems. Using rewards for new behaviours, removing triggers or cues to old behaviours, such as avoiding eating out if intending to lose weight, can help too, along with social re-engineering, which creates or enables access to healthier environments or choices such as access to free or cheap condoms (Prochaska et al. 2002).

There is some evidence supporting the value of this model of behaviour change. Characterising where people 'are at' in terms of readiness for behaviour change can help in the tailoring of interventions to individuals. It has been demonstrated to 'predict' successful outcome of attempts to quit smoking (Ogden 1996) but as Thirlaway and Upton (2009) note, given the complexity of the concepts and theories embodied within this model it is difficult to tease out explicitly the components of this model that contribute to any observed successes. Bandura (1998) asserts that the 'stages' of change are arbitrary in that it is not possible to categorically determine which stage an individual is in, nor the reasons, for instance, for 'pre-contemplation' (Thirlaway and Upton 2009). Resistance to change might reflect various considerations, including lack of knowledge, lack of self-efficacy and underestimation of risk (Thirlaway and Upton 2009). Overall, while the Stage of Change provides some useful insights into the dynamics of change, it is not a model in the same sense as the Health Belief Model because it is a descriptive account of process rather than a causative explanation of behaviour. The HBM, for instance, gives some indication as to why people move into changing behaviours (the forces/factors involved), whereas the Stages of Change model simply describes a process of movement from one behaviour state to another and the characteristic features of each 'stage'.

The final model or theory to be explored is Self-efficacy. Self-efficacy is a key component of the Social Cognition Theory (SCT) (Baranowski et al. 2002), which itself recognises that behaviour, personal factors and environment all interact with respect to health-related behaviour. Self-efficacy is a recognised component of the other models of behaviour change already discussed (behavioural control within the TRA being a similar concept).

Self-efficacy refers to an individual's confidence and belief that he or she has the power to achieve a desired behaviour (Alder 1999; Odgen 2002). It is linked with self-esteem but is based on a realistic assessment (not wishful optimism) of achievement and expectations of personal mastery and success, and helps to determine if an individual will engage in a particular behaviour, i.e. 'how certain am I that I can do that?' (Thirlaway and Upton 2009).

Self-efficacy influences all behaviour and is recognised as the best predictor of behavioural intention and behaviour change (Schwarzer 1992; Bandura 2002).

Perceived self-efficacy will vary 'task to task'. For example, an individual may have a high level of self-efficacy in term of quitting smoking, but not for attempting to lose weight (Wenzel et al. 2002). A belief in a positive outcome and perceptions of self-efficacy will influence how much energy is spent on the task and the overcoming of obstacles (Baranowski et al. 2002).

According to Bandura (2000), people's sense of self-efficacy can be developed in four ways. These involve providing opportunities for mastery experiences (i.e. experiences that improve an individual's skills and confidence to overcome obstacles), vicarious experiences (seeing, or being with, others engaging in behaviour change and taking cues from appropriate role models), using social persuasion (being told they have the capacity) and providing experiences of success and, finally, working to reduce people's stress reactions and correcting misunderstandings around health issues or options for change.

According to Bandura (2002, p. 304), a 'vast body of evidence reveals that belief in one's efficacy to exercise control over health-related behaviour plays an influential role in health status and functioning'. Self-efficacy has been noted to be a consistent predictor of success in adopting health-related behaviours such as stopping smoking (Wenzel et al. 2002). Information alone does not contribute to this success (Jones 2003) but it is gradually attained by achieving competence, and building confidence, at each stage of a behavioural task or goal, such as learning to inject insulin safely (Baranowski et al. 2002).

Value of behaviour change theory

One of the important elements that emerges when considering the theoretical underpinnings of behaviour change is that no one model or theory substantively predicts actions or outcomes. Intentions concerning behaviour seem to be an important predictive component, but fewer than half of the variations in behaviour are explained by this component, or other components, of health behaviour models and theories (Thirlaway and Upton 2009). What these theories do highlight though, is the ongoing nature of behaviour change. Change is not a one-off event, but requires action, often sustained over a considerable period of time. Moreover, evaluation of the risks of a behaviour or admonition regarding lifestyle alone will not achieve the desired results. More active intervention is required, such as motivational interviewing and active support during the process of change (Thirlaway and Upton 2009), and activities to promote healthy lifestyles and behaviour change are often more successful when linked to key transition stages in people's lives, such as becoming a parent or retirement (NICE 2007).

The work of NICE (2007) concluded that no specific model or approach achieved more positive results; instead, certain skills could be applied across the board. The relevant approaches include helping people to develop an appropriate awareness of the consequences of their behaviour, ensuring that

3

information is relevant to the individual, encouraging and helping the development of a positive attitude and sense of self-efficacy, using normative influences, helping people to formulate realistic goals and supporting people through periods of actual or potential relapse.

The importance of accounting for social factors that might influence behaviour was acknowledged too and interventions must be tailored to the specific needs of the individual, group or community, thereby requiring involvement and consultation with the people in question (NICE 2007). As Montaño and Kasprzyk (2002) note, it is vitally important to obtain deep and clear insights into what drives the behaviours of particular groups so that bespoke interventions can be developed.

Work to promote health: the Expert Patient Programme (EPP)

In brief, the EPP is a self-management programme for people with long-standing illness, aiming as a minimum to develop supported self-care, with patients becoming active partners in their own care. The EPP enables individuals to develop cognitive skills and coping strategies such as relaxation and fatigue management and general health promotion-related knowledge, along with information on medications. A key component of the EPP is to increase an individual's health and personal disease management, and improvements in self-efficacy are a recognised outcome of participation in the EPP (Wilson 2002; Rogers et al. 2006; NPCRDC 2007). Mastery skills, via the setting of short-term goals and monitoring achievements, is a key component of the EPP, as is the opportunity for vicarious experiences and role-modelling. All EPP tutors themselves have a long-term condition and previous experience of participating as an EPP group member and the structure of the group enables the exploration and exchange of ideas and knowledge, and active support of group members (Street and Powell 2008).

More recently, behaviour change principles, such as self-efficacy, have become embedded as core competencies in the work of health trainers (Skills for Health 2007; cited in Thirlaway and Upton 2009). The role of health trainers is to work on a one-to-one basis with individuals to encourage lifestyle and behaviour change, provide support and help to signpost individuals to other support options as necessary, and is currently the subject of an evaluation review due to be published in 2010 (DoH 2009).

Limitations of behaviour change theory and behaviour change as a means of promoting health

Despite the assumed capacity for 'healthy' lifestyles to prevent disease and improve health it is recognised that achieving the desired-for behaviours both for individuals and cumulatively across a population is not easy. As already mentioned, behaviour change theories themselves are not fully predictive of outcome and fundamentally rely on rational explanations and constructs of behaviour, and it is acknowledged that habitual, emotional and instinctive drivers shape behaviour too (Thirlaway and Upton 2009). Moreover, behaviour and lifestyle are embedded within social, economic, environmental and cultural contexts (NICE 2007; Thirlaway and Upton 2009) and socio-economic conditions impinge on choices and can reinforce behaviours that are damaging (NICE 2007). These are documented in the NICE report (2007) as access to information, services and resources, exposure to risks, lack of control and the long-term damage created by disadvantage.

As McKeown and Lowe (1974) note, reductions in mortality were influenced primarily by advances in general living conditions, rather than individual behaviour change, and population level interventions, including legislative change, continue to be effective, such as seat-belt laws (NICE 2007). Given this potential, it is asserted in the NICE document that policy-makers and commissioners must take steps to address the social, environmental, economic and legislative factors that affect people's ability to change their behaviour.

Work to promote healthy lifestyles, in the absence of consideration of socio-economic and environmental impacts on health, may also be ethically dubious. It may have the consequence of simply boosting people's resilience to living in difficult circumstances (NICE 2007) and implies that only certain types of 'healthy behaviour' are acceptable. According to Ogden (2000), behaviour change and healthy behaviours are intrinsically, accorded moral, as well as somatic (of the body), value, and this fundamentally asserts that there is a 'good' and a 'bad' way to behave (Gastaldo 1997), which transmits dominant social and cultural norms about the way we live (Leichter 1997). Thirlaway and Upton (2009, p. 2) indeed reference some strong stigmatisation of so-called 'lifestyle' afflictions such as obesity, quoting Liddle (2008): 'Most obesity is a consequence of stupidity and indolence and not of some genetic affliction. It is a lifestyle choice which people would be less inclined to adopt if they knew we all hated them for it.' This polemic expresses *very* strong moral disapproval of people who do not conform to 'normal' weight and, as can be discerned from reading Case study 1 on obesity (see Chapter 4), trivialises an extremely complex matter. Moreover, this assertion points to some worrying trends in discourse around health, behaviour, choices and responsibility, which liberally accords blame to individuals' experiences and conditions and considerably simplifies the notion of choice (see individualism, p. 92; responsibility, p. 115) It is widely acknowledged that all choice is contingent, and strongly influenced and inhibited by socio-economic, environmental, cultural and psychological factors. Choice is not a simple rational matter alone (Thirlaway and Upton 2009), nor is the notion of choice confined to conformity of prescribed behaviours or statistical norms, and to assert such a matter itself fundamentally undermines the very notion of free will (see p. 80) that such discourse calls upon. As Seedhouse (2004) asserts, no behaviour can be characterised as exclusively unhealthy and NICE (2007) acknowledges the contingencies of behaviour.

Finally, others dispute the strength of the evidence accorded to lifestyles, behaviour and health (Fitzpatrick 2001). A study by Boffetta et al. (2010), for instance, concluded that the evidence that eating five portions of fruit and vegetables a day afforded protection against cancer was very weak. It is noticeable too that in documents that explore the impact of behaviour and lifestyles on health, the existence of evidence to support this claim is asserted, rather than cited (see, for instance, NICE 2007), and as Marantz (1990, p. 219) notes, 'No behaviour or lifestyle is guaranteed to produce disease; equally no behaviour or lifestyle can assure longevity.'

Conclusion

Working with people to promote behaviour change may be of considerable importance to the individual, and although it might prevent disease or illness over a given time period and confer improvements in functioning, contributing to a greater sense of control (self-efficacy) as well as other tangible benefits such as saving money on cigarettes, it is not a **panacea**. Understanding something about the psychology of health and theories of behaviour change can help to shape appropriate interventions and actions, and perhaps, more importantly, stimulate a recognition of the limitations of behaviour change as a means of promoting health. Those who critique the theory recognise that we do not fully understand what works.

Perhaps, too, there need to be limits on the extent to which particular behaviours are proscribed and prescribed, particularly when evidence of benefit is limited or weak. As Cribb and Duncan (2002) note, behaviour change might not lead to more health overall and fundamentally any work to prescribe or encourage a certain behaviour, particularly on a population basis, becomes an ethical matter too (because, for example, it can cause harm too). Consequently we should be circumspect in the pursuit of health-related lifestyle behaviour change as a legitimate objective for the promotion of health and make judgements in given contexts rather than adopting a blanket strategy. After all, as Marmot and Mustard (1994, cited in Pitts 1996, p. 1) note, 'The total number of deaths cannot change – one per person'.

Chaos/complexity theory

Chaos theory outlines a way of thinking that moves away from traditional linear 'cause and effect' thinking, established under Newtonian physics (Plsek and Greenhalgh 2001). When Sir Isaac Newton published his *Principia Mathematica* in 1687 the basic message was that nature operated according to specific, and discoverable, laws (Greenfield 2002). According to Newton's view of the universe, problems could be broken down and solved via analysis and rational deduction, contributing to the development of the **reductionist** approach to medicine and health care (Plsek and Greenhalgh 2001; Martinez-Lavin et al. 2008). Chaos theory led to the development of complexity theory (Greenfield 2002). The ideas about complexity come from many different disciplines, e.g. systems thinking, which has taken its inspiration from the non-linear mathematics of chaos theory (Innes et al. 2005). Mathematical chaos, for instance, describes a situation in which a complex system may be unstable, and small changes within, or externally, may create radical change.

Complexity theory relates to the study of complex, adaptive systems, such as those found in organisations of people (Innes et al. 2005), and is often described using the metaphor of a woodland ecosystem. More colloquially it is often described as the *butterfly effect* (a butterfly flapping its wings in New York can cause a hurricane in Tokyo) (Kernick 2006). Complex systems are composed of a network of agents, with each agent of the system (e.g. a nerve cell in the brain, or a person within an organisation) being shaped by itself (its own characteristics) but also via interactions between itself and other agents. It is the sum total of these interactions that constitutes the larger environment, and it is this interactive quality that creates the potential for small changes within the individual components to have significant effects on the functioning of the whole (Innes et al. 2005). The converse is also possible, that large changes within a small component may have little impact on the whole. According to Pslek and Greenhalgh (2001, p. 625) the key difference between Newtonian and complex systems is that 'mechanical systems' boundaries are fixed and well defined ... complex systems typically have fuzzy boundaries'.

Chaos/complexity and unpredictable outcomes

Chaos/complexity theory has contributed to the analysis of human, social systems and organisational dynamics. The relevance of this theory in this context stems, in part, from our contention that humans are individuals who have the freedom to act, that these 'actions' are not always predictable and actions are interconnected (see free will, p. 80). This itself will change the context of actions for all, and reflects human perceptions and experiences of events and experience, i.e. what we experience is more than its individual parts (Plsek and Greenhalgh 2001). In addition, Plsek and Greenhalgh (2001) contend that individuals do not behave according to rationale dictates, e.g. according to the results of evidence-based practice alone, but respond to a complex mix of dynamics, shaped, *inter alia*, by values and circumstances, and actual behaviour is emergent from this dynamic (see behaviour change, p. 58).

Healthcare itself represents a complex system (Trochim et al. 2006) where unpredictable needs and consequences emerge. Smoking, as a public health issue, is an example of a complex system reflecting the unforeseen unfolding of events. The publishing of the Surgeon General's report on smoking in 1964 was itself the product of many events, but it also precipitated unanticipated consequences, including sowing the seeds for future bans on smoking in public places and stimulating the tobacco companies into launching a range of defensive tactics. None of the 'responses' was necessarily predictable from the initial action and some had far-reaching consequences as a result of one 'small' report (Trochim et al. 2006). In effect key stakeholders respond to the changing environment and the actions of others, and while individual agents may follow simply rules, the impact and outcome of these can be highly complex.

Chaos/complexity and organisational change

In terms of planning and organisational change helpful insights that emerge from chaos/complexity theory include a greater understanding of the contingent and developmental nature of the change process (of individual behaviour and within organisations) and the importance of mapping the diversity of social networks within and between organisations that will have a bearing on how change materialises (Trochim et al. 2006). Boundaries between and across organisations are often less rigid than implied by organisational structures, and learning and change are developmental, cyclical and incremental (Kernick 2006):

> complexity theory resonates with the ways in which health service members view the world and offers a framework within which we can articulate and explore our intuitive insights. (Kernick 2006, p. 389).

As Miller et al. (1998) note, rational, linear approaches to change do not work. Literally the process is more complex than would be implied by linearity (that a change or intervention in A will lead directly and predictably to a change in B). Complexity science would suggest that multiple approaches need to be adopted during change, which let a direction appear gradually, towards those actions and activities that seem to be working best rather than those that fit a predetermined plan (Plsek and Greenhalgh 2001). Plsek and Greenhalgh also suggest that a recognition of the complexity and interconnectedness within organisations helps to explain why seemingly simple change can be subject to significant resistance. For example, the 'simple' change of altering the end of the workday by fifteen minutes might have huge knock-on effects on other aspects of people's lives (e.g. collecting children from school).

Chaos/complexity and healthcare

Innes et al. (2005) suggest that in fact the parameters of complexity provide a more accurate description of medical consultations, e.g. with GPs, than rational accounts. While it is not always relevant to describe the pattern of GP consultations in terms of choas/complexity theory, particularly when there is strong congruence between the parties involved, consultations are frequently unpredictable and non-linear. Complexity can be helpful when considering healthcare issues infused with controversy. In other words, the greater the disagreement or the level of uncertainty, the more complex the process becomes, and more prone to disintegration. Mental health disorders, chronic pain and chronic fatigue fit in this category and meeting these types of healthcare needs may require the involvement of a considerable number of healthcare practitioners, and this itself contributes to its complexity.

Reflective activity

Simply list the number of things that influence your behaviour. See how complex this is!

The physical environment may have its own impact too, as will the time constraints of a consultation and wider socio-economic, religious and other matters. 'Feedback loops in the consultation change the practice of the doctor and the behaviour of the patient during the consultation and future consultations' (Innes et al. 2005, p. 49) and the outcome emerges as a consequence of the interaction, not as a result of 'design or external control. ... New information may be inhibited from emerging if the consultation always runs along predicted lines and also creates ...unrealistic and unfair pressure on the doctor to find successful solutions to all problems and denies patients the opportunity to share and understand the uncertain reality of illness and health care' (Innes et al. 2005, pp. 50, 51). Acknowledging the reality of uncertainty, and the complexity of human behaviours and health, can legitimise the taking of risks to facilitate the emergence of more creative solutions. This requires the ability to deal with a certain level of anxiety, with the doctor's role becoming one of many of the agents within the relationship who seek to influence change, not create it.

Chaos/complexity and health

Similarly, complex disease cannot be understood through traditional, linear and reductionist models but is more helpfully conceptualised through theories such as complexity theory (Martinez-Lavin et al. 2008). The reductionist model of medicine supposes that the whole body can be understood by looking at its individual parts, and that disease must have a structural or serological change associated with it. This sophism derives in part from René Descartes's philosophy, which distinguished between res cogitans and res extensa. The former referred to the soul or mind and was said to be essentially 'a thing that thinks'. The latter was the material stuff of the body (Martinez-Lavin et al. 2008, p. 261).

In essence it can be more helpful to think of bodily functioning as a complex system operating within a spectrum of variability, rather than a static organism operating according to predictable rules and patterns. Variation is in fact normal and necessary, as a body that is in stasis is actually less able to respond appropriately to changes within the environment, and certain diseases such as fibromyalgia are a consequence of a degraded performance of the whole organism, not a malfunction of an individual part(s) (Martinez-Lavin et al. 2008). Very few, if any, human illnesses have a single cause or single cure (Wilson and Holt 2001). This way of thinking implies the need for significant changes in conventional medical treatment practices, and the interventions that have worked for complex disorders reflect a holistic and multidisciplinary approach to therapy (Martinez-Lavin et al. 2008).

Conclusion

Choas/complexity theory provides a useful conceptual framework that supports a critically reflective analysis of the difficulties incumbent in change. Organisational change and individual change, particularly individual change directed towards health-related behaviours, are not straightforward, linear processes and require diverse strategies for goals to be attained.

Commodification

The term 'commodification' originates from **Marxist** political theory and came into usage in the 1970s. It refers to giving an economic value to something that has not previously, or normally, been thought of as something that can be traded, i.e something that can be bought and sold (Resnik 1998; White 2002). Sex, for instance, is 'commodified' when traded for money. Radin (1987) suggests that commodification emerges when ordinary events are ascribed monetary value or described using monetary metaphors, even when no money actually changes hands. An example of this might be when we talk about the 'costs' and 'benefits' of certain behaviours (referring not to actual financial costs, but to social or other 'human' costs) (see behaviour change, p. 58).

Reflective activity

- Next time you open your e-mail account, look at your spam or junk mail. Many of these will be offers for 'cheap' drugs to treat or cure a wide range of supposed health problems. Why do you think these companies are out there?
- Make a note of the number of adverts selling products to improve the functioning of our bodies (for example, bio-active yoghurts or constipation remedies) you see on TV or in magazines or papers. Are they primarily aimed at males or females or are they gender-neutral? Why do you think this is?

Health as a commodity

Seedhouse (2001) and White (2002) comment on the increasing 'commodification' of health and suggest that thinking about 'health as a commodity' is a fundamental principle of Westernised medicine and medical practice (which can provide 'health', at a cost, through drug treatment or surgery). Western medicine is based on the concept that equates health to the 'absence of disease' and a quest to restore 'harmony' of body and soul (Dubos 1987). Consequently, health can be 'lost' when an individual becomes diseased or 'worn-out' and is no longer 'perfect'. Commodifying health suggests that it can be replaced in a similar fashion to acquiring a new handbag or item of clothing when these wear out. For example, drugs or surgery can be 'purchased' to cure a person's heart disease, implying that an individual's state of health can be restored or enhanced by the consumption of pills or particular therapies (surgery, physical therapy and so forth) and that essentially medical practice is a business practice (Gorz 1983).

Commodification of health (Seedhouse 1998b) does have an impact on the way we think about health and opens up the possibility for exploitation of bodily concerns. An extreme example of this, is the commercial sale of human organs for transplantation, which was initially regulated under the Human Organ Transplants Act 1989, now replaced by the Human Tissue Act 2004. This Act criminalised the trading of organs and other related activities and was stimulated by concerns over exploitation (e.g. impecunious individuals selling body parts) and the quality of organs or products available (Wilkinson 2000). Such problems are more likely to happen when financial incentives are used to encourage people to donate blood, for example, as marginalised individuals who engage in 'risky' behaviour, such as drug addicts, may use this as a source of income.

Reflective activity

- Think about how healthcare services in the UK are now referred to as 'commissioners' (an earlier version divided this role into 'purchasers') and 'providers' and patients and other service users are often referred to as 'customers' or 'consumers'.
- Look at some recent healthcare policy documents. Is the word 'consumer' or 'customer' used?

On a more mundane note, Churchill (1999) suggests that the nature of funding of healthcare in the USA positions healthcare as a commodity 'for sale', and commercialises healthcare interactions and expectations. Relman (1980) and White (2002) refer to this as the 'medical-industrial complex', which positions medicine in the competitive market along with other forms of purchasable goods. For example, within the USA healthcare has increasingly been being delivered via managed care organisations (MCOs), large corporations ultimately responsive to Wall Street financial markets (Churchill 1999). This inevitably encourages people to think and talk about healthcare in the same way as any other marketable product and stresses the importance of maximising profits as well as assigning priority to choice, and customer-satisfaction, in service delivery and care (Churchill 1999). White (2002) asserts that this creates 'bad medicine' by inducing a 'bulk-buy', 'see-them-quick', approach to service delivery.

Buying a perfect body

This tendency to commodify and commercialise health also encourages the externalisation of health via the quest for bodily (and psychological) enhancement through services such as plastic surgery (Sacks 1973). According to Sacks (1973, p. 22), this debases the richness of human experience by implying that the body is merely an engine that can be 'titrated or topped-up in a mechanical way', and Lupton (2003) argues that this is fuelled by a strong element of narcissism and the powerful connection people make between consumption and feelings (well-being). The body has become 'a fetishized commondy, something to be attractively "packaged" and offered for exchange' (Lupton 2003, p. 40), which at its extremes manifests through the surgeon's knife.

Reflective activity: health and medicine as a commodity

Reflect on the ways in which you can identify health and health care as a 'commodity': for example, buying health or buying the body beautiful.

- Look at how many programmes are shown on the television that look at ways of improving your health and well-being.
- What sort of suggestions are made about how to improve your health?
- Do any of them involve 'buying' something, or fixing parts of the body?
- In what ways does this improve the person's health?
- What are the limitations of this sort of approach to the improvement of health?

Conclusion

Thinking of health as a commodity reflects many Western approaches to health as we are constantly being 'sold' 'fixes' to health problems. While this can indeed sometimes help to 'fix' a problem (such as buying a pair of reading glasses), thinking about health in this rather mechanical manner fails to reflect the diversity of experiences and conceptualisations of heath and has consequences in terms of side-effects, e.g. iatrogenesis (see Chapter 1, p. 14).

Consumerism

Consumerism is firmly rooted in the commercial and private sectors (Almond 2001) and according to Steele (1999) consumerism refers to the manipulation of the consumer by companies and manufacturers in a quest to sell their goods. It involves the use of marketing techniques, appealing packaging and other attractors and incentives to entice the purchasing of goods. The consumerist agenda is increasingly being echoed in health service reform, informed by ideological shifts in the latter part of the twentieth century. 'We live in a consumer age. People demand services tailor made to their individual needs. Ours is the informed and inquiring society. People expect choice and demand quality' (Milburn 2002; cited by Newman and Vidler 2006, p. 195).

Consumerism and healthcare

Choice is central to **neo-classical economics**, with its focus on property rights, individual freedom, competition and autonomy (Dent 2006; Fotaki 2007) (see liberal individualism, p. 44). The market-orientated reforms of the Thatcher era (Margaret Thatcher was UK Prime Minister from 1979 to 1990) set in motion shifts in the relationship between healthcare providers and patients, particularly a growing emphasis on managerialism, patient choice and the patient as active 'consumer' of health care (Iphofen 2003; Richman 2003; Dent 2006; Earle 2007; Fotaki 2007; Newman and Kuhlmann 2007), and embedded this in healthcare policy of the 1990s (e.g. The National Health Service and Community Care Act, 1990; The Patient's Charters, 1992, 1995) (Almond 2001). Positioning the patient as 'consumer' was also driven by the recognition of the emergence of a more sophisticated and demanding public (the discriminating consumer) (Newman and Kuhlmann 2007), the importance of greater accountability in public services (Martin 2008) and the need to reduce paternalism and the scientific, bureaucratic, power of the professional in health care (Almond 2001; Newman and Kuhlmann 2007).

> Consumerism is a belief and attitude, which regards patients as powerful, active and sentient participants in structuring and developing health services. Their opinions and involvement to assess the quality and provision of services are sought and valued, and form a pivotal role in providing optimum levels of care for all. Consequently health services meet the needs of the consumer and not those of the professional.
> (Almond 2001, p. 896)

The quasi-market reforms were seen as a mechanism for achieving greater equity, efficiency (e.g. reducing waiting lists), accountability, governance and responsiveness to real and perceived patient need (Dent 2006; Fotaki 2007) through mechanisms such as direct payment or patient passports, whereby the individual is in receipt of funding that they can move around to different providers (Pitt and Lloyd 2008). The basic objectives of applying consumerist principles to healthcare was to use this as a mechanism for bringing costs under control and to provide incentives to improve quality (Dent 2006).

According to Newman and Kuhlmann (2007) one of the other key drivers behind consumerism in healthcare is to encourage greater personal responsibility around health to reduce the reliance on state services (for example, the development of the 'expert patient'). It is also seen as a mechanism through which to ameliorate the harms and limitations of healthcare institutions on the experiences of patients, e.g. mental health services, through patient choice and involvement.

Problems with consumerism in healthcare

There are various criticisms of consumerism in the context of healthcare. From an ideological perspective, in the UK, Pitt and Lloyd (2008) suggest that this shift represents a means of privatising the NHS. Earle (2007, p. 21) points to the corrupting effect of consumerism and marketing within healthcare, whereby vast sums of money are spent 'marketing' pharmaceutical products: 'drug promotion does not operate with the consumer interest in mind, but rather focuses on generating profits by maximising sales revenue', and in effect 'constructs' notions of health, illness and disease through the production and promotion of products. Palmlund (2006) argues, for example, that the meno-pause has been transformed from a normal physiological process to an illness and disease, which requires intervention and treatment, such as the prescription of HRT (hormone replacement therapy). Newman and Vidler (2006) also suggest that the focus on consumerism reflects the commodification (see p. 71) of the body.

Practically and organisationally, criticism of consumerism acknowledges power imbalances between the agencies involved, and although consumerism functions to ameliorate the extremes of power, through complaint and protection procedures, corporate entities and big business have considerable power to shift and shape options. It has become, as Steele (1999, p. 165) terms, a 'self-elected oligarchy'. Consumer choice within these changes has been marginal and in fact represents the development of a form of 'proto-professional', whereby the public simply take on the language and priorities of the establishment (Dent 2006).

The complexities of consumerism in the healthcare context

The complexities of patient choice have not been fully appreciated either, rendering the simply transference of consumerism from business to public policy a flawed strategy (Fotaki 2007). According to Adams and de Bont (2007) the image of a new type of patient who is highly reflexive and skilled at acquiring information and becoming an active participant in their care is more imagined than real. As Almond (2001) and McDonald et al. (2007) note, the consumerist perspective within healthcare cannot operate in the same way as, for example, in the retail arena and does not necessarily serve the interests of patients (Piterman 2006). To exercise full autonomy requires access to knowledge, the ability and willingness to conceptually navigate between choices and the existence of different 'products' to choose from in the first place (Newman and Vidler 2006; Piterman 2006). Earle (2007) suggests that real choice within public services does not exist, it is a veneer of choice, a fait accompli ratification of options within selected areas of public policy only.

Moreover, professionals will always have superior knowledge (Lock 1996; cited in Almond 2001) and the information with which consumers might exercise choice can be limited and of poor quality. Adams and de Bont (2007) point to the poor quality of a lot of web-based information and the lack of skills people have upon which to judge the substance and validity of what they are reading. Even information from bone fide sources such as the Department of Health or World Health Organisation might not be strictly neutral or balanced as it is also constructed around particular conceptions of health or what constitutes a good citizen (Adams and de Bont 2007) (see also Chapter 1). Moreover, patients are often vulnerable and lack a wider knowledge base from which to convert information into practical decisions relating to a particular course of action (Piterman 2006). 'Patients have a wealth of information at their fingertips through the internet. What most do not have however, is the skill and knowledge to sift useful and valid information and evidence from useless or harmful advice' (Editorial 2005, p. 343). For many, choice is intellectually, financially and practically not available (Piterman 2006).

Additionally, there are negative consequences of consumerism in health-care. Consumerism could undermine the trust needed in the doctor–patient relationship (Dent 2006; McDonald et al. 2007). An editorial in the *British Medical Journal* questions the appropriateness of consumerism in the NHS: 'Naked consumerism will not lead to better health' (Editorial 2005, p. 343) as *both* the professionals and patients should make contributions to the running of the health service.

As mentioned earlier, one of the drivers behind consumerism was to encourage greater personal responsibility for health. O'Cathain et al. (2005; cited by Newman and Kuhlmann 2007) noted that the NHS Direct service has facilitated patient empowerment, while also creating suspicions about the motives behind providing this service. O'Cathain et al. comment that there is some justification for this wariness, as NHS Direct was established to reduce demand on GPs and accident and emergency clinics.

Being more 'consumer-friendly'

Establishing consumerism requires considerable effort in providing opportunities for consultation, representation, responding to difficulties, providing adequate resources and becoming truly patient-centred (Piterman 2006). In addition, Newman and Kuhlmann (2007) assert that, fundamentally, consumerist healthcare reforms were about curbing the power of professionals and challenging paternalism, although Almond (2001) notes that there is not much evidence that consumerism has been established in particular healthcare services such as health visiting.

Greener (2003, p. 104; cited in Newman and Kuhlmann 2007) comments that 'the government appears to wish to pass responsibility for the running of health services to subsidiary organisations and individuals, while retaining strong central control ... the state has perhaps divorced itself from having to take any further blame for the health service's problems'. In reality, therefore, what emerges is a compromise between the extremes of consumerism within public services (with its individualist focus) and the requirement to meet the collective needs of a community, emphasising 'partnership' rather than 'consumer/provider' relationships (Almond 2001; Newman and Kuhlmann 2007; Martin 2008). Public involvement and partnership has come into practice through mechanisms such as PPI (patient, public involvement) and foundation hospitals have been able to elect consumers onto the board and involve them in decision-making: for example, via citizens' juries (Newman and Kuhlmann 2007). Regulatory bodies such as the GMC (General Medical Council) have also increased their lay membership (Newman and Kuhlmann 2007), although Baggott (2005) and Dent (2006) warn against public involvement merely becoming a mechanism through which to legitimise existing choices.

Conclusion

While there are considerable policy drivers and aspirations to incorporate consumer perspectives into healthcare, achieving this remains a significant challenge. Moreover, there are drawbacks to applying consumerist principles within healthcare settings. However, as Baggott (2005) indicates there are benefits too, including the growth in citizen rights, and these can increasingly be established via consultation, partnership and lay control, and are preferable mechanisms to improving healthcare than those embodied in more market-orientated consumerism.

Empowerment

What is empowerment?

> ### Reflective activity: what is empowerment?
> - Write down what the word *empowerment* means to you.
> - Ask two or three of your friends what they think *empowerment* means.
> - Identify the similarities and differences between what you have all said.

This is not an easy or straightforward question to answer. While it is seen as a 'word' with a definable (simple) meaning – 'to bestow power on others' or 'to gain or assume power' (Labonte 1990; cited in Raeburn and Rootman 1998, p. 74) – the word 'empowerment' represents specific values. These include clear assumptions and claims about the nature of people's lives. 'Empowerment ... in the broadest sense [is] the process by which relatively powerless people work together to increase control over events that determine their lives and health' (Laverack 2006).

The origins of the term are in radical politics (Gibson 1991; cited in Leyshon 2002). Essentially it relates to a particular ideological perspective, which considers that socio-economic and 'political' structures of society constrain people's lives and opportunities. 'Empowerment implies that what you see as poor functioning is a result of social structures and lack of resources which make it impossible for the existing competencies to operate' (Raeburn and Rootman 1998, p. 69). Commentators distinguish between different 'types' or levels of empowerment: *personal empowerment* and *social/political empowerment*. Personal empowerment exists when people feel in control of their lives or have control over their own affairs and are able 'to define their own needs and act upon that understanding' (Raeburn and Rootman 1998, p. 65). Social/political empowerment exists when people have 'a raised level of psychological empowerment amongst the community members, a political action component in which members have actively participated, and the achievement of some redistribution of resources favourable to the community or group in question' (Rissel 1994, p. 45). Laverack (2006) describes this distinction as 'power-from-within' (an

3

increased sense of self-determination and self-esteem) or 'power-over' (redistribution of resources and decision-making).

Why is empowerment relevant to health?

Reflective activity: why is empowerment important to health?

From your understanding of what empowerment is, what importance do you think empowerment has for health?

Empowerment reflects the general principles of the Ottawa Charter (WHO 1986, cited in Earle 2007), 'empowerment ... embodies the raison d'être of health promotion' (Rissel 1994, p. 40). Some of this drive for empowerment – both personal and political – stems from criticism of the 'expert-led'/top-down approach, which is seen as *disempowering* individuals and communities because people's needs are being defined for them (see need (needs assessment), p. 101). This is implicitly and explicitly criticised as representing 'a new arena for colonisation' (Rappaport 1981; cited by Raeburn and Rootman 1998, p. 68). Inspiration around empowerment also comes from the work of Paulo Freire (1972). Freire (1972) argued that central to people becoming empowered was the recognition of powerlessness in the first instance – 'conscientisation'. This requires the development of awareness and knowledge, resulting in 'The rise of consciousness of their situation enabl[ing] individuals to identify their own needs, rather than having them prescribed by others' (Wills 2005, p. 60).

These ideas link empowerment with community development. Community development work 'is about building active and sustainable communities based on social justice and mutual respect. It is about changing power structures to remove the barriers that prevent people from participating in the issues that affect their lives' (Standing Conference for Community Development 2001, cited by Wills 2005).

According to WHO (2003), community empowerment is key to sustainable development and addressing community needs. Empowering individuals within communities is fundamental to enabling the development of new skills and knowledge, ideally promoting greater self-sufficiency. This needs to be based on 'the understanding that the community is the best judge of its own problems and possesses the ability to undertake appropriate action for their solution' (WHO 2003, p. 9)

Empowerment essentially involves participation (Raeburn and Rootman 1998) and can involve communities coming together to address underlying conditions that impact on their lives and health. For instance, it can involve action to improve leisure facilities or the condition of housing (Laverack 2006).

The implications of empowerment for work for health

Empowerment has entered popular discourse within public services too

(Leyshon 2002), and for this to become a reality there must be a two-way dialogue at all stages of developing and implementing any interventions. Empowerment cannot be bestowed by others but must be gained by those who seek it and for this to occur those working in health and social care must work together (Laverack 2006).

Labonte (1993, cited in Raeburn and Rootman 1998) suggests that the *empowerment* role of professionals is as advocates around issues such as housing, social welfare and employment policies. He adds that this role extends to 'offering knowledge, analytical skills, information on how the political and bureaucratic structures function and so on' (Labonte 1993, cited in Raeburn and Rootman 1998, p. 76). Fundamentally, empowering communities involves supporting the development of decision-making, planning, resource management and so forth. Active contributions to policy development and future interventions need to be enabled, along with building a confidence within the community regarding the potential of community action (WHO 2003). Both Handsley et al. (2007a) and Laverack (2005, 2009) suggest, therefore, that practitioners have considerable potential in linking communities with 'higher-level' decision-making and can be involved with communities in ways that help people to become more critically aware and skilled and competent to engage in collective action on matters that affect their everyday experiences. However, to fully act in an 'empowering' manner requires an active partnership between health and social care professionals and others, one in which power imbalances between the groups are actively addressed and diminished (Ritchie et al. 2008; Tee 2008).

Empowerment: limitations and difficulties

Solomon (1976, cited in Tee 2008) suggests that empowerment is about promoting individuals' potential to manage their own problems. This might indeed be important and helpful, but it might have the consequences of merely increasing coping mechanisms within intolerable or unacceptable circumstances and creating 'quiescent communities … [and] a means of "gilding the ghetto" – having little impact on major health inequalities and merely focusing on the felt needs in one area or group' (Wills 2005, p. 61). Tee (2008) also expresses concern regarding the dynamic that often emerges around empowerment, which is one in which professionals are seen as being responsible for empowering the client. This can simply have the effect of maintaining the power imbalance, with one group 'bestowing' power on another, and is often jeopardised by inadequate resources, staff changes and lack of continuity. Laverack (2009, p. 79) suggests that the practice of public health work often takes place within the 'controlling sphere of bureaucratic settings … employing top-down approaches to programming', thus limiting the opportunities for empowerment-based activity. Empowerment implies that the voices of the community are heard and their choices are taken seriously. These choices may not echo traditional disease prevention priorities at all and may clash with other programmes that aim to encourage behaviour change rather than improved socio-economic and environmental circumstances as a route to better health.

Conclusion: empowerment and health

Empowerment is an aspirational concept that can contribute positively to individual and collective health. Its value is increasingly being recognised, especially for communities that lack personal, social and economic resources. Fulfilling this aspiration and attaining an empowerment agenda, however, calls for ways of working that are often alien to professionals and challenge professional autonomy (Handsley et al. 2007a). Moreover, it requires considerable reorientation of access to actual power (for example, economic resources) (Wills 2005) and this requires strong practical and ideologically driven action that can harness the skills of those working in health and social care with communities and provide 'clarification of how to make this ... operational in a programme context' (Laverack 2005, p. 112).

Useful resources

The Community Development Exchange website for general information, news, events and jobs around community development (http://www.cdx.org.uk/welcome-to-cdx).

Adams, L., Amos, M. and Munro, J. (2002) *Promoting Health: Politics and Practice*. London: Sage. For a broader, and more in-depth exploration of the political, social and ideological values that shape community development work.

Laverack, G. (2009) *Public Health: Power, Empowerment and Professional Practice*, 2nd edn. Basingstoke: Palgrave Macmillan. For an in-depth account of empowerment and community development work to promote health, including mechanisms for evaluating and measuring this type of work.

Free will

There is a lot of philosophical debate about free will. Essentially free will refers to our capacity to make choices and decisions (see autonomy, p. 55) and there are various versions of what constitutes free will or what it means to have or exercise free will. In essence, it is asserted that human beings are not 'determined' or pre-programmed to do certain things in the same way as, for example, a ripe apple is compelled to fall from a tree due to the power of gravity. Instead, because we have the cognitive and physical ability to act, we have the ability to make choices and exercise free will. There are various ways of explaining the nature of free will. Within the **compatibilist** tradition, for instance, free will exists in the absence of coercion, and when an individual could have (would have) chosen a different option to the one actually selected to achieve a certain goal (Habermas 2007). Other considerations of free will suggest that it emerges from our capacity to introspectively reflect on our actions. In other words we remember previous times, when we acted in different ways under similar circumstances. While John Stuart Mill argues that this freedom is an illusion, as we act only according to our strongest motivation, the principle of free will is said to exist on the grounds that it is implicitly and inextricably linked to notions of personal and moral responsibility (for our actions) (Habermas 2007).

The philosopher Peter Strawson (1919–2006) cogently argues that there is a connection between free will (choice) and moral responsibility, and illustrates this by reflecting on the different responses generated by an accidental or deliberate act, such as accidentally stepping on someone's toe in a crowded room, as opposed to intentionally stamping on someone's foot. In the first example, we would not attribute blame (the person could not help it), but not so in the second example (as it seems they chose to act as they did). Dougherty (1993) further argues that if we deny the existence of free will and the ability to make choices we deny human dignity and encourage passivity and lack of effort and Warnock (1998) suggests that if we treat people as though they will behave in the future as they have always done in the past (i.e. that they are unable to make choices), we objectify and dehumanise them.

Free will and health

For the French philosopher Jean-Paul Sartre (1905–80) free will is elemental. He believed that we 'create' ourselves (who we are) and our options and choices in life, and when we act as though we have *no* choice, by making statements such as 'I had to do x', or act only according to a predefined role, then we are acting in what he calls bad faith (denial of our free will). To Sartre, there is always a choice, and to deny free will prevents us from developing, from fulfilling our full potential and taking responsibility for our behaviour (Seedhouse 1998a) (see behaviour change, p. 58).

Thus the concept of free will is closely bound to discourse around personal behaviour and 'lifestyle' choices, a matter that features in a lot of contemporary health debate. However, the literal extent of free will and choice is not at all clear. For example, Henk ten Have (1994, p. 120) argues that:

> it is not at all clear that lifestyle is primarily an individual affair, nor that each individual is rational in the minimal sense of having certain capacities of understanding and deliberation, nor free in the sense that he is able to choose and act according to his decisions.

Seedhouse (1998a), Waller (2005), Bambra et al. (2007) and Butland et al. (2007), comment on the impact of social, environmental, economic and genetic factors and commercial advertising on choices and the outcome of choices. Waller (2005, p. 183) argues that 'One of the main problems stemming from just-deserts responsibility is the veil it drops on the important social and environmental causal factors.' Moreover, attempts to take control of factors over which they actually have *no* control can be counter-productive and contribute to feelings of helplessness.

It is also argued that different people have different abilities to act and take control, linked, at least in part, to a sense of self-efficacy (Waller 2005), and opportunities to improve circumstances or change behaviours are limited. As Shiu (2001), notes, we have yet to discover a foolproof cure or treatment for addiction to tobacco, for instance, and therefore blaming an individual for being unable to change their behaviour is akin to blaming someone whose chest infection will not respond to antibiotics (Loughlin 1994).

Moreover, arguments about paying for, or denying, treatment to those who have 'chosen' a health-damaging behaviour are often flawed and punitive. In principle there is no difference between someone requiring treatment for a broken leg sustained while rock climbing, or someone needing treatment for lung cancer developed after many years smoking. Both outcomes are consequent to behaviour, but as Ubel et al. (1993; cited in Waller 2005, p. 186) note, there is a tendency to make 'social desirability judgements' and moralise about particular behaviours and not others.

While holding people responsible for their behaviour is an important motivational principle, using blame can be counter-productive. Such action would damage clinical relationships, and trust and honesty between patients and health practitioners. An individual might be discouraged from declaring a particular behaviour if they felt sanctions would be applied as a consequence, or it might, perversely, feed into a type of fatalism, as people fear failure so will disengage from any attempt to take responsibility (Waller 2005). Loughlin (1994) and Waller (2005) add to this the observation that the consequences of many 'lifestyle' behaviours emerge *many* years after the habit became established, or, indeed, after the habit was ceased. People, therefore, do not categorically know or anticipate the certainty of a particular ending when they take up and establish habits, often as vulnerable, malleable, adolescents (Clements and Sider 1987; Loughlin 1994), and these decisions are consciously, or unconsciously, based on an awareness of the contingent nature of outcomes. As Marantz (1990, p. 219) puts it 'No behaviour or lifestyle is guaranteed to produce a particular disease; equally no behaviour or lifestyle can assure longevity.'

Waller (2005) and Loughlin (1994) argue instead that the notion of free will and therefore responsibility for *actions* should be separated from claims about responsibility for *consequences* of choices or actions: 'Any sensible theory of rational risk-taking must allow some rational risks ... we can be held responsible for taking it but not in any sense ... should [we] be penalised for taking it' (Loughlin 1994, p. 126). Moreover, to argue that people should be made to 'pay' (literally, or through denial of treatment or care) for the consequences of their behaviour is 'particularly odious when applied to medical caregiving' (Waller 2005, p. 178), and may enhance inequalities given that the burden of consequences is not equally shared across society (Seedhouse 2001; Waller 2005) (see healthcare rationing, p. 85). What authors such as Waller (2005) conclude is that decisions about treatments should only be made on clinical grounds (diagnosis and prognosis), and have regard for the principle of altruism at all times (Clements and Sider 1987; Dougherty 1993).

Conclusion

The principle of free will is a central component in Western ethical thinking and a construct embedded in many principles of health and social care practice. However, free will should not be regarded as limitless in reality and should not be used to justify punitive health and social care policy.

Globalisation

Defined by Daulaire (1999, p. 22) as 'the flow of information, goods, capital and people across political and economic boundaries', the term *globalisation* is deemed a descriptor of a modern phenomenon that stirs up both positive and negative emotions. Globalisation implies a blurring of national boundaries and diffusion of identities and practices between communities, traditionally disconnected from each other by distance and physical boundaries. Globalisation is not a new phenomenon. For centuries trade has been carried out throughout the world, bringing both opportunities and disasters. For example, the British tradition of our morning cup of tea was only made possible through global trade (and is arguably a positive outcome of globalisation). However, global trade also spread devastating diseases. For example, it is estimated that following Columbus's and Cook's exploration of the Americas and Polynesia, the native communities were devastated (about 90 per cent died) by the 'ordinary' viruses the Europeans brought with them: cold, flu, measles and so forth (Hong 2000; Seedhouse 2001), and such concerns remain today regarding diseases such as SARS (Martin 2005). Perhaps, too, a not so obvious aspect of global trade was slavery. An estimated 24 million (Bilton et al. 2002) to 60 million (Hong 2000) people were taken from Africa to the Americas or Caribbean, contributing to the disintegration of African societies and subsequent under-development of many countries on the African continent (Hong 2000).

Reflective activity

- See if you can locate any newspaper reports on threats of infectious diseases across the world (an example in 2009 was swine flu).
- What are the implications of this threat for you, your family and local communities?
- What actions are being planned to reduce the health impact of this (potential) event?

Globalisation is increasingly reflected in the transgression of boundaries due to political, social and economic upheaval. For example, during the 1930s and 1940s, Jewish people and others fled Nazi persecution in Europe, and the UK continues to offer asylum to those experiencing political or religious persecution. Economic reasons are also a dynamic for migration. Following the dismantling of national boundaries across EU member countries, the UK has seen an influx of people from the old Eastern bloc, with 1.4 million East Europeans coming into the UK up to 2008. This trend reversed due to the recession in the UK and other countries, which started in 2008/9 (BBC News 2009a). It is worth noting that migration *from* the UK is considerable too, with an estimated 136,000 people emigrating in 2008 (an increase of 36,000 over the 2007 figure) (ONS 2009). Migration issues are a cause of considerable tension, and while it is not possible to explore this debate here, it is worth noting that claims that we are 'over-run by immigrants' create a far too simplistic picture of the issues and the fact of migration does illustrate that the UK is part of a global socio-political economy.

In economic terms globalisation frequently represents exploitation and invasion of poorer countries by the wealthier, industrialised nations, in the pursuit of resources (for manufacturing) and markets for goods (buying and selling). This draws forth accusations of exploitation and abandonment: for example, of indigenous populations and resources in the form of payment for cash crops (for example, palm tree groves, for palm oil, a substance used in cosmetics and food products) at the expense of local food production, and mining and processing of valuable raw materials (for example, oil and diamonds) by multinational companies. This nets vast profits for share-holders and owners in Western industrialised countries, rather than within local economies (Hong 2000), and generally reinforces inequalities across the world (Hong 2000; Schrecker et al. 2008). Worldwide economies are intricately interlinked through global financial markets too, and this has profound effects in all countries. The 'credit-crunch' starting in 2008/9 in the USA is an example of this.

Globalisation and health

This transgression and fluidity of boundaries affects health (Woodward et al. 2001; Labonte and Schrecker 2007a) and extends to the 'health' industry too. According to Cornia et al. (2008; cited in Schrecker et al. 2008) and Schrecker et al. (2008) health trends (for example, as determined by life expectancy at birth) have deteriorated in countries such as those within sub-Saharan Africa, and the inequality gap has increased. While options and priorities for improving health have been limited, because of the constraints placed on government spending by debt-serving agreements, and the fact that the amount of gross domestic product (GDP) required to repay the debt often exceeds that spent on health and education (Hong 2000), business opportunities for multinational, private insurance and healthcare companies across the world have increased (Ollila 2005). This can extend choice for consumers in some areas of health such as eye surgery but, as Zarrilli (1998) comments, this can lead to a two-tier system of healthcare, one privately funded and thereby accessible to wealthier citizens, and the other state-funded, for the poor who are excluded from insurance schemes. Recent privatisation in China's healthcare system has reduced affordability and access (Schrecker et al. 2008) and the Trade-Related Aspects of Intellectual Property Rights (TRIPS) have led to an increasing cost of patented drugs and restricted access to cheaper generic drugs (see consumerism, p. 73).

Globalisation has also facilitated the imposition of domestic policy values on foreign policy funded programmes, such as the USA's emphasis on abstinence-based HIV programmes (Ollila 2005, Owen and Roberts 2005). Ollila (2005) also comments on how the national interests of the USA have fragmented public health programmes such as vaccination schemes, and the increasing involvement of the private sector in partnerships with public organisations such as WHO, has resulted in a dichotomy of costs and risks (borne by the public sector) and profits (reaped by business) (Stansfield et al. 2002).

Essentially, there are calls for a reorientation of priorities towards altruism over profit, to counteract the negative consequences of globalisation of world markets. It is argued that this is vital, on fundamental ethical grounds (e.g. to avoid doing harm), but is also of central importance to sustain development and growth itself, and maintain healthy populations (Von Schirnding 2005; Schrecker et al. 2008). Deaton (2006) and Labonte and Schrecker (2007a) comment that economic development alone will not improve health within countries. Instead, policies and markets need to become people-centred (Labonte and Schrecker 2007b), and include consideration of human rights in policy deliberations (Schrecker et al. 2008), and this remains a challenge within countries and across the globe too.

Conclusion

Economies across the world have been interlinked for centuries, creating opportunities for both exchange and growth, but it is increasingly being recognised that globalisation contributes to socio-economic and practical problems and political tensions across the world. Ameliorating and managing these difficulties remains a challenge and requires acknowledgement of the disparate burden, and damage, globalisation can create for countries and communities across the world.

Healthcare rationing

The term rationing refers to fixing or limiting the amount of something given to individuals or groups to facilitate fair and even distribution (Syrett 2007). In economics it relates to the allocation of scarce resources among competing ends (Syrett 2007). Rationing in healthcare involves using some mechanism to 'bring demand into line with supply' (Syrett 2007, p. 27) in relation to provision of healthcare. It is not a new phenomenon, but remains a controversial issue. Overt reference to rationing, especially 'strong rationing' (explicit denial of services), within healthcare is often avoided (Loewy 1999; Redwood 2000), but it has taken place and still does under various guises, such as by ability to pay, as in the USA (Loewy 1999). As Loewy (1999) points out, rather than explicit reference to rationing, euphemisms such as 'priority-setting' are often used, which at best is disingenuous and at worst dangerous because it disguises the true nature and implications of these processes.

Useful resource: the birth of the NHS

For a short, personal, account of the impact of the introduction of the NHS go to http://news.bbc.co.uk/1/hi/events/nhs_at_50/special_report/118693.stm

Why ration? The purpose of and mechanisms for rationing

At the inception of the NHS in 1948, the demand for healthcare was huge, but it was thought, at the time, that once the backlog of unmet need had been fulfilled demand for healthcare would actually decrease as the population became healthier (Syrett 2007). However, by 1951, payment for glasses, for example, was introduced (Gray 1993). Charges for prescriptions followed in 1952. Arguably this represented the emergence of rationing of healthcare on the grounds of cost, but payment remained at the margins of healthcare, and was in effect means tested (those on low income and pensioners are exempt from the charges – up to 88 per cent of claimants) (Politics.co.uk 2005).

The main form of rationing operating in the early days of the NHS has been referred to as the five Ds – delay, defer, deter, dissuade and decline (Leatherman and Sutherland 2003). In this way healthcare was not obviously rationed but provided only when the service became available to those dutifully waiting in the 'queue'. This sort of rationing could be circumvented by those who had the money for a private consultation but private provision in the UK is a small percentage of healthcare coverage, making up 16.6 per cent in 2002 (ONS 2008). In addition, resources were 'rationed' in effect, via the distribution of resources both across the country and across healthcare specialities. For example, fewer resources are distributed to psychiatric care (Harrison and Gill 2010).

Key to the dynamic for rationing is the year-on-year increase in the cost of healthcare. This increasing demand reflects, in part, the ageing population and the success of healthcare. People now rarely die of infectious diseases in childhood, but live long enough to develop, and live with, chronic conditions (Syrett 2007). However, Syrett (2007) also points out that the ageing population itself may account for less of the rise in demand than often claimed. It is not yet demonstrated that the elderly in fact spend more of their years ill, and expenditure on the elderly is related to end-of-life care, and whether this is at the age of 40 or 80 is immaterial (in terms of cost). However, treating and managing the conditions that dominate our morbidity and mortality profile, such as heart disease, diabetes and cancer, is extremely expensive. For example, it is estimated that to implement best practice, as outlined in the National Service Frameworks (NSFs) for cancer, mental health, renal disease, diabetes and coronary heart disease, across services, could cost between £7.5 billion and £9 billion by 2022–3 (Syrett 2007). Overall, it is generally considered that pressures to ration stem from rising healthcare costs (technological changes account for 75 per cent of the increase in expenditure according to Syrett 2007), increased public expectations and economic constraints regarding the ability to fund provision (Loewy 1999; Syrett 2007).

As a brief aside, it is worth noting that, despite these huge and rising costs, the NHS costs less to run than the private insurance and federally funded healthcare system of the USA, which costs $6,719 per person, compared with $2,815 in the UK. Life expectancy at birth is two years higher in the UK than in the USA (80 and 78 respectively), although annual cancer mortality rates are slightly higher in the UK than in the USA per 100,000 population (147 in the UK, 133 in the USA, 2004 figures) (Heslop 2010). Additionally, the insurance-led system in the USA encouraged spiralling healthcare costs and defensive medicine (Weale 1998). The UK system also provides more healthcare provision for the population as a whole (DoH 2000a). Until recent health care reforms in the USA, led by President Obama, 20 per cent of Americans had little or no health care cover (Weale 1998), over 40 million having no health insurance cover (DoH 2000a), with provision being seriously limited for those who fall outside any form of coverage (Redwood 2000), a similar scenario to the pre-NHS time in the UK.

Redwood (2000) comments that essentially decisions about curbing healthcare expenditure are political, to make sure appropriate healthcare is provided to the population within the capacity of realistic resource provision. Obviously, there will always be disagreements regarding how much money is spent on healthcare, and the NHS in particular, as funding comes from general taxation (80 per cent), some from National Insurance contributions (12 per cent) and the rest coming from user charges and private health insurance (Redwood 2000), but it is generally agreed that there has to be some limit (Klein 1984; Leatherman and Sutherland 2003; Ainsworth 2006). Weale (1998, p. 410) refers to the 'inconsistent triad' within current healthcare provision, the triad being the problematic nature of providing a comprehensive, high-quality, healthcare system *to all* within a population. Instead, he suggests that it is only possible to fulfil any two of these aspirations at a time: for example, a comprehensive service to all (forgoing the high quality), or a comprehensive, high-quality service that is *not* available to all, or a free, high-quality but *not* comprehensive service. In other words, some decisions must be made about funding and what is funded within the NHS, and as Klein (1984, p. 144) puts it, 'The issue ... is not whether to ration but how to ration; how best to devise a system which allocates what will always be an inadequate resource ... in the fairest and most socially acceptable way.'

3

Rationing by controlling expenditure on drugs or treatments

Placing controls on spending on drugs or other healthcare interventions is one way of reducing expenditure (reducing demand). However, as Weale (1998) notes, it is extremely difficult to make such decisions, and it is certainly not possible to create an agreed and comprehensive list regarding what NHS money should be spent on. Various committees worldwide have considered this, and have identified vasectomies, sterilisation, tattoo removal, in vitro fertilisation and gender reassignment as options for exclusion, but this will have little overall impact on costs (Weale 1998). Moreover, as Ainsworth (2006, p. 140) notes, 'PCTs and everyone involved in such decisions can never get it right simply because there is no right answer ... because there is no absolute moral or mathematically correct answer [they] will always be influenced by politicians and patients, drug companies and the courts, by nurses, doctors and newspapers'.

Rationing by evidence-based practice (EBP)

A growing mechanism for exploring care and treatment options within the health service is the use of evidence-based practice (Ter Meulen and Dickenson 2002). The notion of EBP is dealt with in more detail in Chapter 5, but in essense it refers to providing care based on evidence of effectiveness and/or cost-effectiveness. In other words, the drug, treatment or therapy actually works and improves health. The recommendations from the National Institute for Health and Clinical Excellence (NICE) contribute to EBP decision-making. The central vindication of EBP is that it reduces expenditure on ineffective care, and substantiates resource utilisation decisions based on clinical, therapeutic grounds, not simply resource/cost considerations. The treatment decision made around Child B, in the 1990s, is an example of such decision-making in the NHS (see Box 3.1).

Offering healthcare based on 'evidence' helps to rationalise the rationing and allocation of resources, in the light of 'cost-effectiveness', and has been used as part of the 'efficiency' claims for reducing healthcare expenditure (i.e. not using resources on treatments shown to be ineffective). EBP also adds to the drive to create protocol-driven healthcare, especially when funding for the treatment comes from a third party such as an insurance company (via managed care packages as in the USA) (Ter Meulen and Dickenson 2002). Despite this, things such as efficiency savings are considered to be of limited value, leading to compromises in quality or options for individiuals (Syrett 2007). For example, those expected to incur limited benefit from a treatment (e.g. the chronically ill or elderly) may be excluded from access to various therapies (Ter Meulen and Dickenson 2002).

Box 3.1 Case Study: Child B

Child B, who had acute myeloid leukaemia, was denied a second bone-marrow transplant on the grounds of its likely minimal effectiveness. Despite a legal challenge from the father of Child B, the decision was upheld. Child B subsequently had an experimental form of treatment paid for by private donation, although Child B died a year later (Redwood 2000). It would appear that the decision was vindicated by the outcome, although this was not conclusively predicted when the original decision was made.

If you would like to read more about this case go to: http://www.bmj.com/cgi/content/full/312/7046/1587. You should be able to get access to this article in the BMJ via your library subscription.

Rationing by lifestyle

Ultimately, according to Redwood (2000), rationing discriminates between patients regardless of need (see assessing need, p. 101), with an obvious example being denial of treatment on the grounds of lifestyle, e.g. smoking, or status, such as being obese or aged. Rationing on these grounds can be attractive from an administrative, bureaucratic perspective, as the characteristic for exclusion is easily identified. This sort of rationing is evident in transplant treatment where, given a list of different attributes of patients (e.g. age, value of patient to society, outcome of the transplant regarding life expectancy, alcohol consumption), members of the public, family doctors and gastroenterologists came up with different decisions regarding the grounds for selection. Medical practitioners, mainly, but not exclusively, selected outcome as the main criterion, whereas the general public prioritised age (the youngest) first (Redwood 2000). Rationing on grounds of lifestyle also emerges around matters such as smoking and obesity (see Case study 1: Obesity, Chapter 4).

Rationing by postcode

Postcode rationing is another form of rationing, whereby bureaucratically constructed boundaries contract or expand options to care and treatment. Certain treatments may be funded by one primary care trust (PCT) but not another (Rogers 2002). A fairly recent headline example of the postcode lottery involved the breast cancer drug Herceptin. Ann Marie Rogers took Swindon Primary Care Trust (PCT) to the High Court over their refusal to fund the drug (Ainsworth 2006) and eventually won the right to the treatment. However, as Ainsworth (2006) points out, this is not a clear-cut case of 'evil' PCT, denying necessary and appropriate treatment, but a badly thought through decision on the part of the PCT. Swindon PCT had developed a policy of funding under 'exceptional circumstances' but had not advanced a case for refusal of treatment on the grounds of either resources (funding) *or* clinical need. The secretary of state had also made an injunction that financial matters could not be used as the sole reason for denying access to treatment (Syrett 2007). The appeal against Swindon PCT was therefore upheld on the grounds that refusal was 'irrational and unlawful' because no grounds, other than those based on 'personal characteristics', could be discerned in the decision. In other words, it was purely discriminatory to the individual because they had not advanced an argument that a distinction could be made between patients on clinical grounds (Syrett 2007).

3

Useful resources: Herceptin treatment

If you would like to read more about this case go to:

http://news.bbc.co.uk/1/hi/health/4677086.stm

http://www.timesonline.co.uk/tol/news/uk/health/article5853302.ece

And read the article by Ainsworth (2006).

However, it is worth noting too that Herceptin is not a 'wonder-drug' that is denied to patients *simply* on the grounds of money. More precisely, it is a therapy that will help to increase survival in some women with a certain type of breast cancer, and information to aid this type of decision-making is vital to ensure appropriate use of resources (Ainsworth 2006). NICE was, in fact, established to address this problem by making recommendations regarding specific interventions to health authorities (Rogers 2002).

Rationing by QALYs

QALYs (quality adjusted life years) are another tool that can be used, as they constitute a mechanism for intervention selection. They are used to compare the effectiveness of various types of interventions (in terms of cost and life years saved) that could be adopted to address a health need. For example, the cost per QALY for smoking cessation has been estimated at between £212 and £873 compared with £4,000 to £8,000 per QALY for the prescription of statins (Tones and Green 2004). Allocating a QALY to various interventions provides general information about cost and effectiveness, or capacity to benefit, on a *general* basis, i.e. X costs more than Y for the number of 'life years' (potentially) saved. However, this cannot be applied on an individual basis, as someone with heart disease may have their heart function improved by a CABG and not be a smoker – hence smoking cessation is an irrelevant option in their case. QALYs do not relate to actual need (Green and South 2006). Instruments like QALYs are best used, if at all, for population-level decision-making around funding choices for treatments (see assessing need, p. 101).

Criticisms of rationing

Redwood (2000) disagrees with the basic claim that rationing is inevitable and Klein et al. (1996) state that 'government parsimony is to blame' (cited in Syrett 2007, p. 29), although as has already been noted the financial demands of healthcare are considerable and require some form of control. However, many of the mechanisms for rationing are flawed. EBP, for example, purports to facilitate the delivery of effective healthcare and treatment but is regarded by patient groups and others as just another tool for rationing at a clinical level (Rogers 2002; Ter Meulen and Dickenson 2002). In addition, some of the fundamental assertions about EBP are open to question and certainly illustrate the emotive component of rationing, particularly for the 'dread diseases' such as cancer (Klein 1984). As Rodwin (2001) notes, 'evidence becomes an instrument of politics rather than a substitute for it' (quoted by Syrett 2007, p. 7) (see Chapter 5, section 5.1, on research, for further discussion of EBP).

With regard to rationing by lifestyle, according to Redwood (2000) and Davis and Porteous (2006), this fundamentally represents discrimination. For example, denial of treatment on the grounds of actual age ignores the real difference that might exist between this and a person's biological age. Given the ageing population within the Western world, denying treatment to individuals on the basis of an age time line does not reflect the actual state of health for many individuals even in their eighties and the benefit that they can confer from certain treatments, such as hip replacements. Clearly, there is a lack of consensus regarding how choices should or could be made and emotional, and potentially discriminatory, choices could be made if medical and healthcare practitioners could select on the grounds of 'lifestyle'.

Rationing on these grounds is ill-supported by evidence too and is ultimately a morally redundant strategy, as Redwood (2000, pp. 26–7) notes: 'rationing conspires with moral condemnation to ignore need. The recalcitrant smoker may not receive much public sympathy, but the principle is dangerous ... discrimination between patients could place the medical profession in the invidious position of a "health police" ... The blacklist could be extended indefinitely' (see Case study 1, Chapter 4, and responsibility and health, p. 115).

Finally, according to Redwood (2000), postcode rationing springs from chronic under-funding, rather than being a fair and sensible option. As Redwood (2000, p. 72) states, 'The postcode route, with or without NICE, is the unintended consequence of a health service that sees rationing, not the reform of funding, as the answer to its plight.'

According to Redwood (2000), the way forward is to rethink through the solidarity principle and the basis of free-care-to-all and to diversify funding. In other words, mechanisms need to be created that enable people to purchase outside the system, with either private insurance or cash. The availability of more resources to healthcare would not completely negate the need for choices but would ameliorate its extreme consequences (Syrett 2007).

How this might be achieved would require careful economic, political and ethical consideration and would obviously differ country-to-country (Redwood 2000). However, consideration of alternatives is vital as, according to Redwood (2000), the dogma of purity of funding in the NHS can only lead to rationing (and its associated iniquities) and if there was a mixed funding economy, e.g. as in Switzerland, the bar, of what is covered for all, could be set high (Redwood 2000).

Conclusion

What can be concluded from this brief discussion of healthcare rationing is that it raises many conflicting issues around cost, funding, demands (meeting needs) and practical and ethical considerations. Each option therefore needs careful consideration (in context) to ameliorate any negative consequences emerging from the decisions. The possibility of exploring other avenues for actually increasing the amount of resources available is another option too. This latter point, however, will inevitably be informed by ideological and political decision-making. As Redwood (2000, p. 119) notes, 'Finance is a key component of the problem, not of the answer. Money could be raised in any number of ways if the political will to do so were firm enough and sufficiently confident of electoral support.'

Individualism

The term *individualism* is obviously associated with the concept of the 'individual', someone or something with a single distinct entity. Broadly, individualism as a word denotes independence and self-reliance, and actions or thoughts centred on 'self'. It also refers to a particular social theory that emphasises the importance of individual freedom of action (see liberal individualism, p. 44). Primary moral value is accorded to individual human beings (Care 1995). Specifically, 'individualism prizes individual human beings' (Care 1995, p. 405).

Most of us will take for granted that we are 'individuals' (we are our own agents and can act and shape things within the world), but the idea of the 'individual' as a free-thinking, acting, agent was not axiomatic. We have not always recognised the centrality of the individual. The origins of the existence of a free-thinking individual emerged, *inter alia*, from the philosophy of René Descartes (1596–1650). Descartes famously believed *cogito ergo sum* – I think, therefore I am (see mind–body dualism, p. 99). These ideas were further shaped by profound social, political and economic change experienced by seventeenth- and eighteenth-century philosophers, such as John Locke (1632–1704) and David Hume (1711–76), who were strongly influenced by these turbulent times, and captured, and contributed to, shifts in our understanding of the individual. Locke, for instance, was born during a turbulent time of British history that included the Civil War, and led to profound shifts in the political and social order (see the Enlightenment, p. 37). The rule of, and unquestioning obedience to, a monarch and the landed gentry was fading, while urban society, with its demand for more communal, liberal democracy, started to flourish (Strathern 1996a). Europe was 'witnessing the advent of a widespread self-consciousness: the birth of an individuality which thought for itself' (Strathern 1996a, p. 51).

Immanuel Kant's (1724–1804) emphasis on the moral agency of an individual contributed to changing perceptions of the individual too. Kant asserted that all human beings should be considered 'ends in themselves', and be viewed as autonomous beings. Other moral and philosophical thinkers, such as Jeremy Bentham (1748–1832) and John Stuart Mill (1806–73), also accord the individual with the autonomous capacity for experiencing pleasure and pain. The notion of the individual as an agent of their own destiny with rights and responsibilities gained credence, and is a core feature within Western capitalist nations.

Contemporary accounts of the individual also emphasise the concept of self-awareness. The 'individual' in the latter part of the twentieth century is seen as being increasingly focused on 'self', an autonomous being, signified by self-control, self-efficacy and introspection (Ogden 2002). 'This individual no longer interacted with their environment but their focus turned inward towards themselves' (Ogden 2002, p. 100). Etzioni (1993) comments on the consequent 'me-ism' that emerges within Western capitalist societies (see communitarianism, p. 33).

3

Reflective activity

Consider how you recognise someone as an individual.

- Is it just that they are 'separate' from you? (what then about co-joined twins)?
- Is it that they have different personalities, backgrounds, ethnicity (what about the common features here)?
- Do you think we are primarily individuals or part of a collective whole?
- What underpins your thinking?

Individualism and health

These changes in our descriptions, and understanding, of the 'individual' have profound implications for health and health matters. Our concepts of 'health' have shifted to include subjective components, thereby also altering the nature of the relationship between 'experts' and 'self' (the individual) and notions of 'agency' (the ability to act as an independent, thinking being). Concepts of health have moved from being based on the biomedical perspective of health, equating health to the 'absence of disease' and identifying the existence of ill-health and disease thorough objective and measurable phenomena, to being based on subjective, socially and culturally situated notions of health. Psychological and sociological explanations stress the importance of psychological and social factors in the causation of illness and disease, encapsulated in Engle's Bio-Psycho-Social model of health (Sarafino 1990; Armstrong 1994; Nettleton 1995; Ogden 2002). Health, illness and disease are no longer the prerogative of medicine alone, but include social and (inter/intra) personal domains too. This broader perspective, however, does not fundamentally challenge the biomedical foundations of health; instead, they offer alternative causal explanations (social and psychological, rather than purely biological) and shape views about the process of health improvement (from objective, expert-driven prescriptions, to subjective, agency and personal action).

Medicine and health and social care have a long history of delivering care at the individual level. Physicians' relationships with their patients were very much concentrated on close personal attention, observation and rigorous interrogation to reach a diagnosis (Porter 1997). This individual focus is spilling over into the domain of action for health improvement, via health behaviour and healthy lifestyles, too (Dougherty 1993; O'Brien 1995; Leichter 1997; Nettleton 1997; Lupton 2000; Ogden 2002; French 2007; Irvine 2010). The first contemporary health document to explicitly raise this issue was the DHSS document *Prevention and Health: Everybody's Business*, published in 1977. The subtitle for the document is *A Reassessment of Public and Personal Health*, and within the document it was asserted that the current health problems (still current today) were related to individual behaviour rather than environmental factors. This focus on the individual continues in *Choosing Health*, the public health **white paper** published in 2004 (DoH 2004a). Within the document it is stated that 'At the start of the twenty-first century England needs a new approach to health of the public, reflecting the rapid and radical transformation of English society in the latter half of the twentieth century, responding to the needs and wishes of its citizens as individuals and harnessing the new opportunities open to it' (DoH 2004a, p. 2).

However, as Gimenez (1999) reminds us, this focus on the 'individual' as the source of health improvement is a contested notion. Even within the government document *Choosing Health*, the role of the government in improving health is acknowledged and, as Gimenez (1999) also notes, recent scientific advances have led to the re-emergence of genetic explanations to the contribution of disease.

Alongside this remains the continuing debate around the impact of social, economic and environmental factors on health. Poor socio-economic and environmental conditions have long been associated with increased mortality and morbidity. Data collected for Chadwick's famous *Report on the Sanitary Conditions of the Labouring Classes* (1842) demonstrated that the death rate differed significantly not only between 'gentry' and 'labourers', but also according to where they lived. Material and structural factors are generally considered one of the main causes of this disparity between different social groups (Black Report 1980; Benzeval et al. 1995; DoH 1998; Earle and O'Donnell 2007) and it is the interplay between biology, lifestyle, direct working and living conditions and wider social conditions that shapes health outcomes (Earle and O'Donnell 2007).

Conclusion

The concept of the 'individual' is a powerful one in modern Western societies, and reflects the organisation of much of our medical, healthcare and public health systems and delivery. We are reminded, though, that reference to the individual as the panacea for the promotion of health is unlikely to be successful (Gimenez 1999; Earle and O'Donnell 2007) given the plethora of factors that shape individual experiences, choices and actions too (see inequalities, p. 95).

Inequalities (in health)

While it was observed in the section on individualism that increasing focus is placed on the individual, individual behaviour and the individual's contribution to health, exploring the issue of inequalities adds an additional challenge to the validity of this focus. Within any study of health and health-related matters, it is essential to recognise that experiences of health (as recorded via morbidity and mortality data) differ across a population. In other words not all individuals, or groups within a society, experience the same level of health. Many factors have an impact on health, including individual behaviour, social circumstances, environment, government policy, education and so forth (Dahlgren and Whitehead 1991; Seedhouse 2001; Shircore 2009). Dahlgren and Whitehead (1991) have produced a well known framework outlining the key factors that influence health. The domains of influence that they identify include: general socio-economic, cultural and environmental conditions; living and working conditions; social and community networks; individual lifestyle factors; and age, sex and constitutional factors.

Reflective activity

Type 'Dahlgren and Whitehead 1991' into an internet search engine to get access to a copy of their framework.
- What do you think about the factors that they have identified as influencing health?
- Can you give your own examples for each of these domains?
- Which do you think are the most important factors that influence health and how do you think they affect health?

There is not enough space in this book to explore all the complex and detailed aspects that contribute to health (many health promotion texts include a chapter, or content within a chapter, on inequalities in health if you wish to read more about this: for example, Naidoo and Wills 2000; Earle et al. 2007), but poor socio-economic and environmental conditions have long been associated with increased mortality and morbidity. We have already mentioned Chadwick's famous *Report on the Sanitary Conditions of the Labouring Classes* (1842), demonstrating differences in the death rate between 'gentry' and 'labourers' and also according to where they lived. For example, the average age of death in Rutland (a small, rural county in the Midlands) among the 'gentry' was 52 and for 'labourers' 38, while in Liverpool for the same groups, it was 35 and 15 respectively (Thompson 1968). Much of this startling difference was explained by far greater infant mortality in the 'labouring' classes (Bynum 2008). However, this social class gradient continues to exist for most causes of death and illness. For example, on average men in social classes I and II (professional and managerial occupations) will live five years longer than those in social classes IV and V (semi-skilled and unskilled occupations) (Hattersley 1997). For specific diseases, inequalities are also noted. Deaths from heart disease were three times greater among unskilled men than among professional men (DoH 2000b) and differences in cancer rates exist between the most deprived and most affluent areas of the country. Other geographical variations exist too, with mortality from CHD in people aged 65 and over being three times higher in Manchester than in Kingston and Richmond (DoH 2000b), and continuing variations between different areas were noted by Hussey (2009). Inequalities in health are increasingly being recorded according to specific diseases or risk factors/risk behaviours such as alcohol consumption, rather than by social class (see Health Improvement Analytical Team – Monitoring Unit 2007), but it is still recognised that generally, 'even where we are seeing improvements, health inequalities are often present' (Health Improvement Analytical Team – Monitoring Unit 2007,

p. 5). Hussey (2009) also draws attention to lower life expectancy experienced by those with a mental illness, and lifestyle-related issues such as obesity are higher in lower social classes (DoH 1998).

Causes of inequalities

In the nineteenth century the common feature noted by public health commentators as contributing to disease and death was poverty (Bynum 2008). Now, rather than poverty per se (Le Fanu 1999), inequalities in wealth and access to other social, economic and structural resources are deemed to be the source of the continuing health gap between rich and poor (Hussey 2009; Hills et al. 2010; Marmot et al. 2010). In other words, the explanations for continuing inequalities are considered to be multifactorial and cannot be explained by differences in behaviours and risk-taking alone (Earle and O'Donnell 2007), with material and structural factors playing a dominant part in the creation of inequalities in the experience of health (Shircore 2009; Marmot et al. 2010). Marmot et al. (2008, p. 1661) claim that 'poor health of poor people, the social gradient in health within countries, and the substantial health inequities between countries are caused by the unequal distribution of power, income, goods and services, … their access to health care and education, their conditions of work and leisure, their homes, communities, towns or cities'. Bourdieu (1986), Coleman (1988) and Putman (1995) (cited in Earle and O'Donnell 2007) comment on the importance to health of **social capital**, social support networks and membership of 'groups', which provide not only support, but also access to resources, goods, facilities and services, such as healthcare and education. Wilkinson (1996) suggests that social cohesion is important to health and that countries, such as the UK, with unequal distribution of wealth have less social cohesion. In other words, the wealth gap contributes to the health gap. It was noted in an OECD report that while income inequality and poverty had fallen faster in the UK than in any other OECD country, it was greater than in three-quarters of the OECD countries (OECD 2008). A more recent report by Hills et al. (2010) identified that inequalities in wealth and opportunities, which began to rise in the 1980s (reflected in health inequalities too), remain as strong now as they were 30 years ago, and for Marmot et al. (2010) health inequalities result from social inequalities per se.

Implications for policy and action around health and health policy

From this perspective, action to improve health must encompass a broad range of interventions. Marmot et al. (2008, p. 1627) assert that work 'on the social determinants of health must involve the whole of government, civil society, local communities, business and international agencies'. Public policy has an important role to play in improving access to resources from health care to safe public spaces, according to Hills et al. (2010), as otherwise individuals have to rely on personal wealth and other resources, which remain unequally distributed.

However, this perspective is ideologically and politically determined as well as being shaped by the 'facts' (i.e. disparate experiences of mortality and morbidity between different classes within a society), and Bynum (2008) recalls the work of the nineteenth-century pathologist Rudolf Virchow (1821–1902). Virchow was a political activist who agitated for significant social change and improvements in the living and working conditions of the poor. From his detailed analysis of a typhus epidemic in Upper Silesia (then part of Prussia), he argued that what was needed to prevent further epidemics was 'education, better roads, modern modes of agriculture, and, above all, universal democracy' (Bynum 2008, p. 1627), not just more doctors.

As with many aspects of health, the sort of social change approach advocated by Virchow, is not considered legitimate by all commentators. As Klein (1978) points out, tackling inequalities requires significant social and structural changes and this degree of state intervention (legislation and fiscal policy regulation) would be deemed inappropriate and potentially damaging by those taking a liberal-individualist perspective (see p. 44). Spicker (1993), for instance, argues that transferring assets from the 'haves' to the 'have-nots' (via taxation or universality, for example) is violating the moral rule of 'respecting the freedom of the individual', and Klein (1978) suggests that tackling inequalities to improve the overall health of the population is not necessarily an appropriate goal. It could in fact result in a decline in overall health improvements as it is the middle classes, making small, more easily achieved changes in habits and so forth, who have the largest impact on overall morbidity and mortality (as they constitute the majority of the population). Marmot et al. (2010) do recognise that attempting to reduce inequalities by focusing on the most disadvantaged alone will be ineffective, but action should be proportional to need – which they refer to as proportionate universalism (see need (needs assessment), p. 101).

However, to argue against tackling inequalities requires *justification* of inequality as a guiding principle for society and this is generally *not* reflected in health policy and other documentation over the past decade or so (DoH 1998, 1999a, 2004a, 2008b; Hills et al. 2010; Marmot et al. 2010). For example, *Public Service Agreements* set a target to 'reduce health inequalities by 10% by 2010' (Hills et al. 2010, p. 37).

Action to tackle inequalities, according to Marmot et al. (2010, p. 9), should involve six policy objectives:

> Give every child the best start in life.
> Enable all children, young people and adults to maximise their capabilities and have control over their lives.
> Create fair employment and good work for all.
> Ensure a healthy standard of living for all.
> Create and develop healthy and sustainable places and communities.
> Strengthen the role and impact of ill-health prevention.

What Marmot et al. (2010) go on to mention is that this will not be achieved without action from government, local authorities, the NHS and the private and voluntary sectors, and requires action to empower individuals and local communities too (see empowerment, p. 77).

Conclusion

The issue of inequalities per se, and the appropriate approaches and focus of work to tackle inequalities will no doubt continue to be a source of debate, with the policy and documents being criticised as 'ideology with evidence' (Marmot et al. 2010, p. 3). What this demonstrates though is the continuing importance of considering ideologies and values when making decisions around health and social care.

Mind–body dualism

This section provides only the most basic outline of the theory of mind–body dualism but it is mentioned because it has been an influential theory for medicine. It has helped to shape, for instance, the distinction we still make between physical and mental illness. Mind–body dualism describes the theory that the mind and the body are distinct, in both substance and nature (Quinton and Porter 1999). In essence they are different types of entities. This mind–body dualism originated from the philosophy of René Descartes (1596–1650), a French philosopher and mathematician. The idea of dualism is classically represented by Descartes's phrase *cogito ergo sum* ('I think, therefore I am'). Descartes's theory, according to Williams (2003, p. 12), 'drove a wedge between mind and body', although it did posit a relationship between the mind and body, in so far as it could causally affect certain actions, such as raising the arm, and was, itself, affected by certain bodily events: for example, the sensation of pain would be registered in the 'mind' if you stubbed your toe. However, in essence the theory holds that mental and physical events are different (Williams 2003).

Mind–body dualism and health

It was an extremely powerful theory and a key premise upon which the biomedical model of health was based. It reflected a shift away from traditional 'spiritual', transcendental, explanations of disease, ones in which sorcery and other supernatural beliefs influenced perceptions of health, disease and healing, to ones based on scientific study and investigations of the biology of the body (Williams 2003). These ideas contributed greatly to the renaissance of medicine, and science study, during the Enlightenment (see p. 37) and the rise in **reductionist** medicine.

Reductionist, biological, biochemical medicine is strongly reflected in contemporary approaches to healthcare in general and has increasingly been criticised for being too limited, particularly with reference to mental health (Williams 2003). Social (and psychological) explanations of health and disease also contribute to our understanding (Williams 2003). Williams warns, though, that biological explanations should not be abandoned for social explanations, as this is as limited as the original divide. For example, 'mental disorder, ... may indeed be a "label" in the sense that, like all words, it is a social construct, but it is not "merely" a label. It has a referent that has an onto-logical reality ... beyond the multiplicity of "voices" to which we must attend' (Williams 2003, citing Busfield 1996, p. 145). In other words, conditions that affect the body and mind do exist and are experienced as dysfunctions by individuals, as well as having social connotations and social constructs (see postmodernism/social constructivism, p. 47, and stigma, p. 118).

Thus absolute mind–body dualism is being abandoned in favour of what seem more productive considerations, namely that the mind and the body are thoroughly intertwined (Ogden 2002). The distinction between mental health and health per se is an artificial, and unhelpful, construct. Our somatic responses are *part* of our mental reactions to events and visa versa (Seedhouse 2002).

> The idea ... is that the way we are wired-up bodily and what happens to us – how we are raised, how we experience each day, where we live, what race we are, what money we have, how our parents treat us – both play an indispensable part in forming our mental lives. Alter the wiring, or take any of the other influences away and our mental lives change as a consequence. (Seedhouse 2002, p. 53)

Reflective activity

- Consider the ways in which your mood (how you feel 'in yourself', emotionally and psychologically) affects how you feel 'in your body'.
- Similarly, consider how a physical illness, such as flu or a stomach bug, affects your mood.

Practically, healthcare and medicine seem to increasingly recognise that people's mental lives are inseparable from their physical being and that psychological, as well as physical, health should be taken into account within therapeutic regimes (Alder 1999) and work to promote health (Handsley 2007b). This particularly extends to 'mental health' and Seedhouse (2002) asserts that it is a mistake to seek to promote mental heath separately from work to promote health per se.

Conclusion

Mind–body dualism has been an important concept, particularly influencing the development of modern medicine. Its limitations are being recognised though, and more holistic concepts of health are increasingly being embraced (see also Chapter 1).

Need (needs assessment)

Assessing 'need' has become increasingly important to healthcare and primary care trusts are required to commission and deliver healthcare for their populations according to need (Lawton 1999; Horne 2003; Cavanagh and Chadwick 2005). However, ascertaining 'need' is not as clear-cut as it might at first seem. For example, there is confusion and controversy regarding the difference between a 'need' and a 'want' and what constitutes a 'health' need, as opposed to a 'social' or general need (Seedhouse 1994; Rawaf and Bahl 1998; Horne 2003). These are pertinent questions and this section explores some of the complexities of this concept, and provides a brief critique of some of the mechanisms for assessing health need – health needs assessment (HNA).

What is a 'need'?

No overriding theory of need exists (Percy-Smith 1996). Gillam et al. (2007) suggest that needs can be classified in terms of diseases, priority groups, geographical areas, services or using a life-cycle approach (e.g. from children to the elderly) but this primarily refers to domains of 'need', not what 'need' itself might be. As Horne (2003) notes, there is a lack of a universal definition of both the term 'health' and the term 'need'. Much of the discussion about what is 'health' has been explored earlier (see Chapter 1) and it would be useful to read this section again. It is particularly pertinent in the context of trying to ascertain what constitutes a 'health' 'need', as it is recognised that disease-based definitions of health are insufficient (Lawton 1999; Horne 2003).

Various attempts have been made to assess 'need' and what is meant by 'need'. An early attempt by Bradshaw (1972), to explore social need, came up with a taxonomy still noted in more contemporary texts (Rowley 2005; Gillam et al. 2007). Bradshaw's taxonomy of need comprises:

> Felt need – what people themselves perceive as being needed.
> Expressed need – this refers to the vocalisation of 'felt' need, i.e. an actual demand for something.
> Comparative need – this refers to the identification of a 'gap' between, for instance, service provision or type and quality of housing in one area, compared with another, according to the judgement of experts.
> Normative need – this is based on expert-driven perspectives based on an agreed or specified 'standard', such as the level of nutrition needed for an adequate diet (Bradshaw 1972).

According to this taxonomy, 'real' need emerges when data from all the domains described within the taxonomy converge (similar evidence emerges). It is therefore a planning tool for service provision and does not itself provide any means of assessing if the services themselves are needed. The problem with this, as Bradshaw (1994) later acknowledges, is that 'need' is driven by service provision, or the resources that are available, rather than being based on *actual* or **categorical need**. The taxonomy does not help us to determine what constitutes a 'need' in the first place. Bradshaw (1994) for instance, suggests that 'need' could be based around an understanding of what is important for survival and effective human functioning, such as the importance of shelter, although this itself is difficult to determine. For example, what constitutes a minimum or adequate standard of shelter, as this is at least in part socially, historically and culturally situated? Furthermore, this taxonomy of need tends to accord too much value to the opinion of experts (Bradshaw 1994).

Doyal and Gough (1991) suggest that need exists where there are goals, and need differs from 'wants', which are merely subjective preferences. In terms of 'need', these are goals, which enable the avoidance of serious harm to an individual or group, such as the 'goal'/'need' to quit cigarette smoking. They use this as an example to illustrate the difference between a 'want' and a 'need' too; an individual may 'want' a cigarette (i.e. have a craving for a cigarette), but they do *not* 'need' a cigarette, as this would in fact be contrary to avoiding harm. Doyal and Gough (1991, p. 51) pursue the notion of 'avoidance of serious harm' as a component of need, by taking harm to mean 'blocked potential'. This in turn they link with 'life plans' and cite Miller (1976, p 134):

'Harm, for any individual, is whatever interferes directly or indirectly with the activities essential to his plan of life; and correspondingly, his needs must be understood to comprise whatever is necessary to allow these activities to be carried out. In order, then, to decide what a person's needs are, we must first identify his plan of life, then establish what activities are essential to that plan, and finally, investigate the conditions which enable those activities to be carried out'.

Avoiding 'blocked potential' and facilitating life plans are themselves dependent upon the existence of good physical health and autonomy. Need exists when someone is not able, or lacks the resources, to fully participate in society. Thus, Doyal and Gough (1991) assert that physical survival/physical health and personal autonomy are preconditions for individual action and engagement in the world and therefore constitute basic needs.

They cite physical survival/physical health as a basic need for several reasons:

1 Serious disease undermines what might be expected of individuals and their capacity to lead active and successful lives.
2 The existence of disease can be universally recognised and objectively assessed (avoiding recourse to fulfilling subjective judgements of needs, in other words, by their account, fulfilling wants).
3 Opportunities to meet these needs, i.e. improve physical health, exist (*inter alia*, via the provision of health care).

On the other hand, autonomy (see p. 55), as a basic need, has three components according to Doyal and Gough (1991). These are:

1 *Understanding*. Certain skills are needed to promote autonomy. Education, for instance, is vital as it facilitates the development of our intellectual capacity and enables us to engage productively within the world.
2 *Psychological capacity*. This refers to cognitive and emotional capacity. Mental health is an essential component of autonomy because without mental health, our ability to make decisions and act is undermined.
3 *Opportunities*. Individuals need opportunities to make choices concerning life goals.

Given that the physical and autonomous potential of individuals will differ, exactly how these capacities are fulfilled is not to be prescribed. However, Doyal and Gough (1991) argue that this does not detract from the assertion that these are basic needs as, at a minimum, all individuals should be able to achieve a 'normal' level of engagement within society.

What is a 'health' need?

Gillam et al. (2007, p. 112) suggest that health needs encompass education, social services, housing, the environment and social policy. This extends the notion of a health need considerably and it is particularly difficult to identify what constitutes a 'health' need as opposed to a 'social' or general need (Sheaff 1996). This is important to determine, though, as policy and service priority setting and delivery are often segregated according to whether something constitutes a 'health' or 'social' need (Horne 2003), and although it is acknowledged that many factors (social, economic, environmental and so forth) affect health, action on these matters certainly does not necessarily fall within the domain of healthcare.

So what might constitute a 'health' need. Need exists, at a basic level, where there is any form of inequality (for example, differential mortality and morbidity) (Bradshaw 1994) or, as Doyal and Gough (1991) contend, some physical disease or blockage that prevents full social engagement. Sheaff (1996) takes this further by proposing that a 'health' need pertains to our *natural survival drive* and *natural capacities*; in other words, what is necessary for human beings to function. *Natural capacity* at a basic level refers to the requirements for survival (resistance to infection, biological capacity for normal longevity) and what supports our capacity to fulfil the basic activities of daily living (ADL), such as our ability to wash and feed ourselves. If we are unable to independently fulfil these functions or early mortality is threatened, then we have a 'health' need, as illness and disease can undermine these *natural capacities* (Sheaff 1996).

Sheaff (1996) includes *chosen potential* in his categorisation of health need, with *natural capacity* also relating to the ability to fulfil various roles within society. For example, if a concert pianist suffers a hand injury rendering her unable to play, this constitutes a health need, as treatment and healthcare enable the individual to return to full functioning. Sheaff (1996) would include

3

palliative and terminal care as a basic health need, on the grounds that avoidance of pain is a significant component of natural capacity too. Thus, according to Bradshaw (1973, 1994), Doyal and Gough (1991) and Sheaff (1996), health need emerges when disease or disability interferes with our autonomy and/or our natural capacities.

Other concepts of need

Other perspectives on need emerge. According to Cohen, need, to an economist, refers to the capacity to benefit from a treatment (Cohen 2008) and need for health *care* is now defined in these terms according to Gillam et al. (2007). However, Sheaff (1996) suggests that technological advances in medicine and healthcare skew the notion of need, because they simply extend what it is possible to achieve (in terms of disease intervention and longevity), rather than relating to any fundamental need per se. Indeed, Gillam et al. (2007, p. 111) acknowledge that healthcare need is often judged in terms of demand, and demand is 'supply-induced'. Therefore, any meaningful interpretation of the concept of 'need' should be divorced from assessment of current service provision or 'ability to benefit' (Bradshaw 1994; Seedhouse 1994; Sheaff 1996).

Seedhouse (1994) and Liss (1998) suggest that this is based on a false understanding of need. Need is often described as need for a particular 'thing'. For example, someone needs treatment in an intensive care unit, or to be prescribed statins, or to undergo bariatric surgery for obesity. However, to talk about 'need' as need for a 'thing' would lead to there being almost no restriction on 'things' people needed, and produce confusion and lack of clarity, i.e. where the distinction could be made between 'things' 'needed' (Liss 1998). Liss contends that the most appropriate way to conceive of needs is teleological, i.e. relating to some action, end-point or utility. For Liss (1998) and Seedhouse (2004) this relates to goals. For example, the need for food is not simply a 'fundamental need' but is related to the goal of survival.

Therefore, Liss (1998) argues that need(s) is not 'fundamental', nor is it possible to identify basic needs. Instead, he would argue that it is the notion of 'goals' that is fundamental to the concept of need because need exists *only if there is a gap between two necessary conditions*. These two 'necessary conditions' are the *actual state (AS)* (of an individual/ community) and the *goal (G)*. Needs, therefore, are not objects or physical things, but emerge when something is missing or something is needed to fill the gap between *AS* and *G*. This means that it is incorrect to talk of the 'need' for healthcare, or the need for drugs or other medical technologies. These things would only be appropriate (needed) if they could 'fill the gap'. The need is in fact to have the gap filled, rather than the need for a specified 'thing', and it is the goal that determines the object of need (Liss 1998). As Liss notes, the goal to live as a farmer generates different needs to the goal to live as a lawyer.

In summary, what the necessary 'thing' is remains unknown until the two necessary conditions are known. See the example in Box 3.2. Hence it would not necessarily be correct to say that 'I needed the central heating to be turned on', unless and until it could be determined that this indeed could 'fill the gap' and was the most appropriate way of doing so in the prevailing circumstances. As Liss (1998) notes, it is the nature of the goal that determines and justifies the need. Something is not simply intrinsically needed or valued, but is valued for its ability to fulfil a particular goal. In other words, 'there is a need when the goal is not realised and there is a need for a certain thing when this is necessary for realising that goal' (Liss 1998, p. 14). Within this conceptualisation of need options available to 'fill the gap' are constrained by priorities/values and resources too. For example, going back to the example regarding body temperature, if I did not have central heating, a woolly jumper (and hat) would have to suffice!

Box 3.2 An Example of the Gap between Actual State (AS) and Goal (G)

AS ———————————————————————————— G

'I am cold'   'I want to be warm'

There is a 'gap' between my AS and my G – hence a need exists

This 'gap' could be filled by several things:

> a woolly jumper;
> exercise;
> food;
> putting on the central heating.

What is demonstrated is that need only surfaces when goals and purpose exist. If no goal exists, no need will exist. Needs are best regarded as means towards ends (Seedhouse 1994) and these 'means' towards ends can encompass behaviours authors like Doyal and Gough (1991) would consider harmful, e.g. smoking (because it fulfils a particular goal to feel relaxed). However, while smoking can be a logical 'means to this end', it is also legitimate to encourage and enable individuals to reconsider this 'means to an end' in the light of other ends/goals that remain unachievable if this course of action is sustained. Challenging passive or potential damaging behavioural patterns might be important and ultimately create more autonomy as other life opportunities emerge and the likelihood of long-term harm to self or others is reduced (Crossley 2000). Seedhouse (1994) asserts that there is an unbreakable link between purpose and need and it is vital to consider what the 'fulfilling of need' makes possible when deciding or advising upon any course of action.

Healthcare need

Need in terms of healthcare follows this same reasoning 'in so far as it is necessary for realising health' (Liss 1998, p. 14), and as Liss goes on to acknowledge, this brings us back to the points raised at the beginning of this section, regarding the necessity for a clear concept of health as the basis for making such judgements, with health being defined by Liss (1998, pp. 15–16) and Nordenfelt (1987, cited by Liss 1998) 'as a person's ability to reach his or her vital goals ... vital goals are related to happiness ... covering such notions as satisfaction, contentedness and pleasure ... health [is not] sufficient for happiness ... [but] is a holistic concept [relating to] a range of abilities to do certain things ... [that may]vary from time to time'. This broad conceptualisation of health is covered, and extended, in Chapter 1. In terms of healthcare, then, it is not reasonable to expect that 'complete' health is possible in all instances, and healthcare should be related to realistic goals (Liss 1998).

How is health need assessed?

What can be discerned so far is that the concept of need and health need is complex but relates to goals and emerges once information about, or an understanding of, an *actual state* and *goal* emerges. This brings us to the question of how these (health) needs are assessed. As has already been mentioned, assessing health need is an imperative for those involved in providing health and social care. This shift towards providing services to meet (local) need spawned many mechanisms for doing so: for example, Rapid Participatory Appraisal and Citizen's Juries (Horne 2003). These mechanisms serve a function in that they provide a systematic framework for gathering data and information about an area or group. Gillam et al. (2007) suggest that the assessment of healthcare need involves knowledge of the incidence of disease, risk factors, disability and the effectiveness of services to address it.

However, Liss (1998) suggests that care needs to be taken with this, as the validity of making inferences of need from descriptive statistics (e.g. age, sex, occupation, income, morbidity, mortality) can be questioned in two ways. For example, it is not clear *exactly* what age or occupation tells us about health status (for example, people are remaining healthier into later years), nor what needs actually emerge from this information. Liss (1998) argues that it is insufficient to infer need from generalised knowledge of morbidity or mortality, for instance, or the demand for healthcare in a given area (demand being driven by supply).

Nevertheless, there are several formal processes of assessing health needs, more commonly referred to as health needs assessment. According to Quigley et al. (2005) there are five main approaches:

> health needs assessment (HNA);
> health impact assessment (HIA);
> integrated impact assessment (IIA);

> health equity audit (HEA);
> race equality impact assessment (REIA).

Details of all approaches are not explored here, but the main principles of HNA, HIA and HEA are noted.

HNA is a systematic method of reviewing the health needs and issues facing a given population, leading to agreed priorities and resource allocation that will improve health and reduce inequalities (Quigley et al. 2005). HNA involves:

> A systematic collection of information and data which enables the health professional to identify, analyse and prioritise the health needs and potential health needs of a given population in order to design and implement appropriate programmes of care. (Naish 1992, cited by Wright 2001, p. 54)

HNA starts with a defined population. The population can be geographical, a setting (e.g. school), shared interest or identity (ethnicity, homeless), disease-based (diabetes, mental illness) or a combination of these, and to maximise its effectiveness, engagement with the population and the involvement of multi-team approaches is important. The intention of HNA is that clear priorities for the population emerge, resulting in programmes for improving health and reducing inequalities. The choice of interventions should be based on effective and acceptable ones.

In contrast, HIA is about exploring the potential health consequences of a proposal, intervention or development (often one that has yet to be implemented) for a given population. **Quantitative** and **qualitative** sources of information are used to determine the health improvement or reduction in inequalities associated with the intervention, or identify if any health harms may occur (Quigley et al. 2005). HIA is often associated with non-health programmes such as transport, education and regeneration initiatives. For example, a HIA of the second runway at Manchester Airport was undertaken and 'HIAs can be utilised to gauge the effectiveness of many different types of community-based projects' (Handsley et al. 2007c, p. 340).

Finally, the HEA. It is a mandatory requirement for PCTs to use HEAs. The purpose of a HEA is to identify how fairly services or other resources are distributed in relation to the health needs of different groups or areas (not to distribute equally but relative to health need). It can be used to help make investment decisions, to commission resources and to support work that narrows inequalities. HEA is primarily concerned with assessing the impact of services on reducing inequalities, and PCTs are expected to carry out a HEA on priority services (Quigley et al. 2005). For more details regarding the process of HNA, HIA and HEA see Quigley et al. (2005).

Another approach to assessing health needs is rapid appraisal. Rapid appraisal sets out to gain an insight into a community's own perspective on need (felt and expressed needs in Bradshaw's terms), and collects information on community composition, organisation, structure, physical environment, socio-economic environment, service provision and 'consumer' perspective. Qualitative and quantitative methods of collecting information are important to attaining relevant information.

Houston and Cowley (2002) suggest that, at least in principle, needs assessment can be part of an empowerment process (see empowerment, p. 77) but none of these approaches replaces decision-making; instead they provide valuable information to inform and influence the process (Quigley et al. 2005). Gillam et al. (2007) also observe that essentially HNA work is about maximising the health of the population as a whole, rather than informing clinical decision-making. Even at the population level, as Dooris and Hunter (2007, p. 109) note, this is often the most problematic stage of assessing health need; in other words, what and how things should be done to improve health, i.e. what can 'fill the gap': 'public health practitioners have been skilled at acquiring knowledge and handling epidemiological information about the state of health of their communities, but they have been less skilled at applying this knowledge and effecting change in local settings'. In addition, despite lengthy descriptions of process, acknowledgment of the importance of qualitative information as well as quantitative detail (such as morbidity and mortality), and statements asserting the value of social and personal resources, the assessment of health needs seems to be explicitly and implicitly locked into a disease-based notion of health, or factors that affect social functioning. This is reflected in the use of terms in HNA documents, such as 'health condition', 'physical ability', 'pain', 'mental illness' and 'vitality', with no other specific concept of health underpinning approaches (Cavanagh and Chadwick 2005, p. 14).

Taking the notion of need as declared by Liss (1998) and Seedhouse (2004), health need can be judged once the actual state (AS) and goal (G) have been determined *and* judgements made about what might 'fill the gap'. Hence, epidemiological, quantitative data can be used to assess both AS and G, but richer, deeper insights are determined by qualitative data (Horne 2003): for example, asking people what their 'goals' are. Additionally, evidence on what works can help decisions and choices between different options necessary to achieve the goals (and 'fill the gap'). This could, and should, include options and interventions beyond healthcare. For example, education or retraining can help someone with a spinal injury to fulfil their goals of independent living, alongside medical and rehabilitative therapy.

Individual or population needs?

According to Gillam et al. (2007, p. 112), 'The need for health care is the population's ability to benefit from health care, which is in turn the sum of many individuals' ability to benefit.' Sheaff (1996) contends that it is not possible for a population to have health needs as only individuals have natural capacities and natural drivers that require fulfilment. Talk of population need has no ontological status (it does not exist), as it simply reflects the needs of different groups of individuals within society. It may, more correctly, reflect common interests, but a blanket appeal to the 'needs of a population' cannot be sustained, as the differences are likely to be as great as the similarities. 'Need', therefore, has to be assessed at a much more local or individual level.

Conclusions

The notion of need is complex and relates to goals. Talk about need for a 'thing' therefore misconstrues the notion of need and can feed into a dynamic that supports the expert-driven status quo. Mechanisms for assessing health need have been, and are being, developed, and in principle acknowledge the importance of going beyond mortality and morbidity to understand need. However, this still remains a challenge and one thing that emerges in the discussion of 'health' need is that healthcare provision alone is insufficient to meet needs (Bradshaw 1994; Sheaff 1996; Seedhouse 2004).

Useful resources

Mittelmark, M. B. (2007) 'Promoting Social Responsibility for Health: Health Impact Assessment and Healthy Public Policy at the Community Level', in J. Douglas, S. Earle, S. Handsley, C. E. Lloyd and S. Spurr (eds), *A Reader in Promoting Public Health: Challenge and Controversy*. London: Sage Publications in association with the Open University

Further reading about health impact assessment

Quigley, R., Cavanagh, S., Harrison, D., Taylor, L. and Pottle, M. (2005) *Clarifying Approaches to: Health Needs Assessment, Health Impact Assessment, Integrated Impact Assessment, Health Equity Audit, and Race Equality Impact Assessment*. London: HDA. This document provides much more detail on the various methods of HNA noted above.

Raymond, B. (2005) 'Health Needs Assessment, Risk Assessment and Public Health', in D. Sines, F. Appleby and M. Frost (eds), *Community Health Care Nursing*, 3rd edn. Oxford: Blackwell, pp. 70–88. Here you will find more detail about approaches to HNA such as rapid appraisal and citizen perspectives.

Normal, norms, normative, normalisation

Statistical norms

These are interesting terms to define. Some, such as 'normal', are used frequently in everyday conversation, but the significance of these words may not always be recognised. The term 'normal' has different specific meanings in different contexts. Normal, in the context of epidemiology and statistical inferences, refers to the clustering around a central value that can be observed when collecting or measuring something such as height, or weight, and what is noted is that many such measurements conform to a 'normal distribution'. For some measurements, e.g. height, this 'normal distribution' may be large, while for others, such as blood sugar, it may be quite narrow (Davey 1994a). A normal distribution, bell curve or Gaussian distribution is a distribution that is symmetrical, with the largest number of values being closest to the midpoint, tailoring off further away from the centre (see Figure 3.1). It visually depicts the usual range of values for a particular measurement within a population or group, and for characteristics with a normal distribution, all but 5 per cent of the values will be within two standard deviations of the mean for that particular population (Last 2007). In other words, most people do not differ significantly in these characteristics from the average within a population. However, what is average, and therefore the normal range, may differ significantly between different populations. For instance, the average blood cholesterol in the 1950s in the USA was 220 mg/dL, whereas in Japan it was 170 mg/dL.

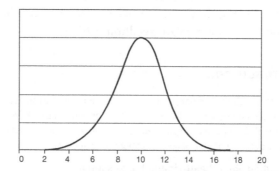

Figure 3.1 Normal Distribution Curve

Although Crichton and Mulhall (2008) note that normal refers to 'disease free' and abnormal to 'diseased', the average and normal distribution of a characteristic or measurement does not necessarily equate with good health (Dent 1995b; Seedhouse 2001). For many such measurements, judgements about what is a 'healthy' measurement can only be determined by epidemiological studies, which measure mortality and morbidity against different values (such as hypertension, blood cholesterol and weight), and even then it can be very difficult to determine *exactly* and *specifically* what constitutes a healthy value, as usually the experience of ill-health, disease or harm is graduated. For instance, the risk of cardiovascular diseases increases progressively throughout the higher range of arterial blood pressure, and thus there is no absolute 'cut-off' point between 'healthy' and 'unhealthy' blood pressure (Appel et al. 2006). Nor does 'normal' always equate with what is considered acceptable. For example, the average life expectancy at birth in 2006 for the UK was 79 and for Kenyans it was 53 (Unicef n.d.) and average reading scores in Finland are 546 compared to 396 in Brazil (BBC News 2002). It could be concluded that the very difference between the UK and Kenyan or Finnish and Brazilian experience is unacceptable although they represent what is 'normal' in the particular country.

the health studies companion

In a social context, the term normal has a specific meaning too. The terms frequently used in this context are *norm(s)* or *normative*. According to Grimshaw (1999), norm refers to implicit social rules that govern and guide expected social behaviour. Émile Durkheim (1858–1917) developed the idea of norms in terms of 'social facts' about standards of behaviour within society. These represent conventions of behaviour, which have a moderating, controlling and coercive effect on individuals, as sanctions are applied to individuals transgressing these 'norms'. Norms are defined in terms of rules or principles, which are used to judge or direct human conduct. Compliance to these rules is required from all social members (Dent 1995b). Normative is a related term, used to describe rules, recommendations and proposals that contain standards or values (they are not 'matters of fact'), and these emanate from a group rather than individuals (Sloman 1999). The social context of norms/normative standards is perhaps the most interesting. For example, its powerful conformist pull has been recognised in health-related conduct, such as Ajzen and Fishbein's (1980) 'Theory of Reasoned Action', which recognises the powerful influence of others on behaviour. Normative patterns are integrated into people's beliefs and used to moderate behaviour in terms of shaping conduct and actions according to what is deemed that others will perceive to be acceptable (see behaviour change, p. 58).

Normative, therefore, has collective connotations and Bradshaw (1972, 1994) uses it in his exploration of the meaning of need. As we have seen, he explores how need might be identified within a social policy context and presents a taxonomy of need, which highlights the mix of judgement and values, which feed into this concept. In particular, he highlights the power of normative definitions of need, these being expert-driven and based on agreed or specified 'standards' such as the nutritional needs for an adequate diet. He goes on to assert that the normative assessment of need alone is insufficient, as it fails to account for personal, social and cultural variations. However, normative values remain powerful drivers of behaviour and health policy priority setting, e.g. identifying matters of (health) concern requiring intervention (see need (needs assessment), p. 101).

In addition, attention is drawn to the social nature and function of norms within sociological dialogue. Behaviours and ideas become 'normal' through repetition, ideology, propaganda and so forth, to the extent that they are seen as natural and thereby taken-for-granted 'truisms' (Adams 2004). Michel Foucault (1926–84) discusses how idealised norms of behaviour, for which punishment is applied if transgressed, become established. Normalisation becomes a mechanism that enables social control with less effort because of its disciplinary power. Crichton and Mulhall (2008) comment on the powerful social construction of normality (versus 'abnormal') within communities linked specifically to behaviours deemed tolerable or not. In other words, values and sanctions are applied to behaviours deemed valuable and socially acceptable, which are essentially conformist. They particularly highlight the power of social norms in the context of identifying and labelling people with a mental illness. The notion of norms and normative behaviour is thus essentially conservative and has pejorative and punitive connotations (see stigma, p. 118).

Normalisation and health

Other discourses position normative ideals as aspirational. This particularly relates to the importance of normalising the life experiences of marginalised groups, such as those with a mental illness or learning disability. While norms and normative patterns contribute to the construction and alienation of those who do not conform (Critchton and Mulhall 2008), they are also considered to be a powerful tool for social improvement. The drivers for this are ideological, but also stem from the scandals surrounding the quality of care and quality of life experienced by those living in large institutions in the 1960s and 1970s (Thomas and Woods 2003). Within the field of learning disabilities, normalisation (the establishment or return to what is considered normal or standard) is seen as a mechanism to help to establish the promotion of independence and autonomy and a means by which people with learning disabilities can live an ordinary (normal) life with access to the same opportunities and choices as others (Viney 1999). This process is also intended to contribute to the increasing acceptance and valuing of people with learning disabilities as normal members of society.

Thomas and Woods (2003) note the contribution of several theorists to the 'normalisation' debate. Wolfensberger (1972; cited by Thomas and Woods 2003), for example, proposed the theory of social role valorisation (closely linked with normalisation) which stressed that people should have valued social roles within the community to counter 'natural' devaluation they might experience, e.g. those with a learning disability. In practical terms this included the employment of people with learning disabilities within ordinary workplaces. Thomas and Pierson (1996; cited by Thomas and Woods 2003) stressed the importance of enabling people with learning disabilities to live a lifestyle as normal as possible, as close as possible to that lived by others in society, so they could live and function within the same structural norms.

Brown (1994) points out, however, that despite principles of normalisations being enshrined in legislation, prejudice and isolation have created a different reality for many marginalised groups, and according to Brown (1994, p. 125) there are several flaws in the notion of normalisation. He cites Szivos (1992), who comments:

> Many of the assumptions about community integration ... may be potentially erroneous and damaging. Dispersal within the community

does not guarantee that people will learn to behave in a way which will overcome intolerance towards them. Instead, people may feel increasingly stigmatized and cut off by social distance from non-disabled people while being physically separated from others who share their difficulties.

Normalisation, therefore, can be difficult to attain in reality and requires persistence of will, effort and resources to ensure opportunities are created, living standards are maintained and prejudice is challenged (Thomas and Woods 2003). According to Whelan and Speake (1979; cited by Brown 1994), the process of normalisation also requires the adoption of socially acceptable behaviour by those hoping to integrate within the mainstream and this itself requires support and management. Not all welcome the idea of normalisations, particularly with regard to sexual relationships (Brown 1994). People with learning disabilities are expected to 'fit into' the social norms of sexual behaviour, which could precipitate opportunities for sexual exploitation (especially of women) (McCarthy 1991; cited by Brown 1994).

People with learning disabilities have many social and practical barriers and may not be able to operate and make choices in the same way as others: for example, poverty and disability create barriers to choice and self-expression (Brown 1994). Tudor (1996), in the context of mental illness, also notes that there may be periods when an individual is unable to operate within the 'normal' way of doing things, and it remains important to treat people differently on occasions in order to ensure their needs are met (see need (needs assessment), p. 101).

Conclusion

The contingent and social nature of 'normal', 'norm' and 'normative' provides a useful foundation for assessing and making judgements about health, specifying criteria that represent 'good' health, and presenting an aspirational framework for social integration for certain groups as a means of life improvement. Concepts of norms, however, remain flawed. Norms are not entirely predictive of good health and when placed in a social context can provide mechanisms for discrimination as well as foundations for greater social integration. Given this potential, discourses on these matters must remain open to scrutiny and what is considered 'normal' should not be taken for granted.

Relativism

Relativism emerges from postmodernist thinking. It refers to the idea that no one theory, idea or value is superior to another (Swingewood 1999), that statements that may be true for one group of people could be false for another (Lowe 1999) and that there are no objective truths about the world (Warnock 1998). Relativism allows for the possibility of pluralism (different cultures, different values) and enables challenges to be raised against taken-for-granted 'truths', 'an openness to new ideas, an ability to criticise what has been taken for granted, and a constant demand for good evidence' (Warnock 1998, p. 117).

However, relativism is heavily criticised on many grounds. While relativism, in principle, enables intellectual freedom, in reality it perpetuates a kind of story-telling, as everything becomes a matter of interpretation. According to relativist principles, no objective, or accepted, truths exists, and therefore it makes no difference if some idea or action is based on evidence or mere fancy (Warnock 1998; Taylor 1999b). Warnock (1998, p. 113) asserts that this can perpetuate a kind of irresponsibility, as it disables any foundations upon which challenges could be made against unfair behaviour, doctrine or tyrannical social or political regimes. 'One would be entitled only to say that it seemed so [unfair] to oneself'. This renders postmodernism and relativism inherently conservative, as the requirement for change, supported by evidence and argument, cannot be conclusively asserted (Swingewood 1999). Moreover, the fundamental assertion of relativism – that no one value, idea or theory is 'right' or better than another – must logically include relativism itself, thereby making it legitimate to dispute the claims of relativism itself.

What re-emerges, then, is an understanding that 'despite the persisting allure of relativist thinking, it fails to instil lasting conviction and sooner or later gives way to some form of objectivism' (Lowe 1999, p. 743). As Warnock (1998) and Pawson (1999) note, individual and societal decisions must emerge from some reference to standards, values and truths that are not oppressive and are useful to individuals and society, but from a relativist perspective it would not be possible to establish what these might be. Philosophers such as Locke and Hume acknowledged the centrality of personal freedom, but they also stressed the necessity of constraint, by law, and the state, to protect the freedom of others (Strathern 1996a, b). It is not possible, therefore, to operate within a society without some assumptions of truths, 'what is', and while evidence is shaped by values this cannot be completely fluid or they would become inoperable (Warnock 1998). Gordon (1992, p. 49; cited by Pawson 1999) adds to this and acknowledges that while it may not be possible to fully discover truth, or be completely objective, 'that these ideas cannot be attained, is not a reason for disregarding them. Perfect cleanliness is also impossible, but it does not serve as a warrant for not washing, much less for rolling about in a manure pile' (see postmodernism/social constructivism, p. 47).

Relativism and health

The concept of relativism pertains to health in several ways: for example, via the acknowledgment of the relativism of human health, i.e. advocating that there is no one definable state of 'health' (Leeuw 1989). As Fenton and Sadiq-Sangster (1996) note, relativist principles accept a diversity of categories of mental health and cultural expression of distress and confirm the possibility of describing phenomena very differently across cultures. However, Fenton and

Sadiq-Sangster (1996) also note that it is still possible to see parallels with disorders such as depression across the diversity of descriptions. Relativism can also be applied pragmatically, in a recognition that approaches to healthcare and work to promote health must account for diversity and utilise flexible approaches to action and intervention. Before options are chosen, different stories and interpretations may need to be extracted to ensure the suitability of any course of action.

However, while flexibility is warranted, work to promote health must not conflate into an 'anything goes' approach. Choices and options for action to promote health must be based on evidence and consider what is acceptable (according to social and ethical values). The challenge inevitably remains to consider what values should operate and influence decision-making and in essence these are based on values that acknowledge or enable the maximisation of human potential and minimisation of harm (Seedhouse 1986, 2000; Warnock 1998). Locating work within a framework and set of values and theories that support reasoned actions and avoid the pitfalls of accepting unacceptable conditions, circumstances or actions (on the grounds that all values and actions are equally sanctioned) is the key and some of the concepts of health discussed in Chapter 1 may help here.

Conclusion

Relativism is a forceful concept in contemporary society, and while it does facilitate the recognition and acceptance of diversity, taken literally it disables the possibility of asserting the validity of any particular course of action. Relativist claims, therefore, need to be considered carefully and counter-balanced by evidence and ethical information and principles.

Rights (and responsibilities)

Some discussion of 'rights' has already been included in various sections of this text, but it is worthy of further deliberation. We do not explore legal rights here, e.g. the Human Rights Act 1998, but focus on the principle of individual rights (and responsibilities). Debates about *rights* and *responsibilities* tend to polarise, and focus around the claims of individuals' rights *vis-à-vis* the rights of others or rights regarding provision of services and so forth, and exploring some of the basic philosophical foundations of 'rights' will help to clarify the practical implications of these assertions.

The concept of the individual, the concept of self-determination and the notion of individual rights emerged from the shifts in thinking associated with Enlightenment (see p. 37) and the philosophical assertions about the rights of individuals remains central to contemporary moral and legal debate (Seedhouse 1988, 1998a, 2009). For example, appeals are frequently made to the *right* to treatment, the *right* to an education, the *right* to life and so forth.

The foundation of rights

Originally the principle of rights, established by Jeremy Bentham (1748–1832), is that a right exists only if there is a law conferring that right. A 'right of way', for example, exists only if a corresponding law confers this right, and once this is established the landowner (in this instance) has a correlative *duty* to maintain the right of way (Warnock 1998). A right is something that should not be infringed, and relates to an area of freedom or entitlement and the conferring of *rights* and *duties* (responsibilities in more modern parlance). This link between rights and responsibilities is important, particularly as others have the responsibility to make rights a possibility (Hoedemaekers and Dekkers 2003). Simply giving someone the 'right to choose', for instance, is insufficient in the absence of information, education, advice and support to enable someone to interpret or act upon choices. Other individuals, and the state, therefore, have the responsibility to enable rights to manifest.

The social context of rights

In addition, a specific right such as the 'right to choose' must be considered in a broader social context. The way the 'language' of rights is expressed frequently fails to acknowledge other considerations that also impinge on 'rights'. For example, one individual's 'right' to choose the type of education they want (e.g. in a public school) cannot be granted without consideration of how this might detract from the 'rights' of others to an education (particularly if resources are diverted from one source to another), or the 'right' of asylum seekers and refugees to free healthcare suitable to their needs may simply not be fulfillable if the resources to achieve this do not exist. Another example is the claim made that an elderly person has the 'right' to live in their own home. For this to be fulfilled, there has to be provision of resources (either their own or the state's) and there will inevitably be competing demands; the rights of others need to be taken into account too. It is clearly not possible, therefore, for every individual to have sacrosanct rights, as these need to be placed in a social and economic as well as moral context, which also takes account of the *consequences* for others. Therefore, simply asserting a 'right' in the absence of an ability to fulfil that rights is empty rhetoric.

The moral context of rights

The relationship between rights and responsibilities has moral connotations too. According to Warnock (1998), if someone claims a 'natural right' they are making a moral proclamation. While a moral claim alone is insufficient to confer a right (this requires a legal status too), morality should underpin such assertions (Warnock 1998). Moral argument can be used to fight for a change in the law, and these moral claims should have substantive foundations too. They must be connected to need and represent 'what is seen to be an intolerable or impossible way to live (i.e. if the need is not met)' (Warnock 1998, p. 59) (see need (needs assessment), p. 101).

However, the language of 'rights' can be so misused that it simply represents everything that is desired or desirable and frequently neglects the correlative of duties (responsibilities) and needs of others (Seedhouse 2009), and as Thompson and Thompson (2008) note, this positions one person's *right* as another person's *responsibility*. Presenting behaviour under the banner of 'rights' undermines the volition behind human behaviour itself. Asserting 'rights' for self, and 'responsibilities' of others, transmutes behaviour into the dynamic of 'rights' and 'duties' only. In other words, an individual would only act if they had the duty to do so and an individual could only expect something if it was a 'right'. For example, there would be no incentive for the act of human kindness, unless it had a utility or legal value.

Reflective activity

Look in your local newspaper for examples of someone taking legal action against another on the grounds of 'infringement of rights', 'duty of care or failure to provide a service' etc. What are the foundations of the claims being made:

- Legally?
- Morally?

If everything is converted to a 'right', what are lost are the moral foundations for behaviour and moral reasoning about what is acceptable (Seedhouse 2009). As Warnock (1998, p. 74) states,

> It is my contention that a civil society could not function if it subsisted only on indignation where rights have been infringed, without the occasion for admiration as well for those, who like the Good Samaritan, go out of their way to display altruism. If justice were the only, or even most fundamental, value, such ideas as compassion, or hatred of cruelty, or shame at dishonesty might wither away. It would be an impoverished … morality that was founded on the concept of rights.

Rights and autonomy

The autonomous foundations upon which a right is being asserted should also be considered, e.g. the right to remain in one's own home. Unless an individual is making a choice based on full, comprehensive information and is able to engage in a rational decision-making process (and this is not necessarily the case, for example, if someone's mental faculties are disrupted), the assertion of the right is flawed. The decision should hinge on the amount of autonomy the individual can truly exercise (Seedhouse 2009) and it might be the case that another course of action is more appropriate, e.g. providing a safe, stimulating, fulfilling alternative living environment.

Limits of rights

Ultimately, beyond the bounds of legal rights it is impossible to show conclusively that 'rights' exist per se and nobody has been able to demonstrate that 'human rights' exist outside of a 'manmade' convention that this is so (Seedhouse 2009). For example, it is not possible to objectively assert that we have a 'right to life'. It is only possible to state that we have 'life' (Seedhouse 2009).

Conclusion

The enactment of rights requires a legal foundation but should also be based on much more open decision-making and public debate than is conferred by a one-sided assertion of a 'right'. What also lies at the heart of 'rights' is the acknowledgement that human beings can make choices, and that these choices require moral foundations and options for autonomous decision-making, without which the notion of 'rights' is rendered meaningless (Law in Action 2009).

3 Stigma

What is stigma?

According to the *Oxford English Dictionary*, stigma means, among other things, a 'mark or sign of disgrace or discredit'. This is the concept of stigma that is relevant in this context. Goffman (1963), in his seminal book *Stigma: Notes on the Management of Spoiled Identity*, asserted that stigma is attributed upon recognition of difference. Stigma is essentially a social and cultural problem (Fink and Tasman 1992) and social construct (Brown et al. 2010; Harrison and Gill 2010) and is attributed to any behaviours that are seen to deviate from the norm. Lai et al. (2000) comment that stigma refers to a trait of an individual or group that attracts punitive responses.

Reflective activity

- Look at the way media reports (TV, radio, newspaper, blogs) describe people with a mental illness or HIV/AIDS.
- Are the words used generally positive or negative?
- What is your reaction to these descriptions?

According to these definitions, stigma is attributed when something deviates from the norm (see norms, p. 109). Normative expectations operate on a subconscious level, but are triggered when meeting someone or something that 'does not fit'. Normative expectations generally facilitate social interactions but a negative reaction might also be stimulated. Once an attribute is recognised as deviant, the group or person is tainted and discredited, and it is realised that 'we had been making certain assumptions as to what the individual before us ought to be' (Goffman 1963, p. 12). Once a matter (behaviour, group, attribute) is stigmatised, interactions and self-perceptions are corrupted – 'The term stigma … will be used to refer to an attribute that is deeply discrediting' – (Goffman 1963, p. 13) and people are disqualified from full social acceptance (Brown et al. 2010). Shame becomes a significant feature of stigma, as both the 'normals' (those who conform to normative standards of behaviour or physical integrity, e.g. are not disabled) and the stigmatised recognise the deviance and absorb the negative connotations. The behaviour of those who are stigmatised can become either overly meek or aggressive (Goffman 1963). Loss of self-confidence and self-respect is common (Sartorius 2002). Behaviour may be overly controlled to maintain the invisibility of the stigmatised attribute, but often, stigmatisation (the ascription of unworthiness or disgrace) can result in literal separation of social groups to avoid any possible contacts where the differences are on view and judgements made (Goffman 1963; Lai et al. 2000). It is not uncommon to advocate that some groups are treated differently to others too, and while the intentions of this might be laudable (e.g. to protect rights), it can have the consequence of heightening awareness of difference (Sartorius 2002). Stigma thus emerges from the recognition of difference and results in discrimination, and consequent to this 'separation', prejudiced expectations regarding behaviour and the negative attributes applied to individuals or groups. Discrimination might be literal in terms of access to employment and other socio-economic resources and opportunities, which others take for granted (Lai et al. 2000; Kobau et al. 2010).

Stigma and health (mental health and HIV)

Commonly, mental illness and sexually related matters (such as sexually transmitted infections (STIs), especially HIV) attract stigma. The origins of contemporary stigmatisation of mental illness lie within medieval times, when mental illness signified possession by demons (Dubin and Fink 1992). While this literal interpretation no longer applies in Western culture, Brown et al. (2010) suggest that stigmatisation of those with a mental illness is still particularly strong. Those with a mental illness are considered weak, dangerous and personally responsible for their condition (Fink and Tasman 1992; Lai et al. 2000; Brown et al. 2010). Their own personal characteristics often become submerged under the label of illness (Lai et al. 2000).

Sartorius (2002), Corrigan et al. (2010) and Harrison and Gill (2010) assert that the stigma attached to mental illness is a major barrier to recovery and attaining a better quality of life. Negative attitudes of the public and health professionals are such that behaviour towards someone is often prejudicial once a mental illness is declared (Sartorius 2002; Brown et al. 2010).

According to Dubin and Fink (1992), the way healthcare systems are structured can reinforce this negativity. Aberrant and out-of-control behaviour is often expected and hospital systems are structured around the assumption of abnormality or danger, and all behaviour is interpreted as a display of illness

(Rosenhan 1973). In fact in a study conducted by Rosenhan (1973), individual had to *prove* they were normal before they were discharged from psychiatric inpatients. In Lai et al.'s (2000) study, they found that the problem of stigma and discrimination stemmed from the psychiatric label, and not the *actual* behaviour of the individual. The impact of stigma can, however, become so internalised that negative attitudes affect engagement with services (Brown et al. 2010).

In the context of other stigmatised conditions, such as HIV/AIDS, Kobau et al. (2010) note that they attract very similar sanctions, health-related problems and socio-economic limitations. HIV/AIDS often attracts stigma because of its association with behaviour that transgresses social norms and concepts of good and bad, such as sex work rather than sex within marriage, or homosexuality (Olapegba 2010; Zaccagnini 2010). HIV/AIDS is also associated with irresponsible behaviour and may be regarded as a punishment for immorality (Olapegba 2010; Zaccagnini 2010). Stigma and discrimination around HIV/AIDS is also linked with racism and misogyny (Zaccagnini 2010). Thus people with HIV/AIDS experience multiple layers of discrimination, including, for instance, restrictions on travel and entry to certain countries (Zaccagnini 2010). Until 4 January 2010 the USA restricted all HIV-positive people from entering the country (Zaccagnini 2010).

Reflective activity

- Do you think TV programmes now present positive or negative images of people with a mental illness or HIV/AIDS?
- What impact do you think this has on your own views and those of your family and friends?

Olapegba (2010) asserts that stigmatisation and discrimination create huge obstacles to the prevention of HIV/AIDS and, as with mental illness, may significantly reduce commitment to treatment and prevention regimes. Denial of the condition might be a consequence of this stigma, further reducing options for treatment and preventative action (Zaccagnini 2010). The national strategy for sexual health and HIV (DoH 2001) highlighted the need to reduce the associated stigma, suggesting that this reduced options for informed decision-making around STIs, including HIV, and inhibited access to services and treatment. Zaccagnini (2010) suggests that this impact extends to deterring government action against HIV/AIDS and public education.

How can stigma be tackled?

Of particular concern is the portrayed link between mental illness and violence and the lack of public understanding about recovery from mental illness, and Lai et al. (2000) comment on the need for increased public awareness of mental illness. This should include basic information about mental illness, as those who are more knowledgeable tend to be less prejudiced (Lai et al. 2000). Olapegba (2010) calls for mass education to increase knowledge of HIV/AIDS, along with programmes to stimulate attitude change, suggesting that there is widespread ignorance and misinformation about HIV and AIDS. Fear of congagion abounds (Zaccagnini 2010) and people, for example, still fear casual contact with a person with HIV/AIDS (Olapegba 2010). Olapegba warns of the necessity for careful consideration of the way messages about HIV are portrayed, though, as they can reinforce the high level of fear associated with the disease (that is, it is linked with death), rather than its potential to be effectively managed.

This shift in awareness may need to be extended to stigmatised groups themselves. For example, for people with a mental illness or HIV the negative connotations of their condition are absorbed into their own self-perceptions (Goffman 1963; Lai et al. 2000; Corrigan et al. 2010; Harrison and Gill 2010; Zaccagnini 2010). Such assimilation of stigma seriously diminishes an individual's self-esteem and self-efficacy (Corrigan et al. 2010). Corrigan et al. (2010) examine the consequences of declaring a mental illness and suggest that it can have a positive effect on the individual. To maximise this benefit they suggest that people should be actively supported and helped to consider the personal advantages and disadvantages of being open, which are likely to vary according to circumstances and place. Access to support from others who have already taken the step of declaring their mental illness to others can be extremely valuable to people considering this option.

Useful resource

Go to http://news.bbc.co.uk/1/hi/health/2116303.stm
and http://www.time-to-change.org.uk/
to learn more about campaigns to end stigma against those with a mental illness.

Between 1998 and 2003 the Royal College of Psychiatrists campaign *Changing Minds – Every Family in the Land* aimed to educate the public and raise awareness and the National Service Framework (NSF) for Mental Health (DoH 1999b) acknowledged the need to tackle stigma and reduce discrimination. In 2001, the World Psychiatric Association initiated a global programme to tackle stigma and discrimination associated with schizophrenia (Sartorius 2002). This programme has long-term aspirations to change the way services and other social institutions serve, and interact with, those who have a mental illness and their families. Sartorius (2002) also argues that the consequences of stigma can be addressed by greater consideration of the individual. For example, he suggests that the rights and duties of people with a mental illness should be considered in the context of their particular behaviour and abilities, not in accordance with the diagnostic label. The NIMHE (National Institute for Mental Health in England 2004; cited by Harrison and Gill 2010) also planned work with different forms of media to address issues of stigma and discrimination. The work of NIMHE included plans to challenge discrimination at all levels and involve service users and carers.

Zaccagnini (2010) identifies that addressing treatment and service provision issues for those with HIV/AIDS can have a positive impact on stigma too, although the complex nature of stigma around HIV means that the solutions are also complex. For example, an important aspect of tackling stigma lies with legislation to protect the rights of those with HIV/AIDS (Zaccagnini 2010), but community-level education and action around HIV/AIDS are vital too.

Media portrayals both reflect and perpetuate negatives views of people with a mental illness or HIV (Harrison and Gill 2010; Olapegba 2010), so they could be used to present more positive imagery (Lai et al. 2000; Harrison and Gill 2010; Olapegba 2010). It is worth communicating the common nature of mental illness and using high profile events to publicise more positive attitudes (Future Vision Coalition 2008). This is also important for redressing myths around HIV/AIDS (Olapegba 2010).

Primarily stigma, discrimination and prejudice should be tackled by demonstrating tolerance and non-discriminatory behaviour by those working in institutions or with people who have a mental illness. Zaccagnini (2010) notes too that the prevalence of negative attitudes towards those with HIV/AIDS requires careful handling, and protecting confidentiality is important to prevent discriminatory practices emerging. For example, Zaccagnini recommends the use of universal precautions (whereby infection control practices are the norm), so that people with HIV/AIDS are not treated as pariahs.

Harrison and Gill (2010) discuss the necessity for work to empower people (see empowerment, p. 77) with mental illness and redress the imbalance between patient and professional that is established within institutions. Developing processes that establish joint decision-making and partnership working is an essential component of this. To achieve these sorts of changes requires significant shifts in the socialisation of professionals, in professionally held negative stereotypes and in the working practices of health and social care practitioners, such as the interpretation of duty-of-care (Harrison and Gill 2010). More resources are needed to enable work with patients and carers to improve self-esteem and increase social support networks. Providing support for people to gain and sustain employment is also vital to redress many of the consequences of stigma (Harrison and Gill 2010).

Essentially, stigma can only be tackled by normalising matters (see norms, p. 109) such as mental illness and HIV, and this itself emerges through exposure and finding ways for people to interact with each other without, for instance, *denying* the existence of an illness (Lai et al. 2000). If people with a stigmatised condition are seen and heard then, in principle, differences reduce (Zaccagnini 2010). The commonality between people and groups can then be established, rather than a focus on dissimilarities, and people can establish and assimilate mechanisms for engagement into habituated practice, rather than being unnerved by the unexpected. Ultimately, actively challenging stigma and prejudice is necessary too (Zaccagnini 2010).

Conclusion

Stigma has many connotations and can seriously harm individuals and families with conditions (or lifestyles) that deviate from the norm. Tackling stigma, therefore, provides an opportunity to liberate potential, reduce harm and create and support a more egalitarian society for all.

3.3 CONCLUDING COMMENT

This chapter has attempted to provide a more detailed discussion of key terms and concepts that abound within the realms of health. While these entries cannot provide a conclusive account of the matters under scrutiny, they do illustrate the contentious nature of some of the debates: for example, around healthcare rationing. Moreover, it becomes evident that many contemporary concerns are informed by, and based upon, key principles. For example, the current emphasis on behaviour change within contemporary health policy makes no sense without an understanding and acceptance of the concept of free will, and the process of stigmatisation within society is, at least in part, constructed upon notions of 'norms'. Other components of this chapter, such as the entries on autonomy, empowerment and rights, provide some detail to clarify what these terms signify. A deeper understanding of these terms is necessary to truly understand what is (or might be) meant when these words are used within policy documents and conversations, as all too often the explicit meaning is left vague or unstated. Finally, having greater knowledge of possible meaning of these terms and concepts will enable you to construct your own critical analysis of contemporary health matters and challenge some of the simplistic assumptions that might be made, for example, about behaviour change, or when people assert their 'rights', or claim that 'all values are equal'.

Key points to consider include:

> Powerful interrelationships exist between certain concepts and principles of action (within health care and policy).

> The key terms and concepts that inform health policy and decision-making can have varied and complex meanings.

> An understanding of a diversity of ideas and concepts is important for informed decision-making.

4 case studies

4.1 INTRODUCTION

This chapter explores:

> Four case studies of contemporary health issues:
> > obesity;
> > artificial reproductive therapy (ART);
> > HIV;
> > dementia.
> A range of discourses that contribute to our understanding of these health issues.
> The relationship between these health issues and the key ideologies, concepts and theories discussed in Chapters 2 and 3.

Within this chapter you will find case studies on four particular areas within health: obesity, artificial reproductive therapy (ART), HIV and dementia. These topics have contemporary resonance and all are matters that have complex biological but also social, cultural, economic and political connotations. Ideologies, concepts, theories and so forth inform our understanding of issues pertaining to health and social care and these case studies demonstrate this in greater depth. As with all the material within this text we make no claim that what we represent here is in any way all that can be written on these areas. Instead we consider it a taster, rather like one of those whistle stop bus tours where you see four significant historical sites in one day – each site deserves more exploration and hence you must return to them to investigate in more detail in the future.

The following case studies offer you our brief takes on these very complex and contested areas. We have attempted to give you some insight into the possible ways of exploring these areas and tried to include biomedical, sociological, psychological, constructivist and critical perspectives. For example, while our understandings of obesity are predominantly informed by medical explanations, non-medical discourses (for instance, those informed by feminism or social constructivism) help to draw attention to the harms associated with the medicalisation of weight in contemporary society. Similar contentions emerge in the discussion on artificial reproductive therapy (ART), and this case study explores the socio-cultural drivers that shape the demand for

ARTs. The dementia and HIV case studies are also equally interested in moving from reductionist, though very powerful, biomedical discourses to a more critically located discussion of the socio-political discourses that inform our understandings. Embedded within these case studies is an exploration of the function of stigmatisation in its many forms, and its implications for practice, policy focus and implementation, and our overall responses in terms of treatment and management.

Overall, these case studies are representative of particular perspectives and interpretations informed by a very small proportion of the enormous amount of research and literature available. It is intended that they are read as introductions and alongside material within the other chapters as well as your own independent reading. Various discourses and concepts that function within health, discussed across Chapters 1–3, are deeply embedded within these case studies, often in ways that are not explicitly acknowledged. In the research chapter (Chapter 5), examples of research carried out in these four fields are accessed as a way of unpacking the research process. These real world 'empirical' research articles highlight even more the contested discourses and complexities of ART, obesity, dementia and HIV.

4.2 CASE STUDY 1: OBESITY

Introduction

Reflective activity

- Make a brief search on the Internet for any news stories about obesity.
- What is the main focus of the stories?
- What sources of evidence do they cite?
- Can you locate any reports that tell a different story about obesity?

We all know that in the early part of the twenty-first century, Western industrialised countries are facing a health crisis of huge proportions. Obesity is a potent example of a modern-day health matter in which medical-scientific declarations have helped to shape the 'production of health' (defining the existence and nature of a health matter). The purpose of this case study is to explore the legitimacy and substance of this perspective, through scrutiny of the medical-scientific evidence itself, and by drawing on other discourses it is possible to reveal how both our understanding of and our responses to a health problem such as obesity are also socially, culturally and morally constructed. What becomes evident is that one epistemological position alone (e.g. medical/scientific) cannot provide the only, or main, set of insights into any given issue, and indeed as Bovbjerg (2008, p. 60) notes, 'the social and medical construct of "obesity" has changed over time'.

Obesity: the growing threat

Tackling obesity is now considered to be a key government priority (DoH 2008a). We are told that the economic costs of obesity are estimated to be between £3.3 billion and £3.7 billion per year and overweight and obesity are referred to as 'the public health burden' (Swanton and Frost 2007). Obesity is defined as abnormal or excessive fat accumulation that presents a risk to health (WHO 2009a) and is usually measured according to height and weight charts, but increasingly by body mass index (BMI). The 'normal' BMI range for women is 21–23 and for men 22–24, with a BMI of 25–29.9 considered overweight, a BMI above 30 considered obese and one greater than 40 considered morbidly or severely obese (Glanville et al. 1997; DoH 2002). However, other categorisations have been used: for example, Shoff and Newcomb (1998) categorised overweight as a BMI of 29.1–31.9 and obesity as a BMI >31.9. This indicates that these distinctions are not scientifically stable categories.

Box 4.1 Your BMI

BMI is used in the DoH (2002) report.

Body mass index is worked out by dividing your weight in kilograms by the square of your height (e.g. 1.53×1.53) measured in metres

$$BMI = W/Ht2$$

For example a woman of average height (168 cm; 5 ft 6 ins) and weight (62 kg; 9 stone 7 lbs) would have a BMI of:

$$\frac{62}{(1.68)^2} = \frac{62}{2.82} = \mathbf{22}$$

In England 21 per cent of adult men and 24 per cent of adult women are considered obese, with a further 47 per cent of men and 33 per cent of women categorised as overweight, which means that two-thirds of men and half of women are now overweight or obese (DoH 2002). The figures cited by WHO (2009b) estimate that 23.2 per cent of the UK population (16 years plus) have a BMI of 30 or above and 38.5 per cent a BMI of 25 or above (in total 61.7 per cent of the population). There was also a rise in the prevalence of overweight from 14.7 to 23.6 per cent and obesity from 5.4 to 9.2 per cent between 1989 and 1998 among pre-school children (Summerbell et al. 2002) and among children as a whole a 2.8 fold increase over ten years in England (the USA has experienced an even higher increase) (Ebbeling et al. 2002). The WHO (2009c) admits that it is challenging to measure overweight and obesity among children aged five to fourteen as there is no standard definition of childhood obesity that can be applied worldwide, although BMI charts for children up to the age of five years have been developed (WHO 2009c).

With regard to the distribution of overweight and obesity, both adult and childhood obesity are more common among the lowest income groups (Scholes 2008) and black and ethnic minority groups (Campos 2004; Singh et al. 2008). In Western industrialised countries, obesity tends to be associated with poverty, not affluence (Campos 2004; Singh et al. 2008).

Health problems linked with overweight and obesity

Obesity is linked to increased mortality. One seminal study by Manson et al. (1995, p. 677) concluded that 'Body weight and mortality from all causes were directly related among these middle-aged women. Lean women did not have excess mortality.' This concern has grown with the Annual Report of the Chief Medical Officer (DoH 2002), highlighting on its cover 'Obesity: the health time bomb' and stating:

> It is well recognised that overweight and obesity increase the risk of this country's biggest killer diseases – coronary heart disease and cancer – as well as diabetes, high blood pressure and osteoarthritis. The National Audit Office (NAO) found that obesity is responsible for more than 9,000 premature deaths each year in England and reduces life expectancy on average by 9 years. Obesity also has significant financial costs, both to the NHS and the wider economy. (DoH 2002, p. 37)

Indeed, in the Annual Report of the Chief Medical Officer (DoH 2002) it is reported that obesity threatens longevity, with some parents outliving their children, and Glanville et al. (1997), Crawford (2002), Ebbeling et al. (2002), Hitchcock-Noël and Pugh (2002) and WHO (2009c) all assert that obesity in adults or children is associated with an increase in premature illness and death (coronary heart disease, some cancers including breast, colon and endometrial, diabetes and musculoskeletal disorders, especially osteoarthritis; WHO 2009c), and with psychological morbidity too (Scottish Intercollegiate Guidelines Network 2003; Muennig 2008). It should be noted, though, that these figures relate to Western industrialised nations. Worldwide, underweight and malnutrition are still considerable problems (Maurer and Smith 2005; Torûn 2005).

4

Why are we getting fatter?

The broad consensus is that we are fatter because we are out of balance. We put weight on when we consume more than we need, while energy expenditure is down (Ebbeling et al. 2002). This positions the problem as a dynamic between 'consumption' and 'production', although it is recognised that latent biological susceptibility plays a part too (Butland et al. 2007).

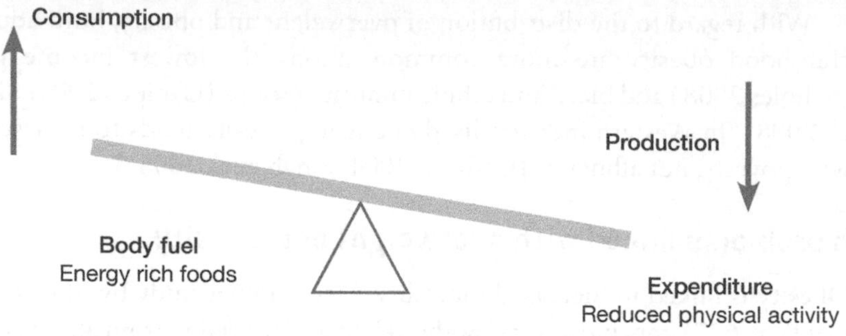

Figure 4.1   *Consumption versus production*

Reflective activity

Make a list of all the things that contribute to increases in energy consumption and reductions in energy expenditure (production) in the population of the UK.

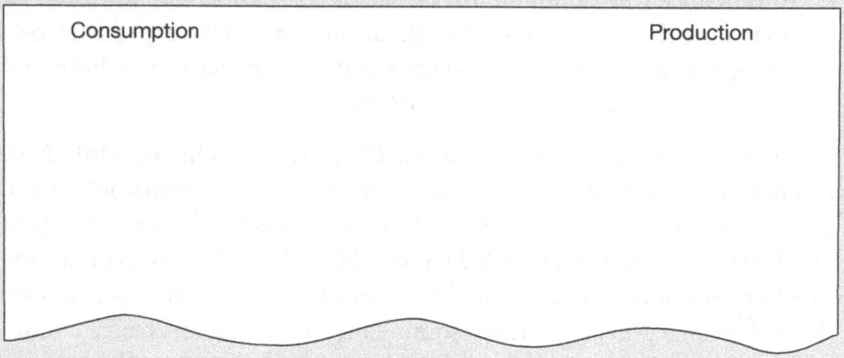

Consumption	Production

Figure 4.2

Shifts in consumption

According to a variety of sources, higher disposable incomes, increased leisure time and access to low cost food in restaurants and other retail outlets mean that we eat out more and that the food consumed on these occasions usually provides a higher calorie, less nutritionally balanced meal (Glanville et al. 1997; NAO 2001; Butland et al. 2007).

Consumer values have also been blamed for this shift in consumption habits, with less time spent on the preparation and cooking of meals. The proportion of income spent on food has declined over recent decades, with the UK approach typified by demand for cheap food at cheap prices (Morgan and Morley 2002), while consumption of convenience foods (which tend to be inexpensive and higher in calories) has increased (Butland et al. 2007). The promotion (via advertising) and availability of foodstuffs has an additional impact on consumption trends (Butland et al. 2007) and Ebbeling et al. (2002) observed that primetime TV for children is associated with heavy advertising of snacks, sweets and soft drinks.

Despite this, there is some evidence of a shift towards 'healthier' food products such as fruit and vegetable, and items such as drinking yogurt (Butland et al. 2007), which arguably represents a 'specialist' food product, rather than a component of an overall balanced diet.

The deregulation of school meals in 1980 contributed to the shift in food consumption habits. Acheson (DoH 1998) comments on the impact of the deregulation of nutritional standards and affordable prices accorded to school meal provision, and the cultural shift towards snacking became a matter of considerable concern (Colquhoun et al. 2001). Nutritional standards have been re-established and Colquhoun et al. (2001) argue that this remains vital for child health and educational engagement.

Shifts in production (energy expenditure)

Reductions in 'production', i.e. energy expenditure through physical activity, are attributed to a variety of causes, including shifts in working patterns and a greater reliance on the use of the car. Populations are more mobile and are frequently located away from sources of employment: travelling long distances to work is now the norm for many individuals, as is using the car to execute the responsibilities of the job. Goodman (2001, p. 51) cited employees' comments: 'It is fairly clear that if using the bike or walking was meaning that they were spending an extra hour or so out of the office as opposed to being in the car, I don't think that would be encouraged by management.'

The absence of acceptable, safe and convenient transport alternatives adds to this reliance on the car and is frequently cited as a disincentive to greater physical activity (NAO 2001; Royce et al. 2003; Butland et al. 2007), although calls for congestion charging to pay for public transport improvement remain unpopular (BBC News 2008). Convenience and safety for cyclists remain contentious issues too (Butland et al. 2007), although some employers are increasingly offering incentives to cycle and disincentives to drive through the provision of cycle hire, showers, cycle sheds and charges for car parking. Many of these initiatives are additionally fuelled by concerns about climate change and form a core part of the 'green agenda' (NAO 2001; Hillsdon et al. 2005) (see environmentalism, p. 40).

Children, too, exercise less. Fewer walk or cycle, with an estimated two-thirds of children aged 5–10 walking to school in the mid-1980s, and more than 6 per cent of 11–16 year-olds walking or cycling. By the late 1990s, just over half of 5–10 year-olds walked to school and fewer than 2 per cent of 11–16 year-olds cycled. Over the same time period, the number of car journeys nearly doubled (NAO 2001). This is partly a reflection of a growth in fears around child safety (NAO 2001; Butland et al. 2007). At school, children exercise less too (NAO 2001). By the time the NAO (2001) report was published evidence had accumulated that the priority attached to physical activity in schools had fallen considerably, with some pupils spending less than an hour engaged in physical activity.

Fears for children's safety have also contributed to this decline in physical activity, along with more reliance on TV and computer-based entertainment (NAO 2001; Ebbeling et al. 2002; Scottish Intercollegiate Guidelines Network 2003; Butland et al. 2007), although Robinson (1999) notes that in many studies this relationship is weak.

What emerges is a complex mix of social, economic and financial drivers that contribute to shifts in normative patterns of individual and community behaviour. Behaviour is situated within a complex social milieu and is not merely an individual concern or uncomplicatedly constructed around personal choice. Choice and opportunities reside *within* a context that makes certain behaviours possible or indeed acceptable (Butland et al. 2007). This awareness is particularly valuable when considering what actions are appropriate (socially, economically and ethically) and achievable to address obesity as a health concern.

What is to be done about obesity?

The solution is simply to eat less and move around more (and more quickly)? A very cursory analysis would indicate that further insights need to be gained concerning what lies behind this 'deceptively simply' (Butland et al. 2007, p. 12) admonishment for shifts in 'consumption' and 'production'. After all, no one wakes up and thinks – 'today I must move less, and eat more, so I can become a fat person'. In fact, the opposite is more likely to be true: we wake up and promise ourselves, 'today I will start my diet/exercise regime'.

Reflective activity

Look at a selection of magazines in your local newsagents.

- How many include diets?
- What claims are being made about these diets?
- How do the diets differ from each other? For example, does one claim that the 'cure' lies with eating only raw vegetables, while the other raves about the benefits of fruit and salad?
- What do you conclude from the myriad of claims?

Dieting

Controlling consumption is vigorously promoted by the diet industry. Pick up any magazine or watch television and a myriad of diets will offer shapelier bottoms, slender waists and smaller dress sizes (Braziel 2001). However, the results of dieting are mixed. At best dieting, particularly calorie control diets, is difficult to sustain (Filiault 2008), and provides only temporary respite from excess weight. No specific diet has demonstrably worked in the long term (Bergh et al. 2008) and commonly leads to 'yo-yoing' between weight loss and weight gain, frequently resulting in a more portly stature in the long run (Bennett and Gurin 1982; Garner and Wooley 1991; Korkeila et al. 1999; Miller 1999; Campos 2004; Olmsted and McFarland 2004). Klein (1996, 2001), Berg (1999) and Campos (2004) comment that cyclical weight gain and weight loss itself is physiologically counter-productive and hazardous. Bovbjerg (2008, p. 62) notes that it is now 'common to point out that individual-level dietary change faces an uphill struggle when attempted in obesogenic environments and societies'.

There is some evidence, too, that the focus on instructing the population about their eating habits per se has contributed to the problem. Traditionally the consumption of fat has been blamed for the increase in obesity because it is the most energy dense of all food substances. However, epidemiological studies do not show a consistent association between fat consumption and obesity and obesity has increased in the USA during a period when fat consumption has declined (Ebbeling et al. 2002). What has increased is energy intake from carbohydrate foods, e.g. breads, cereals, cakes, potatoes and soft drinks, and they may promote weight gain because of their high glycaemic index. For example, the consumption of milk (with a low glycaemic index – but containing fat) actually protects against obesity (Ebbeling et al. 2002).

4

Physical activity

More recent dialogue stresses the importance of healthy, balanced food consumption and refocuses on the importance of increasing physical activity rather than focusing on controlling consumption alone (Filiault 2008). The general consensus is that physical activity is good for health, such as preventing heart disease and promoting psychological health, but is also necessary in the maintenance of 'normal' weight (Filiault 2008). For general health it is estimated that an individual must engage in 30 minutes of moderate activity five times a week, while for those who want to maintain weight loss the target is set at 60–90 minutes of moderate activity a day (DoH 2004b). According to government statistics, few members of the population exercise even to the level beneficial to general health, with an estimated two-thirds of men and three-quarters of women reporting less than the recommended 30 minutes of moderate-intensity activity five times a week (DoH 2004b). The situation in the USA is worse, with up to 25 per cent of adults reporting no planned physical activity in the preceding month (Filiault 2008).

Filiault (2008) reviews the evidence on physical activity and obesity and concludes that it is equivocal. For example, there is less difference between the levels of physical activity for those who are obese and those who are not than might be expected and exercise alone proves to be relatively ineffective at inducing weight loss except if time-consuming, high exertion activity is practised over an extended period of time, generally amounting to an impractical regime for many individuals. Filiault points out that the evidence suggests that fitness mitigates, not eliminates, the consequences of obesity and brings considerable health benefits per se. Overall, success requires both dietary regulation and physical activity and Filiault argues that the emphasis should be placed on activity for health, rather than activity for weight loss.

At the time of writing, a government campaign, primarily aimed at children and families, is being broadcast and encourages more activity and eating less (Change4Life 2010), and many TV programmes are broadcast about people improving their lifestyles, eating less and more healthily, becoming more active and so forth. In terms of physical activity the key admonishments include 'stop using the car', 'get off the bus one stop earlier' and 'take up gym membership'. The challenge is to encourage more physical activity as normative behaviour. We are more likely to exercise in later life if we exercised in our youth, and it is only the activity in later life that confers health benefits, e.g. in terms of heart disease prevention (Thomas et al. 2003).

Reflective activity

Consider the barriers to walking or jogging in an inner-city urban area.

There are several ways this can be done, some operating at the individual level, based on 'cues to action' (see behaviour change, p. 58). These approaches include posters strategically placed in stairwells and by lifts within work environments to encourage using stairs, brief advice from health professionals or referral to exercise specialists (Hillsdon et al. 2005), although the effect is often short lasting.

Instead, Filiault (2008) suggests that it is community-based initiatives that will sustain changes in activity levels and for Bovbjerg (2008) changes in the built environment will contribute to improvement in activity levels. This is supported by a report by the European branch of the World Health Organisation (WHO) (Ellaway et al. 2005), which identified that people were far more likely to walk or exercise locally if that environment was pleasant, with leafy (safe) parks, lower traffic congestion and so forth. Efforts are also being made to re-shift the balance in physical activity levels among school children, including introducing schemes ('walking buses') to encourage children to be more physically active (NAO 2001; Butland et al. 2007).

Action to tackle obesity also includes tertiary level interventions through the use of surgical techniques or drug therapy. These are:

> Jejunoileal bypass. This is an operation used for the purpose of weight loss, whereby most of the intestines are bypassed, although the stomach is kept intact. It has the effect of reducing absorption of food.

> Vertical banded gastroplasty. This refers to the placing of a band around the stomach to create a small pouch. It restricts food intake (as the stomach is literally smaller) but does not affect normal digestion.

> Gastric bypass. This involves both creating a small stomach pouch and bypassing part of the small intestine. This means that only small quantities of food can be consumed and fewer of the food's nutrients are absorbed into the body.

> Drugs, such as fenfluramine and dexfenfluramine, both of which are appetite suppressant drugs. Both have been removed from the market due to concerns about their effects on the cardiovascular system (Glanville et al. 1997).

The problem with drugs (which, for example, affect metabolism and fat absorption) is that they can have potentially life threatening side-effects. The side-effects include pulmonary hypertension and severe cardiac valvular damage (from fenfluramine and dexfenfluramine) and faecal incontinence and flatulence (from orlistat, which reduced fat absorption). They are also only effective while they are being taken and life-long medication might not be acceptable or appropriate, and they only produce modest weight loss (Ebbe-ling et al. 2002).

Surgical treatment has the effect of physically reducing the amount of food (and therefore calories) that can be consumed. While it has been shown to result in a good rate of weight loss (Bergh et al. 2008), surgery can lead to serious complications, such as associated mortality, revision of the initial surgery, vitamin and mineral deficiencies, feelings of fullness, dizziness, nausea and a desire to lie down after eating (dumping syndrome) (Glanville et al. 1997). The general recommendation is that this should be an option of 'last resort', provided for those with 'morbid' obesity and in conjunction with other therapy to support lifestyle changes (Ebbeling et al. 2002), given the surgical risks and other complications, and should certainly not be considered an option for the treatment of obesity at a population level (Bergh et al. 2008).

4

Reflective activity

- Over the next week, try to be aware of how many adverts or articles you see in magazines and papers or on advertising billboards about surgery or drugs to help you lose weight.
- What promises are being made in the adverts and articles?
- Are the limitations or side-effects mentioned too?

Carryer (1997) argues that the concern over obesity as a health problem has resulted in the sanctioning of these medical treatments, despite their limited success and associated harm. There are some regulatory controls on access to surgery (a BMI ≥ 35 (Bergh et al. 2008) but the increasing commodification (see p. 71) of medical therapy, i.e. the availability of such treatments 'for sale' through private clinics, undermines this sort of regulation and increasingly positions surgery and drugs as a lifestyle choice.

The problem with the conflation of business with health (the diet industry, fitness clubs and surgical or drug therapy) is that it becomes difficult to untangle the reason why we are encouraged to engage in a given activity – is it for money (theirs) or for health (ours)? Even if both objectives are part of the 'sell', the profit motive can potentially corrupt the information provided, as in essence the drive is to market a product, or to persuade others towards a particular course of action, rather than to enable free, fully informed decision-making. Nordenfelt (1995) observes that if health promotion messages manipulate the truth in order to persuade people to make certain choices, this breaches the principle of *informed consent*.

Some cautionary notes

The consensus of opinion presented so far indicates that obesity is a considerable health concern but some of the more problematic and contentious aspects of the matter have also been mentioned. It is important to explore this critique further and some epidemiologically and sociologically based studies have challenged the prevailing orthodoxy on the obesity epidemic. The challenge starts with a re-evaluation of the figures purporting an epidemic and presenting a more measured analysis of the health hazards linked to weight.

The size of the epidemic

As mentioned earlier, according to the National Audit Office, at the turn of the twenty-first century (NAO 2001, p. 1) 'over half of women and about two thirds of men are either overweight or obese'. Coles (1999) states that in Wales 55.2 per cent of adults are overweight, or obese, with a Body Mass Index (BMI) of 25 or greater, and it is predicted that by 2050, 90 per cent of today's children will be overweight or obese according to BBC News (2009b). Not only do the figures seem quite startling, particularly the BBC News figure, but they make reference to *both* obesity and overweight in their declarations. Overweight or obese are not the same thing (SIRC 2005). Taken on an individual level this is equivalent to placing someone who is 172 cm (5 feet 8 inches) tall, but weighs 76 kg (12 stone) in the same category as someone of the same height who weighs 120 kg (nearly 19 stone). They are clearly **quantitatively** different but also **qualitatively** different, as evidence of increasing risk of health harm is primarily associated with a state of obesity (Visscher et al. 2000; Flegal et al. 2005, 2007).

Box 4.2 Other Measurements of Weight

Waist measurement

An increased risk to health is present when waist circumference exceeds 94 cm (37 inches) for men and 80 cm (32 inches) for women. Intra-abdominal fat is an independent predictor of risk to health (Hitchcock-Noël and Pugh 2002).

Waist to hip ratio (WHR)

This represents the numerical difference between the waist and hip circumferences: for example, when the waist measures 80 cm and the hips 85 cm, the waist to hip ratio would be 80/85 = 0.94.

A ratio greater than 0.95 for men and 0.85 for women is thought to indicate possible health risks (National Centre for Social Research 2003).

The conventional measurement of obesity, via BMI, has been demonstrated to give an inaccurate picture of potential harmful weight levels. Glanville et al. (1997) comment that interpretation of the BMI is limited by variations in size of body frame, proportion of lean mass and age and gender. Muscle, for instance, weighs more than fat. Thus a very fit and muscular individual may weigh more and therefore, in proportion to their height, have an above 'normal' BMI. Bovbjerg (2008) also points out that the definitions of overweight and obesity are based on norms (i.e. normal/most common) (see norms, p. 109) rather than BMI association with disease risk, and Filiault (2008, p. 243) comments that elevated body mass should be considered *one* of a variety of factors that increase risk of disease, 'not a disease it its own right'.

Other measurements – for example, GHR (waist circumference divided by height) or WHR (waist to hip ratio) (see Box 4.2) – may be more accurate because they measure the tendency for central obesity (apple shape), which is associated with an increased risk of cardiovascular disease, hypertension and non-insulin dependent diabetes (Glanville et al. 1997; Hitchcock-Noël and Pugh 2002).

As mentioned earlier, for children over the age of 5 years, no specific baseline determining 'healthy' weight exists, and this is currently being constructed (WHO 2009c). According to the SIRC (2005) report, the data on childhood obesity, up to that point, had been considerably exaggerated and were an artefact of how the figures on weight gain have been collated. These were collated using the national standard based on UK reference curves from 1990 (children are classified obese if they fall above the 95th percentile relative to the curve for their age) (Zaninotto et al. 2006), as opposed to internationally favoured height and weight measures (which are less arbitrary) (Cole et al. 2000; SIRC 2005). This exaggerates the number of children who are classified as 'overweight' or 'obese', as the percentiles are constructed on data from a cohort of children who were smaller in stature than current generations. Children's heights have generally been increasing (SIRC 2005). Thus, using the UK national standard, around 1 in 6 children are deemed to be obese, while using the international standard the figure falls to 1 in 15 children (SIRC 2005). There is evidence too that the observed increase in obesity in children has 'flattened out' (Scholes 2008, p. 220).

Other claims support the focus on overweight and obese children though as it is suggested that weight problems in children will continue into adulthood. According to Scholes (2008, p. 231), 'Increases in the prevalence of childhood obesity could potentially result in increasing numbers of obese adults in the long term, with serious implications both for individual health and the costs of providing health services.' Up to 50 per cent of obese adolescents are estimated to remain obese in adulthood and health problems in middle age have been directly linked to childhood and adolescent overweight and obesity according to Scholes (2008).

However, the evidence on this matter is mixed. Wright et al. (2001) concluded that there is little association between childhood obesity and adult obesity and no excess adult health risk from being fat as a child (based on data from a prospective cohort study). Instead people who were thinnest as children and fattest as adults experienced most adverse consequences, while a study by Engeland et al. (2003) did identify increased mortality in adulthood particularly associated with adolescent obesity.

Doing harm ... the products of an obsession

4

This dialogue would suggest that linking health risks with weight is complex. For example, being underweight is associated with increased mortality too (a 'J' shaped curve) and risks to health only increase at the higher end of BMIs (Visscher et al. 2000; Flegal et al. 2005, 2007). It is also not possible to make blanket recommendations concerning 'healthy' weights across populations. Evidence from a study by Durazo-Arvizu et al. (1998), for example, indicated that the optimal BMI for black men was 27.1 and for black women 26.8, supported by a later study by Fontaine et al. (2003), who identified that the optimal BMI for this group was between 23 and 30 (23–25 for whites).

Despite this evidence Campos (2004) refers to the continuing preference for smaller body size, including calls for black women to become more dissatisfied with their larger body image. The focus on body size and obsession with weight is associated with emerging levels of body hatred – 'the promotion of thin, is having serious psychological and physical impacts on girls and women' (Orbach 2006, p. 67) – and Davies (1998) noted that overweight women felt that they could no longer declare themselves to be in good health given the epidemiologically based pronouncement on the health harms associated with excess weight.

This points to the power of specific, medical, scientific positions on health, which equate good health to biological functioning and the absence of disease.

As noted earlier in this book, this is a narrow conceptualisation of the nature of health, is not reflective of more holistic descriptions and represents a particular vision, not only of what constitutes health but also of what is described as the 'good life' (Seedhouse 1997, 2004). This vision of the good life is constructed around particular principles, where all things should be taken in moderation, lauds the 'productive' citizen and equates him or her with the 'good citizen' (Seedhouse 1997, 2004).

Population surveillance and rationing access to healthcare

Despite these cautionary notes action is increasingly being taken to monitor weight, particularly among children. Guidance produced for PCTs set out how the National Child Measurement Programme (NCMP) should be carried out (CGOU 2008). School Nurses and others are tasked with developing a programme for weighing and measuring children in primary and middle schools. To fulfil legal requirements parents must be informed about the programme and be sent the results. Parents must be given a reasonable opportunity to opt out of the scheme and evidence from a study by Grimmett et al. (2008) indicates that some parents can find this information distressing. More drastically, a few cases have even been highlighted in the media whereby care orders have been taken against families if a child is obese, this being considered a matter of child abuse. While the concern here is linked to concerns over future health problems and a decrease in longevity (DoH 2002; Fontaine et al. 2003), such drastic action has attracted criticism (Fitzpatrick 2008).

Useful resource: obesity as child abuse

Go to: http://www.spiked-online.com/index.php?/site/article/5797/. Read the article but also click on the audio link 'Should obese children be taken into care' to hear a short discussion about this issue.

Another contentious course of action is the decision (Dehn 2007) to deny access to certain treatments, e.g. hip replacements for adults with BMIs above 30 (three PCTs in East Suffolk 2005). Davis and Porteous (2006) indicate that if this policy was implemented nationally an estimated 8,452 patients would be denied total hip replacements and 12,929 denied total knee replacements, although they found no convincing evidence of clinical contraindications associated with weight. An editorial by Horan (2006) suggested that it is only in the morbidly obese (BMI > 40) that significant contraindications exist. Davis and Porteous (2006) maintain that this policy is likely to result in additional suffering, discrimination against women and additional costs to social services caring for patients whose mobility would remain restricted without surgery.

So why do such policies prevail? It is apparent from the points of critique noted above that reflective scrutiny of the evidence is necessary to inform balanced judgement that minimises harm and avoids victim-blaming, and that the medical-scientific perspective on obesity provides an incomplete and sometimes skewed picture of the nature of the problem. None of this is intended to suggest that obesity as a health problem should be dismissed, but it is puzzling that noticeably prejudicial decisions are made about access to health care when they are unsupported by evidence. Campos et al. (2006a) argue that the issue of obesity evokes, and is imbued with, emotional, social and cultural meaning, as is the consumption of food itself (Crossley 2000; Lupton 2000). Other discourses help to explain the social and cultural dynamics that feed into our continuing concern over obesity, elucidating the origins of our perceptions of, and responses to, obesity as a health issue. As Gard and Wright (2005, p. 168) argue, 'the "obesity epidemic" is much more than a "natural phenomenon" which can adequately be described and explained by science. Instead ... the "obesity epidemic" is, as much as anything else, a social idea (or an ideology), constructed at the intersection of scientific knowledge and a complex of culturally-based beliefs, values and ideals.' It is to these discourses that we now turn.

Why is weight becoming public enemy no. 1? The social constructions of obesity

Klein (1996), Campos (2004), Campos et al. (2006a) and Orbach (2006) suggest that, at least in part, our responses around obesity reflect deeply rooted social and cultural prejudices – 'talk of an "obesity epidemic" is serving to reinforce moral boundaries against minorities and the poor' (Campos et al. 2006b, p. 58) – and reinforce positions of social status, class and privilege (Campos 2004; Gard and Wright 2005). These prejudices themselves are informed by social and cultural beliefs about responsibility, individuality and morality, and reflect the cultural absorption of old religious codes within an increasingly secular society. Obesity now attracts the moral disapproval once labelled gluttony and sloth (over-eating and under-exercising) (Helman 1994), and those who are obese are frequently attributed negative qualities (lazy, lacking self-control, ugly and so forth) (Campos et al. 2006b). Rozin (1997) makes a direct connection between the Protestant focus on self-discipline and control and our consternation about unhealthy lifestyles, and Katz (1994) points out that eating fattening foods is commonly spoken of as a 'sin' – how often have we heard or even said, 'I know I shouldn't but ...', 'naughty but nice ...', when we take a bite of chocolate or eat cake or chips – while, in contrast, dieting and exercise equate to atoning for these sins (Katz 1994).

This secularisation of 'religious' regulatory codes fits comfortably with contemporary societies' emphasis on the individual and personal responsibility for our own state of being (including personal and social achievements and state of health), although the very notion of the individual itself is a social construct. Starting in the seventeenth century, and linked to social and economic concerns (the growth of capitalism and the free market economy), new perceptions of the connection between ownership, property and the self emerged. A new moral culture started to establish itself, which prized autonomy, gave a new importance to self-exploration, featured personal commitment in the vision of a 'good life' and introduced a shift in political language towards egalitarianism and subjective rights. 'Personal interest' thus became the motive for human action (see Enlightenment, p. 37).

Sociologists such as Pierre Bourdieu (1930–2002) and Michel Foucault (1926–84) provide some additional insights into our contemporary focus on the body and individual lifestyles. Broadly, their socio-historical accounts explore the shift towards describing the 'body' in normative terms (through observation and categorisation of 'normal' bodies) and ascribing cultural ideals and moral value to 'flesh'. Thereby, the body has come to represent regions of social and personal control, and symbols of our status and anything out of the 'norm' (e.g. 'normal' body weight) become an emblem of disruption to a stable society (Campos 2004) and moral turpitude (Bordo 1993; Davies 1998). As Huff (2001, p. 45) argues, 'The individual body is subjected to a culturally formed composite picture that reflects not so much an actual average as a cultural ideal.'

The connection between cultural ideals and body weight is clearly present in our current perceptions of beauty. Klein (1996) discusses how images of beauty have changed considerably over the centuries and suggests that until very recent times, large (fat) physiques were considered desirable. Glance at pictures by Rubens, the *Three Graces* (lots of cellulite there!) and ancient figurines of Venus (e.g. the *Venus of Willendorf*) and what will be revealed are images which would now only be used on a 'before and after' cosmetic surgery shot. Historically, fat was linked with power and wealth (Sobal 1995, cited in Gard and Wright 2005; Klein 1996) and it is only in the twentieth and twenty-first centuries (and in Western countries) that very thin people have been regarded as glamorous and beautiful. As Orbach (2006, p. 67) states, the fashion, cosmetic and media industries 'promote thin as the only body to have'.

This promotion of an ideal feeds into the increasing commodification and consumerism of health (see commodification, p. 71, and consumerism, p. 73), whereby 'good health' and perfection are 'bought and sold' through fashion, pharmaceuticals and surgery, encouraging 'a pill for every ill' (Brown 2005). Campos et al. (2006b) particularly point to the high level of funding received from pharmaceutical companies for obesity research and suggest that at the very least this skews the interpretations and intervention choices that emerge.

Conclusion

Some of the arguments that reflect the contested notion of obesity and health have been explored in this case study, although it must be acknowledged that the territorial and contradictory responses to the evidence surrounding obesity are so great that it is not possible to do justice to them all. However, sufficient discussion has been presented that it should be evident that health matters are not merely 'objective' matters of '**fact**' and that 'facts' themselves, and how we use them, can be tainted by social and culturally informed ideals. For example, 'facts' also exist citing the contribution of social inequalities in creating ill health, but this matter does not seem to attract nearly as much public, press and medical attention as obesity. Obesity, on the other hand, pushes many medical, moral, ideological and cultural 'buttons' and it is the non-medical discourses that enable a much more socially and culturally complex picture of the nature of obesity as a health hazard to emerge. From this dialogue it can be concluded that there is substance to the claims of the construction of knowledge and that the variety of views are legitimately held. Other discourses also remind us that interventions to manage the public health 'threat' of obesity have social and cultural consequences too and that circumspect responses are wise.

This case study has highlighted these contradictions and explored some of the social, cultural and moral foundations that inform our thinking around obesity, and from this it is concluded that a balanced response, aimed at promoting opportunities for health-fulfilling lives, is ultimately more productive than focusing on weight per se (Blair and LaMonte 2006; Campos et al. 2006a; Filiault 2008). As Bovbjerg (2008, p. 61) observes, 'obesity is a multicausal phenomenon, not likely the result of a single influence, nor likely resolved by a single approach'.

4.3 CASE STUDY 2: ART AND IVF

Historical overview

Since the birth of the first 'test-tube' baby, Louise Brown, in 1978, the pioneering treatment of *in vitro* fertilisation (IVF), developed by Patrick Steptoe and Robert Edwards in Oldham, and other artificial reproductive techniques (ARTs) have frequently been portrayed as a miracle of medical science and technology. Now approximately 11,000 babies are born through ARTs annually (MacErlean 2008), and in a BBC online news report (BBC News 2003) it is stated that 'eventually no-one would be beyond help. ... At present the majority of men and women with fertility problems have a chance to become parents ... [for] some ... who cannot produce ... eggs or sperm and have none in storage. ... Professor Alan Trounson ... said that progress was being made in this area ... in future we'll be able to take cells and reconstruct the equivalent of sperm and eggs. It is theoretically possible.'

While this might seem like the exciting, humane edge of medical science, ARTs and IVF also raise considerable controversy. Debate is ongoing and includes issues such as equity and entitlement, biological frailty, commercial integrity and consumer exploitation, and public cost and welfare.

Such controversy, and diversity of concerns and interests, illustrates the multiplicity of discourses required to understand the territory of ARTs. Understanding IVF and ARTs merely from a biological perspective fails to provide sufficient insight into the implications of such practices. It is not merely a biological affair but, *inter alia*, has profound social and ethical connotations too. Social and psychological perspectives around ART and IVF provide the foundations for a robust and well rounded critical dialogue and understanding of this contemporary phenomenon. In this case study we show, again, how a synthesis of knowledge and insights from the range of academic disciplines that constitute Health Studies enables a more realistic, balanced view of IVF and ARTs to emerge. IVF and ARTs are not merely a matter for consideration within biological, medical sciences, but are subject to social, sociological, psychological and economic critique. Of particular relevance in the context of ART and IVF is feminist dialogue around issues of fertility, motherhood and the role of women in society (see feminism, p. 43). Critique from all of these perspectives is brought into this case study.

The emergence of IVF and ARTs

The biology of the process is interesting and, given the frequent portrayal of IVF and ARTs as 'medical miracles', an overview of this is presented first. IVF literally means fertilisation outside the body and was the first of a huge number of technological advances to assist reproduction, which now include the ability to implant an egg from one woman into the womb of another, freezing embryos and sperm, and intra-cytoplasmic sperm injection (ICSI) – injecting sperm directly into an egg. Pre-implantation diagnostic techniques have also been developed, whereby embryos with certain characteristics can be discarded before implantation. This latter innovation raises potential controversy around 'designer babies', choosing preferred characteristics, or tissue typing for 'saviour babies', siblings who are sufficiently genetically compatible with each other for organ or tissue donation to take place (Deech and Smajdor 2007). Since 1984 when the Warnock Report recommended a robust system of regulation, the UK Human Fertilisation and Embryology Authority (HFEA) has been empowered to regulate and monitor new developments (Deech and Smajdor 2007), with various parliamentary acts being passed in 1990, updated most recently in 2008 (The Stationery Office 2008).

IVF itself, while long established, is not necessarily a straightforward procedure. Fertilisation of the egg (ovum) outside the body requires the harvesting of a number of eggs to increase the likelihood of success. As a woman normally only releases one egg per menstrual cycle (very occasionally two or more in the case of fraternal (non-identical) twins or triplets), multiple ovum release needs to be stimulated through the inhalation or injection of hormones. These multiple ova are then harvested and mixed with partner or donor sperm (the 'test-tube' bit) and the resulting fertilised ova, by then embryos, are implanted into the woman's uterus. The HFEA and NICE (National Institute for Health and Clinical Excellence) recommended in 2004 that the maximum number of embryos for implantation should be two for women under 40 and three for women over 40 (Ledger et al. 2006). This is judged as the appropriate balance between maximising the chances of the embryos 'taking', i.e. the woman continuing with a successful pregnancy and live birth, and minimising the risks to both mother and babies from multiple pregnancies (Deech and Smajdor 2007).

Risks associated with a multiple pregnancy include increased likelihood of miscarriage, the development of complications such as **pre-eclampsia**, and premature birth, which itself increases the risk of physical or neurological damage (Deech and Smajdor 2007). Added to this is the considerable increase in costs. Almost all of the costs of pregnancy and postnatal and neonatal care, if necessary, are borne by the NHS, and it is estimated that a triplet birth costs the NHS ten times more than a singleton birth, and combined costs from twin and triplet births equate to an extra 3,374 couples being treated for three cycles of IVF if multiple births were reduced (i.e. implantation of fewer embryos) (Ledger et al. 2006).

IVF therapy itself is also not without risk. The hormonal therapy needed to stimulate ovum production and 'ready' the woman's uterus for implantation can result in ovarian hyperstimulation syndrome (OHSS). Mild cases manifest in swelling and abdominal discomfort, severe cases in nausea, vomiting, sudden weight gain and fluid retention, difficulty in breathing, the formation of blood clots and very rarely death. There is also *some* evidence of a very low risk of developing ovarian cancer. The physically invasive procedures to extract the eggs and implant the embryo run the usual risks of minor abdominal surgery, e.g. infection or perforation of the bowel, bladder or uterus (Deech and Smajdor 2007).

An ethical dimension also emerges as a consequence of stimulation of multiple ova and the fertilisation of many more embryos than an individual woman needs. The embryos are initially frozen for use by the individual woman if the initial implantation fails, or they are made available for donation to another infertile couple. Surplus embryos may also be used for research, such as stem-cell research, a matter that raises huge controversy and was banned in the USA under the George W. Bush administration (Pilkington 2006).

These biological advances create, and raise, both opportunities and difficulties, as the potential around ART and IVF is sometimes exaggerated. Overall, the effectiveness of IVF is perhaps surprisingly low. According to Deech and Smajdor (2007) the success rate for the average woman of optimal childbearing age is 28.2 per cent per cycle, and in older women and if frozen embryos are used the success rate is considerably lower. The comparable figures quoted on NHS Choices website (2010a) indicate an even poorer success rate, this being 29 per cent only for women under 35 years, reducing to 26 per cent for those aged 35–37 years, 17 per cent for women between 38 and 39 and 11 per cent for women 40–42 years old. De Lacey (2002) argues that the true paucity

4

of success is obscured in media reports (the stories of women who fail to conceive remain invisible), implying improved odds with continuing treatment, rendering consumers vulnerable to exaggerated claims and diminishing opportunities for informed decision-making (Meerabeau 1998).

As a healthcare treatment, ART raises cost concerns. Birenbaum-Carmeli (2004) equated the cost of three cycles of IVF to that of one hip replacement. Comparisons aside, partly due to the limited success rate, the actual cost of the therapy (fertility treatments range from £4000 to £8000; Walsh 2008), and the non-life threatening nature of infertility, most treatment is catered for by private practice. In 1993 it was estimated that 90 per cent of treatment was provided privately, and the treatment was recognisably low on the priority list of service provision for NHS providers. Following the 2004 NICE recommendations (Ledger et al. 2006), the then Minister for Health, John Reid, stated that by April 2005 all PCTs should offer one full cycle of IVF for all of those eligible, but as Ledger et al. (2006) note, these changes should be cost neutral (through improvements in clinical practice in this area). Despite the aspirations, by 2006 only 25 per cent of IVF cycles were funded by the NHS and resource allocation to ARTs is likely to remain under scrutiny given continuing pressure over the funding of public services (see health care rationing, p. 85).

For some, the lack of provision of ARTs on the NHS constitutes a denial of need although, as discussed in the section on assessing health needs (see need (needs assessment), p. 101), this is not a straightforward claim to sustain. Taking a teleological understanding of need (i.e. goal directed), while it is true that ART does enable childless people to fulfil this goal, it is an expensive means of doing so, and other options are possible too, such as adoption. However, claims in support of providing ARTs are social and cultural and not just technical or biological, pertaining, for example, to the maternal role of women in society and the value placed on having children within many countries. As Sandelowski and de Lacey (2002) note, several cultural, and ethical, discourses inform our understanding of ARTs-related issues, and some of these will now be explored.

ART: social and cultural inequalities and controversies

Normative roles of women: the social construction of motherhood and fertility

The arena of fertility treatment interfaces with socially constructed norms and taboos, particularly around motherhood, the existential nature of the maternal instinct and the 'right' to a family; and all of these contribute to contested values and arguments that emerge around ARTs and IVF (Throsby 2001; de Lacey 2002; Birenbaum-Carmeli 2004). Van Balen (2008) refers to the psychological and social limitations that emerge through involuntary childlessness and the importance of motherhood to women's self-esteem and social position in many parts of the world. Throsby (2001), de Lacey (2002) and Birenbaum-Carmeli (2004), point to feminist discourse (see feminism, p. 43), which attributes this exaltation of reproduction, fertility and motherhood to **patriarchal** social systems. This **patriarchalism**, coupled with other inequalities, and a lack of employment or educational alternatives to the nurturing role, sanctifies motherhood as *the* role for women (hence the impact on self-esteem linked to childlessness), and can seriously limit other opportunities and choices for women (Throsby 2001). According to Birenbaum-Carmeli (2004), motherhood is so valorised in, for instance, Israeli society that IVF attracts unrestricted public funding. The focus of health and social policy is on supporting the development of the family and promoting the growth of the Jewish population and the State of Israel.

A consequence of this predilection for motherhood and fertility, and lack of childless role models, is that women who fail to conceive are positioned as failures (Throsby 2001), and this stance is oppressive to those who cannot or do not want to have children (Birenbaum-Carmeli 2004). Dyson (1995) and Inhorn and van Balen (2002) comment that ARTs, therefore, have the capacity for simply reinforcing women's reproductive status and the normative value placed on motherhood and can open up the possibility of exploitation of vulnerable, desperate, individuals (Franklin 1997).

Ethical dilemmas

The posthumous use of sperm

ARTs and IVF are clearly associated with ethical dilemmas as they involve the creation of life (Meerabeau 1998), but other ethical controversies emerged as a consequence of what the technology makes possible. For example, the technology makes it possible for a woman to request the use of her dead partner's sperm (or embryos previously created and kept in deep-freeze storage). This becomes ethically contentious if the man did not give, or retracted, consent. While the development and birth of a fatherless child might occur naturally for a variety of reasons, the existence of the technology pushes against social and ethical conventions pertaining to consent and family constructs. A case in Australia in the early 2000s illustrates this controversy (Cannold 2004, Oakley 2004, Parker 2004, Spriggs 2004). Following the sudden, accidental death of her fiancé, a woman requested the posthumous removal of his sperm to enable her to conceive his child, but this request was refused by the Supreme Court in Brisbane. Spriggs (2004) argues that this decision was wrong, as prior to his death he had expressed a desire for children, had consented to organ donation in general and had previously donated sperm as part of a university campaign/project, from which Spriggs (2004) suggests that desire for posthumous offspring could be inferred. Cannold (2004), Oakley (2004) and Parker (2004), commenting on the same case, disagree. They argue that *explicit* consent is necessary in order to protect the autonomous wishes of an individual and prevent them being used as a 'means to an end'. Oakley (2004) in particular argues that one's wishes when alive might not reflect what would be wanted following death, so the inference Spriggs refers to could be incorrect. As Deech and Smajdor (2007) suggest, the request for use of sperm in this manner, if granted, implies that the state can legally ignore individual wishes and sanction fatherless families, a controversial issue in its own right. Clearly, then, such issues are not simply technical ones, but also reflect ethical and social concerns.

Designer babies and saviour children

As already mentioned, the principle of not treating someone as a 'means to an end' is important and this applies to a potential baby (one conceived naturally or via ARTs) too. This principle informs the boundaries around which new pre-implantation genetic diagnosis (PGD) (selecting a baby on the basis of their genetic make-up, including sex-selection) operates (Deech and Smajdor 2007). Selecting the sex of a child is not permitted in the UK, on non-medical grounds, and selection of traits for so-called 'saviour children' is allowable only if the condition suffered by the existing child is life threatening, the child-to-be-born is not at risk of any life threatening genetic condition itself and all other avenues of treatment have been exhausted. Additionally, only cord blood, not organs or other tissues, can be harvested from the baby (Deech and Smajdor 2007). The regulation against 'designer babies' is also founded on the principle of non-maleficence (do no harm), because of its potential to be used as a mechanism for eugenics and the state-sanctioning of 'desirable traits'.

Consumer choice or consumer exploitation?

4

Reflective activity

Type 'IVF facilities' into an Internet search engine and see just how many IVF clinics are offering treatment. What do you think are the benefits but also potential harms of this range of choices?

Sandelowski and De Lacey (2002, p. 41) describe fertility services as being where 'commerce meets procreation'. Fertility specialists are among the highest earning medical professionals – even earning more than plastic surgeons (Deech and Smajdor 2007) – and the lucrative nature of fertility treatment provides scope for exploitation of those 'desperate' for a baby (de Lacey 2002). For example, the complexity and uncertainty of ARTs means that the prospective parents are not fully equipped to make informed judgements about the quality, or necessity, of various therapies (Meerabeau 1998). De Lacey's (2002) postmodernist inspired research (see postmodernism, p. 47) identified that women sometimes felt that they were being directed towards treatment that benefited the IVF practitioners rather than it being the most suitable personal option, and they reported feeling duped by over-blown promises of success. They were often persuaded to 'stick at it' and 'remain positive', and that technology 'will deliver' if 'you want something badly enough' (de Lacey

2002). Infertility is 'situated as the bogey' (de Lacey 2002, p. 46), and the actual problems and difficulties inherent within the infertility treatment often remain hidden. Consequently, it is argued that commercially driven fertility treatment should be constrained in favour of social, ethical and technical regulation to minimise the potential for exploitation (Meerabeau 1998) (see consumerism, p. 73).

Throsby (2001) and de Lacey (2002) observe though that those seeking fertility treatment are not entirely passive or naive. Those engaging with ARTs are just as likely to position themselves as 'informed gamblers' or 'calculated risk-takers' (de Lacey 2002) and if fertility treatment fails, to reject the social construct of this representing maternal/social 'failure' and instead actively reframe the decision to cease ARTs as one of autonomy and benevolence (Throsby 2001).

Useful resources

Read the news stories about the birth of octuplets at: http://news.bbc.co.uk/1/hi/7852623.stm

To read about some of the controversy raised by the event go to: http://today.msnbc.msn.com/id/29038814/ or http://www.washingtonpost.com/wp-dyn/content/article/2009/02/03/AR2009020303935.html

Rights of the individual, responsibilities to society?

Fertility treatment raises concerns over social, as well as financial, matters too. Much of the blog commentary, for example, linked to the birth of the octuplets in the USA in 2009 refers to disquiet over the social and welfare impact of multiple births.

Van Balen (2008) notes, though, that addressing infertility can fulfil an important social need because the consequences of childlessness, particularly in developing countries, can be significant. These include the serious loss of social status, and poverty. Poverty results from the cost of paying for traditional, or Western, fertility treatment and from the absence of children to support elderly parents. However, funding for ART in developing countries is usually not high on the government's agenda, with priority accorded to more pressing health concerns (including maternal mortality) and indeed population control (van Balen 2008).

The provision of ART is also restricted in Western industrialised countries, largely on financial grounds, and even those seeking ARTs indicate an acceptance of constraint on the grounds of social fairness. The judicial use of scarce resources is an important consideration, particularly in a publicly funded health and social care system. As one of the participants in Throsby's (2001, p. 24) study stated, infertility 'wasn't going to kill me', and greater priority was placed on fairness of access, rather than unlimited access (Throsby 2001).

The legitimacy of any restriction of access to ARTs is sometimes challenged on the basis of 'rights', i.e. the 'right to have a child' (for instance, the Human Rights Act 1998 included the 'right to found a family'). The notion of rights (see rights and responsibilities, p. 115) in this context though is actually an assertion of individual need (or want) and, according to Seedhouse (1994) and Liss (1996), a 'need' cannot be described as an entity in itself, or a specific, objective, 'thing', i.e. the need to have a child via fertility treatment (see need (needs assessment), p. 101). Instead 'need' exists when there is a gap between an individual's (or group's) actual state (e.g. childlessness) and a desired, goal, state (e.g. becoming a parent), and even where this gap is determined it does not automatically imply that ARTs *are* needed. What is determined as being appropriate to 'fill the gap' must include reference to what is ethically acceptable, practically possible (bearing in mind resources and so forth) and socially tolerable (Warnock 1998). 'Rights' must therefore be considered against the backdrop of individual, and social, responsibilities too. 'Rights rhetoric tends to focus on the individual, perhaps to the detriment of legitimate social concerns' (Deech and Smajdor 2007, p. 149). The HFEA has taken the stance that there is no right to a baby per se (Deech and Smajdor 2007) as even with the Human Rights Act, the state has no specific obligation to facilitate reproduction; instead the State has the responsibility to not interfere with the right to reproduce naturally (Deech and Smajdor 2007).

Conclusion

ARTs raises considerable social and ethical issues and demonstrate that competing interests and drives are never entirely resolvable. What is clear though is that technological advances alone cannot determine future options and service provision. Instead they require constant review in the light of evidence of effectiveness, or harm, and shifts in social and cultural values (Deech and Smajdor 2007). Serious consideration must be given to the balance between private and public rights and responsibilities and difficult, and sometimes unpopular, decisions about public service provision will have to be made. Scientific, social, economic and psychological matters all contribute to the discourses around IVF and ART and the acceptability of what is actually provided has to emerge from a synthesis of perspectives and debates about what is acceptable and affordable. These debates should also include challenges to the dominant normative constructs, particularly around the role of women in society. Part of this should include advancing opportunities for women and promoting positive role models of womanhood without motherhood (Throsby 2001).

Useful resource

Deech, R. and Smajdor, A. (2007) *From IVF to Immortality: Controversy in the Era of Reproductive Technology*. Oxford: Oxford University Press. This text provides a comprehensive overview of ART and associated legal and ethical issues

4.4 CASE STUDY 3: HIV

Introduction and terminology

The purpose of this case study is to provide you with an insight into how HIV and AIDS are located nationally and internationally. It gives a range of perspectives and concerns, starting with epidemiological and biomedical definitions and meanings, and then opens up the discussion to address a wide range of differing discourses and theories. This is in effect a snapshot of a hugely contested area, the debates, approaches, treatments, responses and meanings are ongoing and it is worth noting that throughout this case study the material presented is a mere drop in the ocean.

Despite the enormous significance of HIV worldwide, the main focus in this case study is primarily HIV in the UK and the Westernised world. This is for three reasons: first, to try to cover the 'whole world' in this brief exploration would not do any of it justice; second, the discourses and understandings of the virus, as well as the history and responses, vary enormously across the world; third, discourses concerning HIV and AIDS as separate but associated conditions need to be clearly delineated.

Medical definitions and meanings of HIV and AIDS are explored further into this section, but for our immediate purposes it is worth briefly clarifying that HIV and AIDS are not one and the same thing. HIV is a virus, and in the UK can be controlled by medical treatment and managed through 'lifestyle choices'. Thus, in the UK people who have HIV are not necessarily going to 'get' AIDS or indeed die of the virus. AIDS, on the other hand, is a range of syndromes that can develop from having the HIV virus; the syndromes and symptoms of AIDS are multiple and people in the UK do die of AIDS. In the UK more people live with HIV, many for a considerable time, than die of AIDS. Indeed, in the UK HIV is no longer classified as a life threatening condition, but more of a chronic, manageable 'health' condition.

For the purposes of this case study, unless we specify otherwise, the vast majority of the issues explored are concerned with HIV. Very often people will be divided between those who have been diagnosed with HIV, i.e. HIV+/ HIV positive, and those who have not been diagnosed with HIV, i.e. HIV–/ HIV negative.

Epidemiological perspectives

The area of HIV/AIDS is globally as well as nationally significant and concerns are such that HIV/AIDS is now positioned as a global **pandemic** (Schoub 1999; Pratt 2003; Barnett and Whiteside 2006). It is the first global epidemic for over 60 years (Barnett and Whiteside 2006), and HIV/AIDS is a 'disease' that, according to Schoub (1999, p. 18), has four central features that make it a powerful disease with which to contend:

> ❯ it is infectious and transmittable from person to person;

> once one acquires the infection it follows a particular disease trajectory that will eventually lead to death in most cases;
> all people with HIV remain infectious, to a greater and lesser account, throughout their life;
> the number of people with HIV, and therefore the source of further infection, is ever growing and expanding.

Two-thirds of all adults and children with HIV live in sub-Saharan Africa (Barnett & Whiteside 2006; Joint United Nations Programme on HIV/AIDS (UNAIDS) and WHO 2006; Scambler and Paoli 2008). International figures recorded by the Joint United Nations Programme on HIV/AIDS (UNAIDS) and WHO (2006) state that just under 40 million people worldwide are living with HIV, of whom 740,000 are in Western and Central Europe. According to the Health Protection Agency (HPA) and Avert's (2009) figures, there are around 83, 000 people in the UK living with HIV, with over 27 per cent of these being 'unaware' of their status. Official recordings of death due to AIDS also vary widely from country to country. In 2006 sub-Saharan records showed that 2.1 million people died of AIDS, while the figures for Western and Central Europe were 12,000. These figures continue to fall as ART (anti-retroviral treatment or therapy) is increasingly available and effective.

A historical picture of the prevalence of HIV in the UK is provided by Avert (http://www.avert.org/uk-statistics.htm2009). According to its recorded figures, in 1999 and 2003 there was a steep increase in the number of HIV diagnoses. A peak of 7,975 new diagnoses was observed in 2005. During 2008, 7,298 people were diagnosed with HIV in the UK, the third successive year there had been a decrease in diagnoses, though this is still far higher than the pre-2003 rate and also obviously clearly indicates that the number of people in the UK living with HIV is still growing. A major component of this recorded rapid increase over the past 15 years has been the rise in heterosexually acquired infection. Avert (2009) suggests that while only about 20 per cent of heterosexual infections were, or possibly were, acquired in the UK, they are still, overall, on the increase (more on the category of origin of infection later). The second significant factor in this recorded increase has been the introduction of clinician reporting, which was only introduced for HIV diagnoses made after the beginning of 2000 (Avert 2009).

Reflective activity

- Type into your search engine 'who is most at risk to HIV/AIDS' and explore what the various sites say about this.
- How has this changed over time?

One area of interest in the way figures are collated and recorded is that within HPA figures, new categories around whether people were infected abroad or at home have appeared, as have differentiating ethnicities. As with obesity and the manner in which BMI has been both defined and recorded, viewing statistics over time does not always reflect the complete picture (see also literature review and documentary research for issues of credibility and dependability in recording techniques in Chapter 5). The change in the recording of HIV is reflective of findings that claim that over 65 per cent of women in the UK diagnosed with HIV came originally from the sub-Saharan countries (Doyal and Anderson 2005). What is worth bearing in mind when you look at these, and any, figures is that these can only represent people who have had their diagnoses officially recorded. Therefore, estimates given of the numbers of HIV+ cases who are 'unaware' of their status can only be just that – estimates – though they are often based on deductive reasoning (see p. 248) and previous epidemiological research.

Biomedical discourses

One place to start, and certainly a very powerful place to start, is in your understanding of the biomedical definitions of HIV/AIDS. These definitions are generally similar, across the board, though it is worth noting that increasingly there may be different strains of HIV (Scambler and Paoli 2008; Avert 2009; Nam 2010) and that while HIV and AIDS are generally considered in tandem they are positioned and experienced differently. Historically our understanding of HIV/AIDS has become increasingly sophisticated and informed but, as with dementia, original understandings still have relevance to how we engage with the detection, prevention, treatment and cure of the virus. In this instance its initial detection and definition was seen as 'a gay plague' or 'gay cancer', and the stigmatisation (see stigma, p. 118) and resultant early responses were informed by discourses of homophobia and particular versions of sexual morality (Wilton 2000) – factors that Tamsin (2000, p. 93) believes 'were a significant obstacle to infection control and disease prevention'.

Reflective activity

- Type 'gay plague' into an Internet search engine and explore the various sites.
- Note down the definitions given to this term.
- How do you feel that these definitions might still be pertinent today?

HIV (Human Immunodeficiency Virus) is a retrovirus, and like any other virus it attacks and infects cells within the human body and replicates itself within those cells. HIV specifically attacks the cells that make up the immune system. Our immune system is a group of cells that protects us from, and attacks, viruses and bacteria. HIV targets in particular our CD4 cells within the immune system (Avert 2009). It can very rapidly mutate and once your body has it there is no way to get rid of it. In some ways HIV is no different from other viruses like herpes, as both stay in the body and cause 'silent infections'. 'When it first infects it may or may not cause clinical disease, ... but soon settles into its latent or silent phases which usually lasts for many years'

(Schoub 1999, p. 21). The length of time can vary widely between individuals. Left untreated, the majority of people infected with HIV will develop signs of HIV-related illness within 5–10 years. However, the time between HIV infection and an AIDS diagnosis can be 10–15 years, sometimes longer (WHO 2010). The life of the virus can continue for some time and as the damaged cells replicate the individual is more and more vulnerable to diseases that may or may not eventually progress to AIDS. There are considered to be different strains of HIV: the one we know as HIV-1, and a second less virulent and slower acting one, HIV-2 (Schoub 1999; Barnett and Whiteside 2006). Within each of these types are sub-types, which mean that the viral variants can have a wide variety of characteristics (Pratt 2003).

AIDS (Acquired Immunodeficiency Syndrome), like dementia (see Case study 4), is a syndrome, which essentially means in biological terms that there is a collection of different signs and symptoms that are all part of the same underlying medical condition (Aidsmap 2009). It is, according to Schoub (1999, p. 20), 'the end-stage disease manifestation of an infection with a virus called the human immunodeficiency virus (HIV)'. The damage to the immune system caused by HIV means that our bodies are less and less able to protect us from opportunistic (those that would otherwise be controlled by our immune system) infections. So depending on what stage of HIV one is in, one's general health and the state of the immune system, different clinical problems may, and do, develop (Schoub 1999; Pratt 2003; Aidsmap 2009). Eventually our immune system can be so compromised and our bodies so weak and infected by various infections that we are unable to sustain it and, therefore, people die of AIDS.

The most 'at risk' populations in the UK to HIV are gay men (who are often defined in statistics as 'Men who have Sex with Men', MSM), sub-Saharan people, heterosexuals who contracted HIV in other countries and intravenous drug users (Joint United Nations Programme on HIV/AIDS (UNAIDS) and WHO 2006; HPA 2008; Aidsmap 2009; Avert 2009). While with the last the risk, and therefore prevalence, has been hugely reduced with policies about providing free needles etc. (Aidsmap 2009; Avert 2009), Davis (2008) questions the reliability and validity (see p. 251) of this finding, as there have also been recent reports of increased risky injection practices in both England and Wales (Hope et al. 2005). Ridge et al.'s 2008 study found that the groups most affected by HIV in the UK were also gay (mostly white) men and black African heterosexual men and women, with most of the latter having acquired the infection in Africa. Ridge et al. (2008) go on to to say that the majority of gay men acquire their infection in the UK, as does the growing white HIV+ heterosexual population. All reports indicate that MSM and heterosexual populations are increasing in their diagnoses of HIV. The number of heterosexually acquired HIV infections diagnosed in the UK has risen hugely over the past 15 years. In 1999, for the first time, the rate of heterosexually acquired HIV diagnoses overtook the rate of diagnoses in MSM. The peak was 4,921 in 2004, since when there has been a moderate decline. A total of

4

45,947 cases had been reported by the end of June 2009 and this is set to increase (Aidsmap 2009; Avert 2009; WHO 2009; HPA 2010).

A reminder: it is worth pointing out that simply giving epidemiological spread and biomedical data is not sufficient to try to 'understand' HIV/AIDS. The spread, management, experiences, response and treatment of HIV/AIDS are informed by social, political, sexual and psychological dimensions that are increasingly the concern of researchers. The implications abroad, as well as nearer to home, need to be explored much further.

Biomedical definitions of causes

There are various ways in which HIV/AIDS is transmitted and what is 'known' is that it can only be transmitted through contaminated bodily fluids (Wilton 2000; Shafer et al. 2002; Barnett and Whiteside 2006). However, it is worth noting that what is 'known' (see positivism, p. 227, and deductive reasoning, p. 248) in terms of biomedical fact and what is believed and understood by the general population are not always the same thing at all.

Reflective activity

- List as many 'causes' for HIV that you can think of; include here ones that you 'believe' as well as ones that you have heard.
- How has your behaviour, sexual and otherwise, been influenced by these beliefs?
- How has the behaviour of others you know been influenced by their beliefs?

Barnett and Whiteside (2006, p. 41) list the following, in order of importance, as the main methods of transmission:

1 Unsafe sex.
2 Transmission from infected mother to child.
3 Use of infected blood or blood products.
4 Intravenous drug use with contaminated needles.
5 Other modes of transmission involving blood: for example, bleeding wounds.

The vast majority of HIV infections are from sexual transmission (Schoub 2001; Pratt 2003; Barnett and Whiteside 2006). HIV can be present in 'seminal, pre-ejaculatory, vaginal and cervical secretions, and in saliva (and other body fluids, especially blood) in affected individuals, a variety of sexual behaviours can efficiently facilitate viral transmission and these behaviours can occur in both heterosexual and homosexual encounters' (Pratt 2003, p. 33). Barnett and Whiteside (2006) and Pratt (2003) both explain that anal penetrative sex has a higher risk of infection than vaginal; hence gay men – in the Western world – were the group that was first identified with HIV and have the highest risk of infection. Cohen (2004) found that male-to-male transmission was 1:10 to 1:1,600, while male to female transmission was 1:200 to 1:2,000, and female to male transmission 1:7,000 to 1:3,000. Cohen (2004) and

Barnett and Whiteside (2006), however, add a proviso to these figures in terms of the limitations attached to the routes of transmission and their estimations. What they want you to consider is that how people report their sexual history may impact on these statistics (see stigma, p. 118; free will and health, p. 180; challenges to epidemiology, p. 195; norms and normalisation, p. 109).

There are a number of conditions that can increase the risk of transmission and again the definitions provided reside in the biomedical model. What becomes apparent is that transmission is not simply isolated to one informing variable, i.e. a partner, or indeed both, being HIV positive. A number of other possible variables can make the transmission of HIV more probable:

> the likelihood that the sexual partner is infected with HIV;
> the type of sexual activity;
> the disease stage of the infected partner;
> the presence of other sexually transmitted infections;
> the frequency of partner change;
> biological factors;
> the lack of male circumcision;
> viral variants;
> host infectiousness (Pratt 2003, p. 35).

Other informing conditions for transmission

The huge over-simplification of positioning the transmission of HIV into non-contextual, non-political, non-power contexts has been, and continues to be, challenged by a number of researchers and research results. Social constructivists and feminists (see also Chadwick's *Report on the Sanitary Conditions of the Labouring Classes* (1842) for an exploration of the impact of social context on our health as a way of both challenging and developing your ideas about reductionism and positivism), for instance, believe that poverty and living or life conditions can also cause and facilitate the spread of disease. Added to this are issues of gender and women's reduced power to negotiate, malnutrition, stigma, education and opportunity, discrimination, people's notions of responsibility and duty to themselves and others and, finally, shame and fear.

The discussion of Seedhouse's (2001) theory of 'foundations for achievement' of health (see Chapter 1) presents the notion that in order for an individual to achieve their optimum potential they must be enabled to achieve both their 'chosen and biological potential'. Interwoven within these five conditions are theories of liberal individualism (p. 44) and creative autonomy (p. 55). Basically, what Seedhouse (2001) suggests is that what an individual needs to achieve this 'state' includes meeting their basic needs of shelter, food, warmth and purpose, information, education (to make reasoned decisions), community and medical services. Looking at health inequalities (p. 95) you will see that not everyone has equal access to treatment provision, and this too needs to be considered when exploring conditions for transmission.

Shefer et al. (2002) and Klunklin and Greenwood (2006), in their studies of South African and Northern Thai populations, clearly demonstrate how we not only 'other' (i.e. put outside the experience of 'ourselves' and our own identity) people at risk, but can also 'other' our understanding of how the disease is transmitted and understood to not include us. Shafer et al. (2002) distinguishes between our biomedical knowledge and what actual meaning is given to HIV, i.e. shame, being diseased, dirty, promiscuous, sick and evil etc., and how that can function to potentially increase the risk of HIV through discourses of denial, shame, silencing and stigma (see poststructuralism, p. 49, discourse analysis, p. 329, social constructivism, p. 49, and postmodernism, p. 47).

Reflective activity

- How have you heard people with HIV/AIDS described?
- What are some of the beliefs about who 'gets HIV' and how we or they get it?
- What aspects of the above beliefs could also describe your behaviour and characteristics?
- What do you believe does not relate to you?

Klunklin and Greenwood (2006) also talk about how HIV is seen in terms of meanings rather than simply its pathology – so shame, disgust, dirt and disease form part of the discourse around HIV/AIDS and have implications for how we behave and often situate it as being outside of ourselves. The meanings and moral positioning that we attach to HIV/AIDS and its transmission can, and do, have a direct effect on how we treat, manage and respond to the virus. Hughes et al. (2008) in their study of the urban poor in US nursing homes point out that in the early part of the epidemic nursing homes wouldn't even admit people with HIV/AIDS. Nearly all the research, and indeed health promotion and public health campaigns (see Chapter 1) acknowledge the stigma of HIV/AIDS. Scambler and Paoli's (2008) research particularly focused on how stigma can act as a barrier to the effective prevention and management of safe sex practice; their research focused on female sex workers (FSWs), who are seen by the Joint United Nations Programme on HIV/AIDS (UNAIDS) and WHO (2006) to be one of the four key populations globally that need to be targeted with HIV health initiatives and interventions.

Evans and Lambert (2008) (see ethnography, p. 233) provide an example of the recommended community-based approach to HIV prevention, with its focus on participation and mobilisation. The success of this project was largely informed, among other things, by working *with* FSWs and the political and social context in ways that, rather than positioning FSWs as deviant, simply pragmatically worked with what was in ways that were designed to empower the individual to be 'mistress of her body' in realistically contextual ways. Scambler and Paoli (2008, p. 1849) consider that one of the main impediments to successful work with FSWs (and clearly this can be broadened to include any HIV+ population or individual) is the 'shame and blame ubiquitously applied with FSWs', which 'enhance their vulnerability, impair their human rights, and impede attempts by third parties ... to contain the HIV/ AIDS epidemic'.

The impact of these discourses of shame, gender and stigma on the complexities of how to practise and/or negotiate safe sex (defined here as with the barrier method of the condom) is complex and imbued with discourses of power, politics, gender, sexuality, individuality, autonomy and rights and responsibilities (Schrimshaw and Siegal 2002; Shafer et al. 2002; Doyal and Anderson 2005; Klunklin and Greenwood 2006; Davis 2008; Evans and Lambert 2008; Lee and Sheon 2008; Persson and Newman 2008; Scambler and Paoli 2008).

Reflective activity

Consider the following for either yourself or people you know:
- When you have sex do you use any barrier methods, e.g. condoms or femidoms?
- What conditions impact on your decision as to whether you use a condom or not?
- How (if at all) would having sex with a 'casual' partner differ from having sex in a long-term relationship?

Prevention of transmission

Prevention of transmission, in simple biological terms, is the condom, which provides a physical barrier between the penis and either the vagina or anus. The focus for prevention campaigns has been to encourage condom use or even practice abstinence (Avert 2009). How these campaigns have been devised and targeted is another area of interest in terms of research; at a very prosaic level, as Wilton (2000) suggests, the use of condoms is the most straightforward, cheap and available method of safe sex in the UK and is 'known' to protect people from the transmission of STIs, yet clearly people are not availing themselves of this. Recent statistics on STIs within the UK population generally would indicate this, as could the continual increase in the numbers of HIV+ individuals.

4

Reflective activity

- Why do you think people don't use condoms?
- Using either Google Scholar or Web of Knowledge (to check if your institution has access to this search engine go to http://wok.mimas.ac.uk/), search for 'risk taking behaviours and sex'. You will find a plethora of articles and material that discuss the many manifestations, understandings and meanings of risk taking.
- Now type in 'risk taking and personal fable' and read some of the articles here too.

Let's talk about sex

Given that the main transmitter of HIV/AIDS is seminal fluid, sex has a lot to with HIV/AIDS. Our attitudes, beliefs and practices regarding sex are absolutely connected with the way in which we have sex with other people and the way we think about it. Sex can be an incredibly difficult area to talk about and clearly issues of negotiation and openness impact on how, if at all, we disclose our status or ask other people about theirs. If sex is imbued with meanings of embarrassment, shame and secrecy, excitement, desire, thrills or risk and spontaneity, then all these discourses need to be added to the melting pot of HIV/AIDS management and interventions. Within our sexual encounters there can be notions of trust – e.g. we trust our long-term partners and therefore don't practise safe sex; we trust that people will tell us if they are HIV+; we trust that people won't have HIV – or, when sex is linked to risk, danger and immediacy, we may not want to think about safety and responsibility.

Risk taking

Risk taking theories, touched on in individualism (see p. 92), liberalism (see p. 44) and stigma (see p. 118), are relevant when considering this issue. It also maps across to obesity (see Case study 1) and our eating habits. The idea being that simply because we 'know' that something is 'good' for us, e.g. condom use, healthy eating, that does not mean that we practise this. The theories that attempt to 'explain' this are multiple and can include risk taking behaviours, personal fables, personality, social conditioning, choice and values, to name but a few. Rhodes's (1997) research on meanings of risk taking makes a number of very useful points to consider, not least that behaviours that for public health reasons are considered risky 'may be viewed in different terms ... [and] appreciating what "risk" and risk behaviour actually mean ... assists in developing interventions to reduce the a variety of harms' (Rhodes 1997, p. 223). Alberts et al.'s (2007) more recent study of adolescent risk taking behaviours suggests that the personal fable (i.e. the belief of invulnerability) and the function of egocentric decision-making, informed by a variety of variables including gender and the idea of the 'imaginary audience' (i.e. everyone is watching me) has a great impact on behaviour too.

The question here is risk taking behaviour, and its link to discourses of choice impacted upon by other confounding variables: for instance, gender, with women having less power to negotiate and/or being problematised in particular ways when they are 'in control' of their sexuality and sexual behaviour (see feminism/feminist methodologies, p. 43, and inequalities in health, p. 95). We also need to consider discourses of risk in relation to sex and our sexual behaviours – once again how we situate risk in terms of our sexual behaviour may very well be linked to our meanings of masculinity, desire, femininity and 'being in the moment'.

The focus of prevention

The focus, it is argued, has been on endeavours to contain and problematise the 'at risk' populations as being outside the 'norm' (see norms/normalisation, p. 109), an early example of this being the title of 'gay plague', which both the USA and the UK used to define their response. Along with intravenous drug users, the health promotion campaigns particularly targeted these populations, positioning them as the problem outside the mainstream and therefore positioning HIV as outside the norm. Persson and Newman (2008, p. 632) posit that a 'key cultural production of HIV/AIDS' has been 'as a disease of the "other", making possible the idea that infection was linked to identities located outside the "mainstream"; outside "proper" heterosexuality'. Thus, demonisation of 'outsider' populations not only informed media reports but also impacted on campaigns and even funding for research in HIV. There is an interesting parallel with dementia (see Case study 4) in terms of how particular populations are valued and seen, and this can impact on how monies are organised and indeed how care is managed (see health care rationing, p. 185).

Persson and Newman (2008, p. 632) go on to say that media representations and campaigns have changed, particularly since the global pandemic has continued. Their rather cynical, though not unfounded, contention is that 'international recognition that HIV is transmitted through particular practices, not particular people ... [means that] HIV has become repositioned as a global crisis and as a heterosexual epidemic'. However, once again, one needs only to look at how the media reported on the spate of convictions in the early and mid 2000s of individuals for 'recklessly causing grievous bodily harm' by giving someone HIV (THT 2010) to see that demonisation is never far from methods of representations.

4

Reflective activity

- Using an Internet search engine, look for the following: 'Convictions for HIV transmission, UK'.
- Read the various reports, as well as the various comments on individuals who have been charged with 'recklessly causing grievous bodily harm', and see how they are presented.
- Note down the descriptions of those being 'accused'.

Interventions and treatments

It is in the area of sexual transmission that there is the most research and contention. Transmission through blood transfusions has been reduced drastically in the UK (and other countries) by the screening of donated blood. This has been the most successful achievement in terms of prevention and reduction overall. Mother to child transmissions have also been reduced in the UK (Sherr et al. 2006; Aidsmap 2009; Avert 2009). EBP, including RCTs and systematic reviews (all discussed further in Chapter 5), demonstrated that the likelihood of vertical transmission can happen in the prenatal period, at delivery and/or in the postnatal period via breast feeding (Barnett and Whiteside 2006; Avert 2008). The use of anti-retroviral drugs (ARDs), which are designed to decrease the viral load and increase the CD4 count, has contributed to the reduction in numbers, as has the support for bottle feeding and, more contested, caesarean sections (Schoub 1999; Barnett and Whiteside 2006; Avert 2009). Clearly all these interventions will be impacted upon by cost (see health care rationing, p. 85), availability and potentially opposing views informed by culture, religion and necessity. Simply 'knowing' something is not enough to implement changes and, indeed, may not always be transferable across all contexts.

For instance, what happens to women who are HIV+ in a cash poor country where malnutrition is rife? It may well be more contextually relevant to continue to breast feed their infants, as: it is free while formula food may not always be; formula food may not be readily available; the water supply can be unsanitary; instructions for using formula milk are not in the woman's mother tongue, or she has not been taught to read (a condition that many women exist in due to patriarchal power and cultural norms). Finally, breast feeding as a preferred option for the child's health has been supported throughout countries in Africa and greatly supported by the WHO in terms of education and health promotion activities. Information on vertical transmission through HIV+ women's breast milk has not been long in existence. Read the links below to get some of the current thinking on this issue.

Useful resources

http://www.uniteforsight.org/women-children-course/breastfeeding
http://www.who.int/features/factfiles/breastfeeding/facts/en/index.html

Anti-retroviral therapy

Treatment of HIV in the UK is largely with anti-retroviral drugs, which are designed to increase the CD4 cells and reduce the viral load, i.e. how much of the virus is in your body. The more CD4s you have, the more your immune system can combat the virus. This is also known as combination therapy for this reason. In the UK we have access to this therapy and as a result the positioning of HIV has changed from being constructed in terms of AIDS and mortality to it being 'reconceptualised as a manageable chronic illness' (Persson and Newman 2008, p. 633). This is a very important point for ongoing treatment as well as 'living with HIV'. The HPA's 2009 Report (http://www.hpa.org.uk/web/HPAwebFile/HPAweb_C/1259151891830) gives a very brief estimate of HIV-related lifetime costs and clearly the NHS's priority will be to reduce the numbers of people creating those costs – thus prevention will be a priority.

Approaches to prevention

Where does that take us in terms of how we understand, position, treat and live with HIV? As previously said, research in this area is often separated in terms of looking at quality of care and interventions (very often supported by **EBP**). A good example of this is Sherr et al. (2006), whose research looked at HIV testing in pregnancy. HIV testing during pregnancy is seen as a primary way of preventing vertical transmission, because the earlier mothers who are HIV+ are identified, the earlier preventative measures can be put into place. Research dating back to the early 1990s, such as Ades et al. (1991), found that the majority of women with HIV either didn't know or didn't disclose their status during antenatal care. At this point, we need to briefly consider the nature of stigma more explicitly in the case of HIV/AIDS. While we have throughout this case study directed you to the section on stigmatisation in Chapter 3 for further elaboration, we want to touch on it more explicitly here as a way of clearly positioning its power to impact on lives.

The function of stigma in mediating responses to treatment and prevention

Bond et al (2002, p. 347) state that 'HIV/AIDS-related stigma, and its associated discrimination, is known to negatively affect all aspects of HIV prevention, diagnosis, treatment and care'. Their research is particularly concerned with HIV+ mothers accessing treatment but is equally applicable to any population or group who have to run the gamut of healthcare services. What they, along with many others, claim is that stigma in relation to HIV is interwoven with pre-existing stigmas of sexual conduct and morality, gender roles, patriarchal norms, drug intake, position of power and placement in society, i.e. being within marginalised or disempowered populations (Wilton 2000; Shafer et al. 2002; Klunklin and Greenwood 2006; Sherr et al. 2006; Persson and Newman 2008; NAM 2010). Bond et al. (2002, p. 248), citing the work of Bharat et al. (2001), consider that HIV/AIDS stigma can be identified on a multiple of levels but could include the following:

> Self-stigma is manifested in self-blame and self deprecation.
> Perceived stigma is manifested in the fears that people have around being stigmatised if they are HIV-positive and choose to disclose their HIV status to others.
> Enacted stigma is when people are actually discriminated against because they have, or are thought to have, HIV.

Bogart et al.'s (2008) research on stigma experienced within families also discusses the multiple meanings given to stigma, both from within families themselves and in the wider public arena. Their research was intended to measure what they defined as categories of stigma. Their categories are not dissimilar to Bharat et al.'s (2001) definitions, and while clearly there are difficulties in, for instance, measuring children's understanding of the concept of courtesy and adults' understanding of it, what is useful with this breakdown is the ongoing implications of stigma in our understandings of HIV.

Useful resource

Access and read the research carried out by Bogart et al. (2008) to explore the meanings and implications of stigma:

Bogart, L. M., Cowgill, B. O., Kennedy, D., Ryan, G., Murphy, D. A., Elijah, J. and Schuster, M. A. (2008) 'HIV-Related Stigma among People with HIV and Their Families: A Qualitative Analysis', *AIDS and Behavior*, 12, 244–54.

As with many researchers Bogart et al. (2008) recommend that more work needs to be done in order to reduce the prevalence of the resulting discriminatory behaviour informed by stigmatising attitudes and beliefs. Although researchers have indicated that stigma has indeed reduced as more positive role models and depictions of HIV+ people are more widely circulated, there needs to be more work done on both the external and internal impacts of stigma. Wolitski et al.'s (2009) research suggests that continued media positive representations are needed, as evidence shows this has considerable impact on reducing stigma and discrimination.

Given the complexities and very real constraints that HIV stigma can enforce, preventative approaches have endeavoured to address these discourses in various ways, rather than negating their impact.

4 Government responses to HIV risk

The UK introduced various strategies to encourage women to take the HIV test. In 2003 it was suggested that all pregnant women as a matter of common practice should be offered the HIV test – a sort of universal opt out approach. Research would seem to indicate that there was an increase in uptake and a subsequent uptake in treatment, thereby reducing infant transmission (Sherr et al. 2006). The government more recently put together UK National Guidelines for HIV Testing in 2008, which further endeavours to 'normalise' HIV testing as a part of common healthcare practice in all relevant areas, including GP surgeries and any medical admissions in areas that already have a prevalence level of greater than 2 per 1,000 (HPA 2009).

Early testing is considered to be one of the major strategies for prevention and treatment and can be very effective in treating HIV early on. In 2008, an estimated 55 per cent (3,970/7,218) were diagnosed with a CD4 count of less than 350 (the point at which anti-retroviral treatment is recommended). It is now one of the main targets to reduce, along with testing the undiagnosed, of the HPA, not least for reasons of the economics (see healthcare rationing, p. 85), as well taking on the role of 'positive libertarians' in terms of reducing perceived risk. Normalising the HIV test in healthcare is also a route that the UK sees as a way of working with HIV as a chronic long-term illness, and identifying the large portion of people accessing healthcare who either don't know or don't disclose, informed by the belief that once you 'know' then you are then responsible for ensuring that you do not spread it any further. The 2008 Guidelines take this all into account in the following ways:

> A significant number of people are unaware of their HIV+ status.
> Late diagnosis is the most important factor related to morbilidy and mortality.
> Testing in a wide range of healthcare settings is to be encouraged and offered.
> Patients with specific indicator conditions should be routinely recommended to have a HIV test.
> All doctors, nurses and midwives should be able to obtain informed consent for an HIV test in the same way that they currently do for any other medical investigation (British HIV Association 2008).

A similar approach is also being taken in USA policies with regard to normalising HIV testing. The theory is that 'routine testing can be seen as a strategy to reduce the stigma associated with the decision to test and redefine HIV testing as a routine clinical procedure' (Lee and Sheon 2008, p. 167). Lee and Sheon's 2008 research looks at why people choose to take the test. They found that MSMs make up the population that has most taken to a routine of screening and can often go for repeat testing, particularly in publicly funded centres. Stories of why they took the test were constructed around responsibility and the right thing to do, at the same time minimising any notion of risk taking behaviour – this latter arose partly because the HIV test counselling was constructed around taking preventative action. Sherr et al.'s 2006 research found that while take-up of HIV testing increased over the two years, often the very populations most at risk were most likely to refuse the test – they propose that in order for the blanket approach to be more effective, approaches need to be focused in terms of routine and targeted offers of testing for everyone, rather than paying only lip service to 'normalising' testing for all populations (including heterosexuals).

Disclosing

Schrimshaw and Siegal's (2002) research focused on the difficulty of mothers' disclosing to their uninfected children. Bogart et al.'s (2008) research found that the fear of being stigmatised by their own children, as well as the impact for children of having an HIV+ parent and being identified as having HIV, impacted on the ways in which parents chose to, and chose not to, disclose.

However, legal frameworks that imply a link between non-disclosure and increased sexual risk behaviour are not conclusively supported by research (Wolitski et al. 2009). What research does show is that concern regarding the stigmatising reactions to disclosing does indeed impact on to whom people choose to, or choose not to, disclose.

Doyal and Anderson (2005) consider the impact of living with HIV for African women in London, and how it positions them in terms of their community, identity, fears around responses, immigration status and so on. Findings indicate that fear and concern about disclosing their status to others were informed by the stigma attached in their community as well as in the majoritised community, and the fear around having a relationship where their status may need to be disclosed.

The gendered experience of being HIV+ is an important aspect explored in research, in terms of both how men's sexuality can be located within 'heterosexual ideology that essentialises and priorities an uncontrollable male sexuality over safety, in particular safe sex technologies perceived to constrain or compromise male sexual pleasure' (Persson and Newman 2008, p. 638), and how women are often being located in terms of being to blame (Shafer et al. 2002), having less of a power base in terms of negotiating safe sex and having control of their own sexuality (Shafer et al. 2002; Doyal and Anderson 2005; Evans and Lambert 2008).

Disclosing to others an HIV+ status is another area that is widely researched. The fear attached to disclosing, how we want to be seen, issues of responsibilities and rights all interweave in how and when we feel able to disclose.

Reflective activity

- If you were HIV+, how would you disclose your status?
- What would 'get in the way' of you telling?

Responsibilities and rights

Persson and Newman (2008) and Davis (2008) both explore the implications of an increasing individualisation (see individualism, p. 92) within how we manage our health and well-being. This links to responsibility and opens up questions about who is responsible for ensuring HIV is not spread. And, indeed, what is our duty to each other's, and our own, well-being? Our location of sex as a 'private affair' between consenting adults means that we consider its negotiation to reside with the individuals involved. This means, in essence, that we either trust each other to practise safe sex or knowingly engage in consensual risky sex. Does the responsibility for ensuring 'protected sex' reside with the individual who knows they are HIV+ (and by know we mean both those who have been tested and those who suspect or don't want to know their status), with both sexual partners or with the individual who believes they are not positive? The huge debates around this are evidenced in the literature and health promotion materials, some of which imply 'look after yourself and don't depend on others to do that for you', while others encourage abstinence and still others a consensual negotiation of sexual practices. For truly balanced negotiation to take place all partners concerned would need to be of equal power status and, it has been argued, have equal access to shared information (informed consent). The practice of negotiation is also informed by working towards a common goal, albeit often a compromised amalgamation of these goals.

While Westernised approaches to health promotion have increasingly drawn on human rights, choices and the protection of the rights of the individual to have sex etc., the media and legal representations are increasingly drawing on old and familiar discourses of blame and 'victimology'. Persson and Newman (2008, p. 639) say that 'although unprotected sex is mentioned as the mode of transmission … the focus is decisively on deception and criminal excess'. Thus, it is the not telling that is being increasingly seen as deviant, although establishing that in the law in terms of intentionality is incredibly difficult. Instead the law in England is concerned with 'reckless behaviour causing HIV' and a number of prosecutions have resulted from this. The focus here is on the person with HIV either not telling or lying about having HIV and/or not using a condom during sex. Clearly for the law to 'invade the bedroom' once again (and it does have a history of this so it is not unusual, particularly concerning practices that have been socially constructed as deviant) the ostensible intention is the setting up legal frameworks for safe and responsible sexual practices. Given that HIV is on the increase, and most people who get it 'claim' they didn't know the other person had HIV, the reasoning behind this legal practice is situated in 'punishing' this behaviour.

Useful resource

See the Terrence Higgins Trust website link to explore the implications and meanings of the law for sexual practices. Within this link are further discussion papers that challenge and consider issues of discrimination, stigmatisation and the inappropriate use of the law when considering the criminalisation of HIV transmission.

http://www.tht.org.uk/informationresources/prosecutions/

The complexities of disclosing and people's responses to HIV+ status can be related, as well as how people take responsibility for themselves and others. Discourses of individualism (see p. 92) and autonomy (p. 58) also play a part in this and it is no wonder that the field around this is so politically and personally dynamic and contested. If health policy is endeavouring to normalise the taking of the test, to destigmatise HIV, it is interesting that prevention, as in safe sex practices, is still an area that is contentious (see rights and responsibilities, p. 115).

Reflective activity

- How do you 'know' that your sexual partner is not HIV positive?
- How do you 'know' you are not HIV positive?
- When having sex who is responsible for practising safe sex?

Conclusion

The ongoing debates concerning HIV/AIDS indicate that there is no finite understanding of its complexities. Different discourses and theoretical positions clearly have an impact on the concerns of researchers, policy-makers, economists, moralists and the individual. Accessing the research chapter, as well as the chapters on theories and concepts regarding health, will give you further insight into this contested area.

Useful resources

Health Protection Agency: http://www.hpa.org.uk. The HPA provides data, from ongoing surveys, on UK HIV prevalence (defined as the proportion of people in a population who are infected with HIV) within various and particular populations, new diagnoses and treatments. It is also useful to get insight into how HIV is being positioned and prevention, management and treatments that are available in the UK. It is worth noting that the data available are based on that which is recorded and collected – see the survey discussion in the research chapter for a discussion of this.

NAM: http://www.Aidsmap.com/cms1038153.aspx. NAM produces and distributes accurate, up-to-date and evidence-based resources (printed, electronic, audio and on-line), covering both the medical and social aspects of HIV, to people living with HIV and to those who work to treat, support and care for them. Information on prevention, treatments and issues of living with HIV is provided.

Avert: http://www.avert.org.uk. This is another source of information, statistics and up-to-date news on areas affecting people living, or working, with HIV/AIDS. A good source of international statistics.

World Health Organisation (WHO): http://www.who.int/topics/hiv_aids/en/. This is a source of international and national statistics as well as information on what is happening worldwide in terms of responses, as well as recommendations for practice.

http://www.who.int/pmnch/MTT8pressrelease.pdf. This is a publication by the International Treatment Preparedness Coalition (April 2010) detailing the effects of government budget cuts and moratoriums on spending on the developing world.

Also look at the Terrence Higgins Trust (http://www.tht.org.uk/) and George House Trust (http://www.ght.org.uk/). These are two of the organisations that work with, and for, HIV+ populations.

www.sigmaresearch.org.uk. A social research group specialising in the behavioural and policy aspects of HIV and sexual health.

See also:

de Zulueta, P and Boulton, M. (2007) 'Routine Antenatal HIV Testing: The Responses and Perceptions of Pregnant Women and the Viability of Informed Consent. A Qualitative Study', *Journal of Medical Ethics*, 33, 329–36.

Elford, J. and Hart, G. (2005) 'HAART, Viral Load and Sexual Risk Behaviour', *AIDS*, 19, 205–7.

Lee, S. H. and Sheon, N. (2008) 'Responsibility and Risk: Accounts of Reasons for Seeking an HIV Test', *Sociology of Health and Illness*, 30(2), 167–81.

Leonard, L. and Ellen, J. M. (2008) '"The Story of My Life": AIDS and "Autobiographical Occasions"', *Qualitative Sociology*, 31, 37–56.

Scambler, G. and Paoli, F. (2008) 'Health Work, Female Sex Workers and HIV/AIDS: Global and Local Dimensions of Stigma and Deviance as Barriers to Effective Interventions', *Social Science and Medicine*, 66, 1848–62.

Sontag, S. (1991) *Illness as Metaphor and AIDS and Its Metaphors*. London: Penguin Books.

4

4.5 CASE STUDY 4: DEMENTIA

Introduction

We have chosen to look at dementia as it is once again a topic that is current within UK health policy as well as a concern for the UK more generally. The demographics of the country are such that the older population is growing, and it is the older population that is most vulnerable to dementia. The ways in which dementia are positioned, researched and considered vary widely and as health study students you will find that the material available for you to consider is vast. As with HIV, the most powerful discourse, that of biomedicine, is presented first. We look at what have been 'identified' as the signs of this condition and its impact in terms of cognitive, mental and physical impairment. Interestingly, research and discussion in dementia focus on both individuals with dementia and their carers, largely separately and occasionally together; though the approach has been historically somewhat different. Informal carers, i.e. family or friend carers, make up the bulk of those who offer and provide care for people with dementia, so the amount of research on this area makes sense. Given too how healthcare rationing (p. 85) informs care, as well as discourses of capitalism, communitarism and individualism, the continued emphasis on justifying informal care givers as a main resource needs to be explored further. What you will see is that when researching people with dementia the positivist school of **paradigms** dominates, while very often when researching carers there has been more emphasis on their experience, i.e. phenomenological and/or **social construction** paradigms. Research has been and is continuing in all areas, looking at how individuals cope, manage and understand the experience as well as looking at **EBP**, nursing home care and increasingly the experiences of people with dementia themselves.

4

Reflective activity

- Look up in at least three dictionaries the definitions of 'demented'.
- What are the connotations of being described as demented?
- Consider the following sentence: 'She was demented, absolutely demented – throwing things around, yelling and shouting – well out of order.' What ideas do you form of this woman who has been so described?

Biomedical definitions of dementia

First, dementia is a broad term used to describe a clinically identified condition (DoH 2007), of which Alzheimer's disease (AD) is the most common (Cunningham and Archibald 2006). The term dementia is an umbrella term used to connote symptoms that emerge when the brain is affected by various and specific conditions (DoH 2007). NHS Choices provides the following definition: 'Dementia is a syndrome (a group of related symptoms) that is associated with an ongoing decline of the brain and its abilities. These include: memory, thinking, language, understanding, judgement.' (NHS Choices 2010b). Tolson et al. (1999, p. 1128) define it as 'a non specific label, which is usually used to describe a progressive and chronic loss of memory'. Zwakhalen et al. (2007, p. 494) define it as 'a syndrome characterized by progressive decline in the cortical functions'. They go on to say 'there is no such thing as a typical patient with dementia'. The WHO (2009) also describes dementia as a 'syndrome due to disease of the brain, usually of a chronic or progressive nature'. The commonalities between these definitions seem to be:

> syndrome;
> progressive and/or chronic;
> related to the brain;
> loss of memory;
> impacts on mental abilities.

Detecting and measuring dementia

What is also worth noting is the comment that Zwakhalen et al. (2007) make about there being no typical individual and/or patient. **EBP**, epidemiology, **RCT**, systematic reviews, experiments and deductive reasoning are central to how dementia is understood, as well as informing and reflecting practice priorities. Valid and reliable research using these methods has had to find ways of ascertaining the level or degree and specific 'type' of dementia in the individual and have devised all manner of tools to do just that. What can be used is an interview based rating scale and screening tool, and many of these exist. Their purpose is to bring together the research evidence and utilise this as a way of measuring and ascertaining whether or not an individual has dementia – the most popular or widely used is known as the Mini-Mental State Examination (MMSE). There are, and continue to be, tests developed to identify dementia and its stages, aspects and so on. Dementia funding largely focuses on 'finding the cure', 'managing the condition', 'reducing/slowing down its progression' and finally developing tests that will identify dementia as early and effectively as possible.

Finally, the third source of information is located on the Alzheimer's Society (2010) website and discusses the most popular and commonly used assessment tool, the MMSE.

Reflective activity

Take a five-minute dementia test. Follow the links below:
http://www.timesonline.co.uk/tol/life_and_style/health/article6469784.ece
http://www.alzheimers.org.uk/site/scripts/documents_info.php?categoryID=200292&documentID=121
What did you think of these tests? Would you consider them accurate?

Biomedical range of dementias

The field of biomedicine is very complex, and within the space available here it is impossible to fully explain, or unpack, the vast area of neurological science associated with each of these conditions. Presented below is a brief summary of the wide range of material available. In order to have a far more detailed understanding you will need to read further around the topic and engage with the vast amount of literature available.

Alzheimer's disease (AD)

This is seen as most common form of dementia, making up 50–55 per cent (Killeen 2000; McKeith and Fairbairn 2001; Cunningham and Archibald 2006). AD affects the structure of the brain and leads to cell death. The onset of the disease can be gradual and the decline is often slow and gradual (DoH 2007). Cunningham and Archibald (2006, pp. 52–3; McKeith and Fairbairn 2001) define it as follows: 'it is a degenerative disease affecting the brain. As a result of the changes in the structure and function of two proteins ... plaque and neurofibrillary tangle form in areas of brain tissue, which destroy them ... the temporal and parietal lobes of the brain are generally affected ... which can result in significant memory loss and an inability to recognise people and places.' McKeith and Fairbairn (2001) emphasise the progressive and global nature of AD, citing loss of memory, language skills, practical abilities, social judgment and insight, with personality and behaviour being altered, and these are all accumulative.

Lewy body dementia (DLB)

Lewy body dementia is another common form of dementia: estimates range from 4 per cent (Alzheimer's Society 2009), to 20 per cent (McKeith and Fairbairn 2001; Cunningham and Archibald 2006) and possibly 36 per cent (Del Ser et al. 2000). It is often hard to diagnose and identify as DLB; the Alzheimer's Society (2009) indicate that it has similarities with both AD and Parkinson's disease (Cunningham and Archibald 2006). McKeith and Fairbairn (2001, p. 15) write that 'The central characteristic of dementia with Lewy bodies ... is fluctuating cognitive impairment with periods of increased confusion and windows of relative lucidity ... as the disease progresses more persistent cognitive impairment and neuropsychiatric features become apparent.' Cunningham and Archibald (2006) describe it in very similar terms and go on to say that it can also result in hallucinations, delusions and falls.

Vascular dementia

This is seen as the second most common form of dementia (20 per cent according to Cunningham and Archibald 2006) and occurs both as a distinct condition (10 per cent: McKeith and Fairbairn 2001) and in conjunction with AD (10 per cent: McKeith and Fairbairn 2001). It is often caused by mini strokes, so it can be quite sudden in onset and lead to what is known as 'cell death' (DoH 2007) and to cognitive impairment (Sander 2002; Cunningham and Archibald 2006); again the parts of the brain that can be damaged are those related to speech, language and memory (Cunningham and Archibald 2006). Cantley (2001, p. 327) provides a fairly broad definition of vascular dementia 'due to stroke disease or impaired blood flow in the brain. Onset is often sudden and symptoms may be focused on a specific area of functioning rather than a more global impairment. Deterioration may be stepwise.' Finally, McKeith and Fairbairn (2001) indicate that vascular dementia is not the single cause of dementia but is often found in association with other pathologies, such as AD.

Other forms of dementia are as follows:

> Pick's disease;
> Huntingdon's disease;
> Creutzfeldt-Jakob disease (CJD).

Biomedically defined symptoms of dementia

Alongside the symptoms that are mentioned above, the DoH's (2007, pp. 11–12) publication *Who Cares? Information and Support for the Carers of People with Dementia* lists the following:

> Be very forgetful, especially of recent events and people's names.
> Be muddled about time, day, place and unable to find their way around familiar surroundings
> Have difficulty in talking, and often repeat themselves.
> Be unable to make sense of what is said to them.
> Have difficulty with carrying out household tasks and neglect personal hygiene.
> Put themselves at risk by leaving pans to boil dry or gas fires unlit.
> Behave inappropriately, like going out in their nightclothes or wandering around the streets at night.
> Hide or lose things and accuse others of stealing them.
> See or hear things that are not there.
> Become angry, upset or aggressive very easily.

In the later stages of the disease people may:

> Be unable to remember things they have just said or done.
> Not recognise known faces and familiar objects.
> Be unable to express themselves.
> Be unable to understand what is said to them.
> Be very restless, especially at night.
> Try to carry out actions or re-live events from their past.
> Be unable to carry out household and personal hygiene tasks without a lot of help and supervision.

> Have bladder and bowel incontinence.
> Have to use a wheelchair.
> Be bedridden.

Reflective activity

Choose three of the 'symptoms' from the list above:

- How many people do you know have displayed these behaviours?
- How many people over the age of 60 or 65 have displayed these behaviours?
- Why do you think, or know, they behave like this?

The point of the exercise above is to touch on the difficulties associated with identifying particularly early signs of dementia. Many of the early signs are similar to those of stigmatised stereotypes of getting older, as well as being descriptors associated with mental health issues, stress and depression (Victor 2005; Age Concern and Mental Health Foundation 2006).

Demographics and spread

Dementia is very common in the UK population and the most vulnerable to it are the elderly (Sweeting and Gilhooly 1997; Tolson et al. 1999; McKeith and Fairbairn 2001; DoH 2009). Tolson et al. (1999) and Ott et al. (1995) consider the increase in prevalence of dementia as people grow older and McKeith and Fairbairn (2001) state that at 75 this prevalence is about 10 per cent and thereon after every five years this prevalence doubles. Cunningham and Archibald (2006) state that dementia affects one in every 20 people over the age of 65, and at 90 years and over this rises to one in every three people. According to DoH figures as of 2009, about 700,000 people in the UK have dementia, and of these at least 15,000 are under the age of 65. The DoH (2009) estimates that as the proportion of our overall population increases in age so will the number of individuals with dementia; so by 2038 there will be at least 1.4 million individuals living with dementia.

4

Reflective activity

Access the two documents below for further information on demography and its implication for future practice:

http://www.kingsfund.org.uk/document.rm?id=8277 [A 2006 publication that provides demographic details of spread.]

http://www.publications.parliament.uk/pa/cm200910/cmhansrd/cm100316/halltext/100316h0001.htm [This is a Hansard report of a debate on the government's dementia strategy, which took place in the House of Commons on 16 March 2010. Note the consideration of demography, costs and concerns regarding research spending and finally the dominance of biomedical models as a way of framing this discussion.]

Context as an important informer to all fields of dementia

The word dementia itself is Latin-derived, meaning 'without mind' (McKeith and Fairbairn 2001). The historical and cultural understandings of madness and mental instability were such that individuals were not considered to be human, the very essence of being a human being our ability to think, feel and be self aware and conscious (see mind–body dualism, p. 99, Kitwood's model of personhood, p. 177, citizenship, p. 115, and Descartes, p. 38). Thus, individuals with any form of mental impairment were often sectioned away and separated from the rest of society (being unwanted and, therefore, better off unseen). Their treatment was informed by the notion of them being 'diseased' and subhuman; they were considered a danger to the rest of society and something to be feared. To have a relative who developed such behaviours was often seen to be shameful and something to be shut away.

Reflective activity

In what ways do you think our treatment of people with dementia now differs (and from when)?

Challenging meanings and responses

Our responses to how we may understand dementia are still informed by these discourses – Sweeting and Gilhooly (1997) undertook a fascinating piece of research on the notion of social death – such that older people with dementia, having increasingly compromised abilities to be 'productive', are positioned as lacking in value, being seen as a burden and therefore excluded from everyday life (often put away into homes, separate from the rest of society and reducing their ability to interact and engage in that world). This is an interesting response given that research clearly indicates that isolation, lack of a sense of purpose and reduction in meaningful social interaction can further impact on the experience and indeed development of dementia (Gilliard et al 2005; Parker 2005; Age Concern and Mental Health Foundation 2006; Gould and Kendall 2007).

Alternative views to biomedical cause and effect responses can start from a position that considers present responses to dementia as being the antithesis of Maslow's Hierarchy of Need (1943), except perhaps the basic provision of food, shelter and concepts of safety, i.e. as being often interpreted as for their own good (Parker 2005; Bartlett and O'Connor 2007; Baldwin and Bradford Dementia Group 2008). The question here is: whose concepts of safety are these? Positive and negative meanings of liberty, in particular the government's role in deciding 'who knows best', are a useful point from which to explore this issue. Kitwood's (1997) notion of personhood – which emerged as a result of the hegemony of biomedical science – saw that responses removed practices of creative autonomy and reduced the freedom, and questioned the capacity for free will, of individuals with dementia. Seedhouse's five foundations for 'good health' can also be seen to be negated in favour of cause and effect practice, which measures intervention and outcome on pre-tested tools that cannot take into account individualised experiences of dementia (see challenges to RCT, p. 292, EBP, p. 192, epidemiology, p. 194).

The function of stigma in making sense of dementia

Goffman (1963), a main theorist concerning the function of stigmatisation (see poststructuralism, p. 49, **social construction**), wrote about the active power of being given a title or label. First, it can be the central way of describing and understanding self and others; second, it can also act to subsume all other aspects of the individual so that all they become is that stigmatised identity. There are links here too to symbolic interactionism (see p. 242) and the article, which is discussed in the research chapter, may be of further use to you.

According to Milne (2010), 'stigma against older people with dementia ... is widespread and its consequences [are] far reaching ... stigma accentuates and deepens the distress experienced by the person with dementia, adding to their existing disability' (Milne 2010, p. 227–8; citing WHO 2003; Thornicroft 2006).

The Alzheimer's Society and Mental Health Foundation (2008, p. 5) also centralise the function of stigmatisation in the field of dementia. For them it acts in a multiplicity of ways, echoing Goffman's (1963) thesis that stigma is both a construction and an active force. For them 'The stigma of dementia is very pervasive. Media representation of dementia often did not help but the research indicated that the reaction of people close to them, as well as the responses of professionals, had a more detrimental impact on people with dementia and their carers.'

The National Dementia Strategy (DoH 2009) explicitly acknowledges the role of stigma in dementia and one of its core policy aims is 'addressing stigma and raising public awareness'. Link and Phelan's (2001), Grahame et al.'s (2003) and Milne's (2010) discussion of stigma sees strategies that are needed to tackle stigma head on as needing to be informed by demystifying it, openly talking about it and endeavouring to demonstrate the 'humanity and capacities' of people with dementia, which challenge the 'disaster scenario attitudes', recognising that dementia has a number of stages and that people within the mild and moderate stages can function relatively normally and independently.

Talking about it and getting dementia out into the open, instead of locating it in the shadows, seems to be strongly supported by biomedicine as well. However, the focus of some biomedicine, in terms of the manifestations of this stigma and resultant discrimination, is more on finding cures, causes and reduction or management interventions, as opposed to improving the quality of care and interactions, and this has been a very powerful voice. Thus Wilkinson (2005) challenges the discrimination and stigmatisation of people with dementia as being evident in funding of research. Figures from 2005 indicate that the costs of Alzheimer's disease in older people outstrip those of CHD, cancer and stroke combined, but the research funding is 10 per cent of that on heart disease and

4

only 3 per cent of that on cancer. Interestingly Milne (2010) writes about dementia research as being 'big business', often focused, as previously suggested, on cures. Wilkinson's (2005) claim, while probably still holding true in terms of proportion, has developed from there – not least, as some cynical commentators have suggested, because of fears around the growing cost of care.

Pulsford et al. (2000), Cunningham and Archibald (2006), Clare et al. (2008), MacRae (2008) and Parsons et al. (2008) are among many researchers who position stigma in terms of how we understand dementia as a 'disease'. For them the progressive nature of dementia is often elided into the final stage, when independence and cognitive abilities are more fully compromised, with a significant effect on the course of dementia itself. Their research is with individuals with dementia themselves, in the various stages of dementia. Their findings indicate how many of the individuals know they have dementia and know they are going to get worse, and how very often they are treated by carers, health professionals and their families as if they are already in the acute stage.

According to Wilkinson (2005), Poole (2006), the Alzheimer's Society (2010), Milne (2010) and Age Concern the result of stigma (as well as the complexities of identification), similarly to HIV, can result in a slowness of the individual to present for diagnosis, for the family to recognise the potential signs, for doctors to identify it and for it be responded to in ways that allow options and approaches to be explored. Given that the construction of dementia is largely defined by the last acute stage, and often responded to with horror, pity, fear and disgust (Behuniak 2010), as well as there being seen to be no possible cure and the symptoms being seen as inevitable, it is no wonder that delays and denials proliferate.

4

Reflective activity

Given that dementia is often also positioned in discourses of mental health:

- What are the popular characteristics of people with mental health issues?
- What similarities are there with how we describe people with dementia?
- What are the stigmas attached to both?

Discourses of ageism

Stigma within dementia interweaves with stigmas of mental health as well as our attitudes to age. Ageism is a hugely powerful and all-pervading form of stereotype and discrimination in the UK. Milne (2010, p. 228) defines age discrimination as representing 'an important element of the way in which older people experience later life and gain access to socially-valued roles and resources. It functions to reinforce age-related norms and perpetuate assumptions about old ages and ageing as a process.' Research carried out by Age Concern and the Mental Health Foundation in 2006 found that age discrimination impacted on overall **well-being**, and acted to exclude older people from everyday life and opportunities. They also found that age discrimination had a multiplicity of impacts on older people, including contributing to feelings of worthlessness and despair. It impacts on self-esteem in terms of both lowering it and lowering their expectations, and finally it was found to create practical barriers in terms of service delivery and opportunities – all of which was informed by an often pervasive attitude of disrespect.

Reflective activity

- What do you feel about getting old?
- What are your fears and concerns?

One response to this has been the Employment Equality (Age) Regulations (2006), which in the first instance focus on addressing ageist discrimination in employment, education and training. This is to be rolled out to include 'banning' unfair discrimination against adults when providing goods and services, including health and social care services, when the relevant part of the Act comes into force – which according to Age Concern (2009) (now called Age UK: For Later Life; see http://www.ageuk.org.uk/) is anticipated to be 2012.

Challenges to the dominance of biomedical meanings

What has already been made clear even in the reductionist and epistemologically positivist approaches to biomedical science is how very complicated identifying, and treating, symptoms of dementia is. Given the complexities of measuring a syndrome that is so multifaceted, there are various models of practice considered appropriate to work with people with dementia. The most widely used in healthcare is epistemologically informed by the medical model (Gould and Kendall 2005), one that sees dementia as a progressive neurodegenerative disease (Parker 2005; Zwakhalen et al. 2007; National Dementia Strategy 2009). Thus interventions are designed around **EBP** and are largely evidenced through experimental, cause and effect **RCTs** and systematic reviews (see p. 288). Clearly, these measures are limited in many ways and standards of practice in nursing homes, as well as outside nursing homes, have been criticised for being substandard and lacking in diversity and humanity.

4

Useful resource

Look at the reports on the Alzheimer's Society website based on research carried out in 2009 on quality of care:

http://alzheimers.org.uk/site/scripts/news_article.php?newsID=579

http://www.pronurse.co.uk/news/articles/2173-dementia-care-standards-in-england-criticised

The two reports are particularly focused on hospital care.

Using your own search strategies and engines find five media articles, over the past four years, which report on poor care in nursing homes.

A more humanistic and holistic model, the enriched model of care/dialectic model (Poole 2006, Gould and Kendall 2007, Thomas Pocklington Trust 2009), has its roots in the work of Thomas Kitwood (1997). While this is intended as an integrated model, addressing social and physical health, individual personality, personal biography and cognitive impairment (Thomas Pocklington Trust 2009), the challenges to both care homes and informal care givers to provide this quality of interaction are great. Gould and Kendall's (2005) paper on developing guidelines for NICE/SCIE looks at these difficulties, particularly informed by the contrasting **epistemological** approaches informed by healthcare and medicine, and the social model of care that informs social work. Their paper gives useful insights into the process of endeavouring to bring these together, as well as suggesting that the guidelines are just that – that interpretation and implementation are far more relevant when considering how practice is carried out.

Despite the acceptance, by government and various health bodies, of Kitwood's work in terms of 'informing the rhetoric of care', researchers challenge the idea that this is actually what is happening in practice (Gilliard et al. 2005; Parker 2005; National Dementia Strategy 2009). The difficulty here is that healthcare rationing (see p. 85), capitalism (see p. 32), stigmatisation (see p. 118), discrimination and contested notions of personhood (more of that later) are clearly acting as mediators (Grahame et al. 2003, Bartlet and O'Connor 2007, Behuniak 2010, Milne 2010) to how practice is carried out.

Equality

Wilkinson (2005, p. 6) states: 'A major obstacle to developing more effective treatments for dementia is that society does not value its elder citizens, even though our current prosperity and freedom are based on their sacrifices and on the back of their labour.' Not only is Wilkinson positioning ageism as a powerful force in determining funding, he is also, usefully, considering healthcare equality as being implicit within the debates. Forder (2008) discusses the impact of equality on health and social care provision, unpacking it in terms of equality of resources, outcomes and opportunity – the idea, in theory, is that everyone will have access to equal resources, to ensure that outcomes, i.e. well-being and a good quality of life, are achieved. But what if equal quality of life is mediated by ageism, discrimination and stigma?

Forder (2008, p. 5), in her report on 'The Costs of Addressing Age Discrimination in Social Care', considers that equality in health and social care is informed by a capabilities approach that 'focuses on ensuring that people have the same substantive freedoms, that is the capability to achieve the same outcomes should they choose to do so. In this way equality of capability requires account and compensation for all factors ... apart from preferences and effort.' Underpinning this model are ideas of choice and the market forces of capitalism, as well as a complex interweaving of free will (see p. 80), body–mind dualism (see p. 55), health as a personal strength (see p. 18), liberal individualism (see p. 44) and the role of the government; and of course creating and respecting autonomy (see p. 99).

Kitwood (1997), Graham et al. (2003), Davis (2004) and Milne (2010) consider the function of 'normalising' (see p. 109) and stigmatising stereotypes as a way of informing this approach. Who decides what is 'normal' for an older person to achieve?' What is a 'normal' level of capabilities for someone with dementia? The challenge here is that research clearly shows that care provided can indeed be informed by this principle, but the principle is informed not by 'objective and deductive reasoning' as would be claimed, but by ageism, stereotypical ideas of older people and their needs, and discrimination in the treatment of mental health. Forder (2008, p. 7) indicates that 'per head' the elderly (and the definition of this population varies, but is usually considered to be within either the old age pension definitions, or aged 65 and over) have less spent on them than any other age group category. One of the reasons for this is 'the result of discrimination, that is, a state of affairs whereby older people receive support which allows them to achieve lower levels of capability than younger people'. What is interesting is that, according to results published by Individual Budgets (IBSEN), which take into account differing needs and levels of capabilities, older people (over 65) would require a 25 per cent increase in support to meet the qualitative age differences in spending across ages 18–64.

The cost of care

Deciding to discuss costs and healthcare rationing so early on in this case is deliberate. It plays a huge role in the way dementia is responded to, and indeed how it is managed. Discourses of capitalism (the valuing of the individual based on their productivity), autonomy (our ideas about what makes someone autonomous), considerations of free will, the government's role and personal liberty, as well as individualism, play a part in the healthcare rationing of dementia. Given not only that our population is ageing but that we are living to greater ages, it is not that surprising that the number of, and therefore the cost of caring for, people with dementia will increase. This is a cause for concern for the government. The estimated current spending on caring for individuals with dementia is £17 billion, with this expected to increase to over £50 billion in 2038 (DoH 2009).

The Care Services Improvement Partnership – Older People's Mental Health Programme produced a document in 2007 (as part of the National Dementia Strategy), 'Strengthening the Involvement of People with Dementia', which looked at how individuals with dementia and those involved in their care can improve and inform practice, particularly focused on the quality of care received. Part of this concern is influenced by Kitwood's (1997) work on the importance of actively engaging with people with dementia as persons (as opposed to positioning them as bodies in need of particular interventions to maintain baseline standards of life). Drivers to health care rationing will also be informed by our current political climate and the market approach to providing healthcare, as well as ageism and stigmatisation.

The National Dementia Strategy (2009) is also indicative of the government's concern regarding the costs of dementia – its main aims are to raise awareness, increase early diagnosis and intervention, and improve the quality of care. These three areas reflect much of the areas of research themselves. There is, as of yet, no cure for dementia but research has tested, and provided, a number of pharmaceutical interventions that may facilitate and even slow down the impact of the syndromes on the individual. Given that it is at the acute/final stage that care costs are the greatest (Wilkinson 2005), early diagnosis would enable these interventions to be put into place earlier. As many researchers note, the difficulty with diagnosis is that symptoms can be very gradual and are often connected with our stereotypes and typified understanding of ageing. For instance, it is 'known' (Tolson et al. 1999) that the most definitive diagnosis of AD can only be made on a brain biopsy. Often otherwise it is a matter, as has already been mentioned, of symptom identification or indeed symptom and disease exclusion.

Reflective activity

- Compare how the NHS and media represent the future predicted cost of obesity with the future predicted cost of dementia.
- What are the similarities and differences?

Challenging contexts and understandings of dementia

We hope that what you will be realising as you read through this chapter is that the area of dementia knowledge and research is ongoing and vast. The approaches used vary from purely biomedical – increasingly looking for a cure as well as pharmacological ways to reduce its effect and manage it (Wilkinson 2005) – to sociological, psychological and political models of understanding.

Living with dementia: alternative models of understanding

The DoH (2009) in 'Living Well with Dementia: A National Dementia Strategy' provides an overview of the difficulties people with dementia will have and includes 'thinking clearly, remembering things, communicating, doing day-to-day things like cooking or getting dressed'; it also explains that people may have problems with 'being depressed, mood swings and aggression, wandering or getting lost' (DH 2009, pp. 7–8). Zwakhalen et al. (2007) in their research on assessing pain in older people with dementia consider how compromised communication ability, and a varied range of behavioural and response 'repertoires', impact on individuals' ability to communicate their experience of pain. Given that very often tools for measuring pain tend to be reductionist and limited to proscriptive scales and categories, it is not that surprising that individuals who do not have recourse to what is construed as 'normalised' functioning may be excluded from these measurements.

McKeith and Fairbairn (2001) found that parts of the brain can be impacted upon by dementia and these include the areas that inform our moods and memory, our ability to learn and retain information, our language, speech, motor, balance and body awareness skills, and our engagement with meanings, judgements, decision-making and complex behaviours to name a few. Kitwood (1997) and others have found that symptoms can be impacted upon by how we experience and understand the progressive nature of dementia – McRae (2008) is one of many researchers who call into question the notion that dementia (or to be specific in terms of her research AD) is simply a biomedical progressive syndrome and instead posit that how the individual and the people around the individual respond, and treat, the individual with AD can have a profound impact on the progression and experience of dementia.

Kitwood (1997) is a seminal researcher in the area of dementia and introduced the notion of personhood in individuals with dementia; that is, that dementia was more than just a neurological anomaly but related to the whole person. His premise is built on and around person-centred theory (Rogers 1957) and the treatment of individuals with dementia in terms of quality of life and well-being. For Kitwood (1997) the understanding of personhood and dementia rested on interactive and interpersonal relationships, believing that some of the deterioration in people with dementia was not from the disease itself but was from their treatment and loss of independence, purpose and worth. Kitwood and subsequent theorists went a long way to improving care of older people (Bartlett and O'Connor 2007), and have encouraged a widening of the lens in terms of the progressive nature of dementia. So, rather than it being situated only in very clearly defined, measured and sequential stages of decline, he helped to broaden it to include recognitions that personal history, interactions with others, how one is perceived and situated in a social context, freedom and respect also impact on quality of life, performance and behaviour (Kitwood 1997; Bartlett and O'Connor 2007).

4

Kitwood's work was very important in moving the work and understanding around dementia from the simple biomedical model to one concerning personhood – the focus of Kitwood's work and indeed the DoH (2009) Dementia Strategy is on the recognition of the individuality and humanity of the individual with dementia. It also recognises that respect, trust and compassion should be integral to all care offered to people with dementia. In Kitwood's person-centred approach to dementia care he 'contends that the maintenance of personhood through the promotion of subjective well-being should be the principal aim of such care … well-being is a function of the quality of the interaction between the person with dementia and his or her professional carers' (Pulsford et al. 2000).

Brannelly (2006), referring to Kitwood's ethos, writes about the ethic of care, as a way of assessing the quality of care offered to individuals with dementia. Research around the quality of care given can be found to focus on either institutional care (incidental acute and ongoing care in care homes as well as care provided in the community) or informal care. Informal care can be defined as 'unpaid care (financial support for full time carers is available though this can be very patchy), ranging from round-the-clock tending to occasional acts of assistance, provided by family members of friends to individual' (Adamson and Donovan 2005, p. 37). Research clearly shows that informal care by the family is by far the most important and indeed available care for older people (Pickard et al. 2000; Adamson and Donovan 2004). It goes without saying that the government takes full advantage, drawing on discourses of rights and responsibilities and communitarism as a way of packaging support and information for informal carers.

Reflective activity

- Follow this link for people talking about their experiences of living with Alzheimer's as part of the 2008 Report 'Dementia: Out of the Shadows': http://www.alzheimers.org.uk/outoftheshadows
- How do you feel after watching this?

Personhood and beyond

Kitwood's model has been challenged, interestingly enough very much along the same lines that feminists challenge interpretative (see p. 226) and positivist (see p. 227) research, as being depoliticised. Bartlett and O'Connor (2007) do not doubt the importance in Kitwood's personhood model in terms of challenging the dominant biomedical responses as well as stigma and discrimination in dementia, but question its framing of people outside discourses of rights and citizenship. Baldwin and the Bradford Dementia Group (2008) consider that the link between the personal and political has to be made obvious and then acted on to inform policy and care. Baldwin and the Bradford Dementia Group's (2008) research is on the narratives of people living with dementia, and was done with the respondents, using their own frameworks and ways of communicating. It is well known that communication is impacted upon by dementia, and given the short amount of time in terms of intervention, and the propensity to 'render abnormal' the modes of communication, and as a consequence the content, it is little wonder that people with dementia's voice is so seldom, if at all, heard in any policy development (Baldwin and the Bradford Dementia Group 2008). Moore and Davis's (2002, p. 263) research on giving a voice to people with dementia found that 'the person with moderate or moderately severe dementia may be able to present only fragments of a performance story. The more a nurse knows about narrative components or the different sections of a story, the

4

more easily he or she can identify and follow up on a story fragment offered by a persons with dementia.'

Notions of citizenship have been used to understand other marginalised and discriminated again groups (Bartlett and O'Connor 2007; Baldwin and the Bradford Dementia Group 2008). When related to dementia it essentially positions people with dementia as having agency, power and citizenship (rights and responsibilities). It considers, as do social models of disability (Gilliard et al. 2005; Parker 2005), that discriminatory, often socio-political, structures exist that act as barriers to the full citizenship and personhood of the individual. These barriers can be received understanding of dementia, the function of dismissal and our belief that everyone with dementia is 'off their heads'. White (2008; cited in Behuniak 2010, p. 7) also talks about the function of responses to the vulnerable, contending that there is 'resentment that arises from the stress of the burden placed on the stronger to respond to the needs of the weaker; pity that is born of noticing the suffering, but that waives the responsibility for addressing it; and compassion that stems from recognizing shared, mutual vulnerability and that is rooted in equality and autonomy'. For Behuniak (2010) the first two responses do not particularly reflect values of equality or democracy, and could clearly be added to the barriers that exist for people with dementia to live as fully engaged lives as possible. Clearly another barrier to thinking of people with dementia as having citizenship, beyond name only, is the 'ability to think' (Bartlett and O'Connor 2007). This opens up a huge debate about what it is to be a person and what it is to think, and if you would like to explore this further then the writings of René Descartes (see p. 38) would be a useful starting point.

However, citizenship in conjunction with personhood, and taking in the social and political context, could be developed to be 'unconditional and inclusive rather than dismiss the concept out of hand' (Bartlett and O'Connor 2007, p. 114). One has only to remember that in the UK neither women nor people of 'the non-property owning' classes were at one time considered citizens: they had no right to their income, their bodies, the vote, their freedom – concepts of citizenship. Thus these concepts are not fixed but always in flux.

> the citizenship model ... suggests that people with dementia have a unique contribution to make to our society ... Many people with dementia go through a period of great creativity if they are given the opportunity to express it. Other contributions such as emotional veracity and humour, as well as an example of fortitude in the face of major trauma, are often undervalued. (Marshall 2005, p. 18; cited in Baldwin and the Bradford Dementia Group 2008, p. 226)

The role of compassion

Behuniak's (2010) work looks at how compassion can be and has been lost in how we have responded to and positioned people with dementia. Our responses, often fuelled by fear and pity, function to further stigmatise people with dementia. Like Bartlett and O'Connor (2007) and Baldwin and the Bradford Dementia Group (2008) she considers the necessity of developing a political model of care, but one that openly acknowledges our vulnerability. 'This would mean responding to the challenges of individuals with dementia by addressing their dependence, their gradual cognitive decline, their continued humanity, their rights as adult members of society, and their vulnerability to those who would use power over them' (Behuniak 2010, p. 8). The role of compassion – defined here as 'compassion that stems from recognizing shared, mutual vulnerability and that is rooted in equality and autonomy' (Behuniak 2010, p. 7) – needs to be deeply embedded in a political model of ethical care.

Carers and caring

Research around home care is often focused on the experience of being a carer and indeed the impact of caring on the individual(s) involved. Briggs et al. (2003) carried out an observational piece of work that looked at how carers organised care and developed routines and interactions with their relatives. Cooper et al. (2007) provides a systematic review of interventions for anxiety for people caring for dementia patients. It is well known that anxiety and depression are two of the most common mental health problems that carers of people with dementia experience (Russo et al. 1995; Mahoney et al. 2005). Adamson and Donovan (2005) were particularly interested in looking at South Asian and African/Caribbean relatives' experiences of care giving, and Sweeting and Gilhooly (1997) were interested in exploring the perceptions of carers regarding how they related to and saw the person they were caring for. They all acknowledge the amount of work it requires, particularly as the dementia progresses and becomes more acute. McRae (2008) discusses how very often an individual with dementia is related to and treated as if already in the acute stages – that the power of the term itself can result in particular interventions from all sectors that are designed to manage and reduce the impact on others rather than enabling individuals to find ways of managing their condition.

Certainly the intention regarding institutional care (and indeed the information and support given to informal carers) is increasingly built around person-centred care philosophy and practice; this locates the patient as an individual deserving of respect, compassion, dignity and being treated as a person with all the aspects that that entails. Kitwood (1997) and Brannelly (2006, p. 199) define this care as follows, and central to this is the quality of the relationship and engagement between the person with dementia and the practitioner:

> reciprocity, bodily and spiritual care, biography (Sabat 2006);
> relationship-based care (Nolan et al. 2001);
> practitioner knowledge;

> power;
> personal and contractual involvement;
> initiating, building and sustaining relationships (Peplau 1988);
> interdisciplinary working;
> resources;
> quality of care provision.

These aspects form a part of how care is intended to be managed and certainly how strategies of care are planned and considered. Much of the focus of this type of research has been on the quality of care, the role of the carer, interventions and awareness – the National Dementia Strategy (2009) very much reflects this too. On 21 July 2009 a pilot scheme (with the intention to roll it out nationally) was commenced whereby dementia specialists will be introduced to 22 areas in the UK, with the eventual plan being that such specialists would be available to every general hospital and care home, with mental health teams to assess people with dementia (DoH 2009).

Range of care

The range of symptoms and behaviours that accompany dementia, and the challenge to provide care that is individually designed, cannot be underestimated. Looking at the organisation of caring for people in nursing homes (Gilliard et al. 2005; Parker 2005; Gould and Kendall 2007) the emphasis could be argued to be more concerned with control, management, making things easy (for the workers) etc. People with dementia can be very challenging to nurse and care for, particularly in the acute stages. Tolson et al. (1999) researched the challenges of providing care for people with dementia who were also acutely ill; they noted that nursing care for individuals with dementia was seen by the 'consumer' (i.e. patient) to be at its best when delivered in tandem with dementia care. Thus, much of the nursing was done without holistic care and the chronic confusion was not part of the care plan. Cunningham and Archibald (2006) also researched the challenge to practitioners of nursing people with dementia – while research is very clear about the relationship between communication and personal interactions and the well-being of the individual with dementia, what can and does happen in acute (and not just acute) settings may differ depending on what the individual without dementia believes. While it has been found that people with dementia can indeed communicate and contribute to their care, 'the opportunity for this sort of communication is largely dependent on whether the person without dementia believes that communication is possible … these patients can become disempowered, infantilised and intimidated, and the likelihood of this is increased in busy hospital settings' (Cunningham and Archibald 2006, p. 53; Goldsmith 1996; Cheston and Bendar 1999).

Pulsford et al. (2000) found that when working with moderate and severe dementia within a care setting, using sensory motor therapies proved most effective when the practitioners were themselves very active and directive and able to empathise with their individual patients and with their limitations. Clare et al. (2008), in their research with residents of a care home, found that many individuals' psychological health, well-being and need to retain their own sense of identity were still very much in evidence. Many of them were able to express their sense of isolation, confinement, loneliness and lack of self-determination and self-control. Often attitudes towards people with dementia are that they are unaware of what is happening around them – therefore potentially leading to beliefs that this lack of awareness results in no felt feelings or psychological repertoire. Go back to the history of dementia and what Sweeting and Gilhooly (1997) and Kitwood (1997) talk about in terms of personhood. If an essential core to being seen as a person is our ability to hold information and remember and recognise and indeed communicate our experience in what are considered appropriate ways, then when we stop being able to do this are we considered to be socially dead?

Sudnow (1967, p. 74) provided a definition of this phenomenon in terms of 'that point at which socially relevant attributes of the patient begin permanently to cease to be operative as conditions for treating him, and when he is essentially regarded as already dead'. Kalish (1966) divides this into 'self-perceived social death', where individuals see themselves as being as good as dead, and 'other perceived dead', where it is the other person who sees the individual as to all intents and purposes dead (Sweeting and Gilhooly 1997). So Clare et al.'s (2008) research feeds into this symbolic interactionist view by finding that the way in which the practitioners in a nursing home treated, cared for and managed dementia residents was informed by their understanding of dementia; this in turn impacts on the resident in ways that contribute to feelings of disempowerment and dependency. This is an intriguing conundrum to try to unravel – particularly as the notion that as dementia progresses and cognitive abilities are increasingly compromised the ability of the individual to contribute in some way to their own care becomes more contentious (Tolson et al. 1999; McKeith and Fairbairn 2001; Cunningham and Archibald 2006; Zwakhalen et al. 2007)

Ongoing debates

The contrast between what the intentions of dementia care are and what research shows people within homes to experience can be seen (Ballard et al. 2001, Clare et al. 2008) and headlines in papers over the past few years, e.g. 'Elderly people suffering abuse and neglect in residential care homes' (*The Times* 15 August 2007), 'Thousands of elderly abused in care homes' (*Daily Telegraph* 4 May 2008), offer up worrying examples of areas for concern.

But what informs care in residential homes for older people, acute care, our treatment and understanding of age generally speaking? How may our beliefs and attitudes to disabilities, mental health illnesses, getting old, becoming physically less able etc. impact on how we position age and dementia? What happens when getting old and being chronically ill elide – how may our discourses around these inform how we treat and manage care? In Western societies people are valued largely on their productive output and/or potential. Older people can be devalued, stereotyped and excluded by institutional, societal and structural forces that render older people a burden (Sweeting and Gilhooly 1997). Evans (1997) talks about the rationing of health care according to age, and Falconer and O'Neil (2007) write about the impact of meanings attached to older people and how this may and does inform healthcare.

Funding for dementia research has been notoriously poor. According to an open letter published in *The Times* (17 June 2008) and signed by 30 eminent gerontologists and researchers, it accounts for only 3 per cent of the overall research budget. Given the demographics of our population and the fact that dementia is expected, according to predictions, to double within a generation, the need to increase funding into looking at ways at preventing and/or treating dementia is considered imperative.

Conclusion

The above exploration of dementia is only the tip of the iceberg in terms of presenting research, knowledge and information on and around dementia. We hope it gives you some insight into some of the areas that could be further unpacked. It also tells you something about the concerns and interests of the writer. It is, as we said in the introduction to the case studies, a snapshot of a topic, taken from a particular viewpoint. While there has been an attempt to consider as many angles and perspectives as possible, this still only represents a particular representation. What data you collect, and how you decide to use the data will also be a reflection of this; while information about particular aspects of dementia itself may be similar, it is what you do with it and how you use it that gives a topic its particular slant. Kitwood (1997) challenged the focus on dementia being positioned as simply a neurological impairment, with its resulting poor care and treatment, and reasserted the personhood of the individual, contested some of the frameworks by which dementia was understood and, while recognising the huge difficulties in all aspects, posited the possibility of a better quality of life for people with dementia.

Useful resources

Alzheimers Society: http://www.alzheimers.org.uk. Good source of up-to-date research, service user group insight, as well as 'People Living with Dementia' data from and for people living with, and affected by Alzheimer's. Includes *Out of the Shadows* (2008), a report exploring the impact of stigma on people with dementia and their carers.

Centre for Policy on Aging: http://www.cpa.org.uk/information/reviews/reviews.html. Four reports were published in 2009, based on an extensive literature review of ageism discrimination in primary, secondary and community healthcare, social care and mental healthcare.

http://webarchive.nationalarchives.gov.uk/+/www.dh.gov.uk/en/SocialCare/
Deliveringadultsocialcare/Olderpeople/OlderpeoplesNSFstandards/DH_4071271.
This is an NHS 2008 report on Standard 1 – Rooting out Age Discrimination, as part of
the National Service Framework for Older People.

http://www.library.nhs.uk/LATERLIFE/ViewResource.aspx?resID=87878. A report from
the Kings Fund on age discrimination in health and social care. This was written in
2000 and is up for review in 2010, so while it is useful to refer to this document (and
we have here) please also keep a look out for a more current edition.

http://www.pssru.ac.uk/pdf/dp2538.pdf. A Personal Social Service Research Unit
document called the 'The Costs of Addressing Age Discrimination in Social Care'
(2008); an interesting document that defines equality in a number of ways, looks at
the capability model of assessment and is largely based on quantitative research.

DoH (2009) *National Dementia Strategy*. London: Department of Health.

Kitwood (1997)

Link, B. G. and Phelan, J. C. (2001) 'Conceptualizing Stigma', *Annual Review of Sociology*,
27, 363–85

Victor, C. (2005) *The Social Context of Ageing: A Textbook of Gerontology*. London:
Routledge.

Wilkinson, H. (ed.) (2002) *The Perspectives of People with Dementia. Research Methods
and Motivations*. London: Jessica Kingsley

4

5 research

5.1 INTRODUCTION

This chapter explores:

> the main stages and process of research;
> the critical reading and assessment of research;
> empirical research articles related to the four health areas covered in Chapter 4.

In this chapter we take you through the process of research as applicable to health and social care. We have separated this process into the following four sections:

> Introduction to research – understanding research in health studies.
> Introducing the research process and design – the purpose, the topic and literature searching.
> Principles and core aspects to the research process – paradigms, design, literature review, sampling and ethics.
> Methods, analysis and writing up.

How to 'read' this chapter

Our intention in writing this chapter is for you, the reader, to be an active learner in the research journey. Rather than simply discussing what research is in health care (although this is an important element that runs throughout the chapter), we have written it so that you can apply your own research topics and questions as you go along. We are asking you to join us in an applied research journey – in other words we are going to take you through some of the steps that are involved in engaging with critical and rigorous research. We would ask that you engage as fully as possible with this journey, participating in the activities we suggest and constantly applying the knowledge you accrue from here to your own research journey. What you will find is an introduction to research as we give you our critical take on engaging with thorough and systematic research.

Independent reading alongside this chapter

There are a plethora of research texts and materials to be accessed and perused, some of which we recommend at the end of this section. Occasionally we also suggest material for particular aspects of research as you go along. We would recommend you have a read through some of these texts in order to choose ones whose writing style feel the most accessible and helpful for you.

You will find texts that are overarching: that is, they try (with varying levels of success) to cover all aspects of the research process, from the conception of the research topic to the write up and completion e.g. Bryman (2008), Bowling (2009), Gray (2009) and Matthews and Ross (2010). Other texts focus on specific aspects of research – so they may well be solely concerned with a particular method (e.g. Morgan 1997, on focus groups) or school of methods/analysis (e.g. Silverman 2006, 2010, on qualitative research), or they may look at a particular feature, such as the literature review (e.g. Hart 1998). As ever, choosing just one text as your only source is not advisable, as authors all have a particular take on and understanding of research and you must explore and expand your knowledge beyond the 'one book, one perspective' approach that so many students take.

Your role

We would strongly suggest that as an undergraduate student you start as early as possible in considering how crucial knowledge (and experience) of the research process is to all facets of your studies. Your ability to reflect on how you understand your world will form part of that exploration. It will help you develop a more critical eye and the ability to engage in greater depth with all aspects of work and life.

Recording the reflective activities in this chapter

We have already touched on the general purpose of the reflective activities in the introduction to this text, but what we suggest you do when you engage with these during your research journey is to avail yourself of a notebook/journal. Researchers are often required, to enable a critically engaged process to emerge, to record their process as they go along. Thus, the exercises here are also designed to enable you to do this; writing and recording this and keeping it in one place means that it can become a resource for you to reflect back on both during your reading of this chapter, as well as for your research journey more generally.

The use of real world empirical research articles in this chapter

Within some of the sections within this chapter we have used research examples from the areas of the four case studies discussed in Chapter 4, as a way of critiquing and exploring various elements within research. The foci that are taken within the articles are as wide ranging and diverse as the case studies themselves, and this in of itself is indicative of how complex and contested HIV, dementia, obesity and ART are within the research and/or practice arenas. The dates of these articles range from early 2000 to 2010, and when reading through them it is worth taking this into account when considering their timeliness. The approach we have taken, by engaging with these articles, is one we would encourage you to do as well – that is, question, critique, engage and reflect on your research journey.

Useful resources

Recommended texts for the overarching research process

Bowling, A. (2009) *Research Methods in Health: Investigating Health and Health Services*, 3rd edn. Maidenhead : Open University Press.

Bryman, A. (2008) *Social Research Methods*, 3rd edn. Oxford: Oxford University Press.

Davies, M. B. (2007) *Doing a Successful Research Project Using Qualitative or Quantitative Methods*. Basingstoke: Palgrave Macmillan.

Denzin, N. K. and Lincoln, Y. S. (eds) (2008) *Collecting and Interpreting Qualitative Materials*, 3rd edn. Thousand Oaks, CA: Sage.

Denzin, N. K. and Lincoln, Y. S. (eds) (2008) *The Landscape of Qualitative Research*, 3rd edn. Thousand Oaks, CA: Sage.

Gray, D. E. (2009) *Doing Research in the Real World*, 2nd edn. London: Sage.

Green, J. and Thorogood, N. (2009) *Qualitative Methods for Health Research*, 2nd edn. London: Sage.

Matthews, B. and Ross, L. (2010) *Research Methods: A Practical Guide for the Social Sciences*. Harlow: Longman.

Neale, J. (ed.) (2009) *Research Methods for Health and Social Care*. Basingstoke: Palgrave Macmillan.

Ritchie, J. and Lewis, J. (eds) (2003) *Qualitative Research Practice: A Guide for Social Science Students and Researchers*. London: Sage.

Robson, C. (2007) How to Do a Research Project: A Guide for Undergraduate Students. Oxford: Blackwell.

Saks, M and Allsop, J. (eds) (2007) *Researching Health: Qualitative, Quantitative and Mixed Methods*. London: Sage.

Sarantakos, S. (2005) *Social Research*, 3rd edn. Basingstoke: Palgrave Macmillan.

Silverman, D. (2006) *Interpreting Qualitative Data*, 3rd edn. London: Sage.

Silverman, D. (2010) *Doing Qualitative Research: A Practical Handbook*, 3rd edn. London: Sage.

Internet resources

The Qualitative Report, an online bimonthly journal: http://www.nova.edu/ssss/QR/index.htm

Qualitative Social Research Forum, an online peer reviewed journal: http://www.qualitative-research.net/index.php/fqs

Web centre for social research methods: http://www.socialresearchmethods.net

Social Psychology Network, providing research, methods and statistics links: http://www.socialpsychology.org/methods.htm

Social research update, based at the University of Surrey: http://sru.soc.surrey.ac.uk

Free resources for programme evaluation and social research methods: http://gsociology.icaap.org/methods/

5

5.2 INTRODUCING AND UNDERSTANDING RESEARCH IN HEALTH STUDIES

This section explores:

> the role of research in healthcare;
> reflection and reflectivity;
> evidence-based practice (EBP);
> epidemiological study.

What is research?

According to Clark and Hockey (1979, p. 4), 'research is an attempt to increase the sum of what is known, usually referred to as "a body of knowledge", by the discovery of new facts or relationships through systematic inquiry, the research process'. Leedy et al. (1996) understand research as a way to increase our understanding, answer a question or even resolve an on-going problem.

As a point of reflection the use of the term 'fact', in Clark and Hockey's (1979) understanding, is an intriguing one and one that is always useful to critically consider. What is a 'fact': when does something, a bed of knowledge or belief or understanding, become a 'fact'? Is it something that is universally positioned as a fact or is it something that might be contextually informed, socially derived and ongoing in terms 'there's more to know out there?' Part of this discussion is considered when we look at **paradigms** (see p. 221) and the nature of knowledge, but as a starting point try out the reflective activity.

Reflective activity

- What is your definition of a fact?
- List five facts about HIV.
- How do you know these to be 'facts', i.e. what is your evidence and source?

Bailey (1991, p. 1) locates research in terms of it being 'any activity undertaken to increase our knowledge; it is the systematic investigation of a problem, issue, or question', while Fox et al. (2007) emphasise its role as 'generating new knowledge'. Research, then, is an activity; it is something we do mindfully, systematically and thoughtfully. It has a purpose, and is driven and engaged in, by you the researcher, as a way of exploring, explaining, describing, elucidating and expanding upon areas of interest. Wood et al. (2006) develop this notion of research as an engaged activity by situating it in terms of being a continual ongoing process and one that is informed by a continuous commitment to developing and clarifying, or as they position it 'making things better'. This would seem to imply that research is never finite and that it often raises even more questions. According to Walliman (2001, p. 20), the role of the researcher within this is to 'make new discoveries, to change our perception of the world, and to point to ways of improving life'. Whether this is indeed our objective may be informed by our approach and our own belief systems. But clearly the understanding here is that in order for us to undertake a piece of research that does indeed open up a field of study or knowledge, we need to know what is already out there and what is already understood and perceived, i.e. contextualised.

Box 5.1 Key Characteristics of Research

> It is thorough.
> It involves systematic engagement with the process of research.
> It asks questions.
> It is contextualised.
> It has a purpose, relevance and intention.
> It requires the researcher to explore, expand, investigate and engage with what, why, how, where and when – and the 'so what factor' (this being the rationale for embarking on this piece of research).
> It is ongoing and continuous.

The role of research in healthcare

The role of research within healthcare is central and is used to inform, develop, question, improve and evaluate past and present practice. Bowling (2009, p. 1) states: 'Ultimately it aims to contribute to a scientific body of knowledge. More specifically … it aims to improve health, health outcomes and health services.'

The NHS has a department dedicated to managing and developing research – the (NIHR) National Institute for Health Research (see http:// www.nihr.ac.uk/Pages/default.aspx) – and has clear directives regarding the role of research. You, as a student of health studies, will not only find yourself engaging in practice that has been informed by research, you will be, as a reflective practitioner, required to both constantly evaluate and assess your own practice and ways of doing things, as well as probably being asked to participate in and/or contribute to research.

Starting your journey

Critical reasoning

When engaging with research, reading about research, reading **empirical** research articles and indeed writing about research the ability to evaluate and assess are important. The skills of critical reasoning therefore need to be employed throughout. Cottrell (2005) has produced an entire text dedicated to 'critical thinking skills' in which she unpacks the meanings and applications of critical thinking – what is of pertinence here, she feels, is your ability to 'look

5

at the evidence in a detailed and critical way. In particular … weigh up the relative strengths and weaknesses of the evidence, pointing these out … so that it is clear how the writer [in this case you] has arrived at judgements and conclusions' (p. 168).

Essentially we are asking you to recognise and work through your ideas and be able to reason through your understandings, beliefs and attitudes. This should also apply when you are reading research. Critical thinking requires you to see beyond the 'taken for granted' assumptions you have and provide evidence, explanations and a logical train of argument to coherently present your understanding and analysis.

Reflection in research

Related to critical thinking is the ability to be 'reflective'. According to Gomm (2009) reflective inquiry is closely associated with **practitioner research**, which encapsulates the practice of constantly considering, exploring and questioning yourself and research in order to gain insight and inform your working practice. Fox et al. (2007) see reflection as 'a way in which people explore and clarify their experiences in order to lead to new understanding and as a result adapting and developing the research practice' (p. 184). They explore the notion that you can engage with reflection in an informal and ongoing way throughout the research process, and/or follow a more structured approach where you ask yourself particular questions in order to gain insight into 'what you have done, why you did it like that, how did you feel while engaging in the practice, what have you learnt from the experience, how do you make sense of it and finally what are your plans for future practice' (Fox et al. 2007, p. 184). While both texts are particularly referring to practitioner research and practice, the same skills can be applied to you when engaging in research.

Reflective activity

Johns (2009) has written a text on becoming a reflective practitioner', and defines reflection as 'awareness of self within the moment, hav[ing] a clear mind so as to be open to the possibility of that moment. It is the wisdom that helps us see things clearly. Only when we can see things clearly, for what they really are, are we able to make the best decisions mindful of the potential consequences' (p. 4).

- How many different definitions can you find for reflective practice?
- What are the overall themes of these definitions?

Useful resource

Johns, C. (2009) *Becoming a Reflective Practitioner*, 3rd edn. Oxford: Wiley-Blackwell.
This is useful as a text from which to extrapolate to research as well as providing a particular structured model that may be of use to EBP and practitioner research.

Gomm (2009) locates the practice of reflexivity within qualitative research as being a 'self-aware and self-critical attitude and practice where the researcher ... monitors his or her own activities ... how the research was done' (p. 290). Bryman (2008) clarifies this even more by considering reflexivity of the social researcher being about acknowledging and working with their values, approaches, decision-making processes, **subjectivity** and mere presence; considering their relevance to the meanings of the 'social' world they are endeavouring to explore – so he doesn't necessarily simply locate it within only **qualitative** research. Fox et al. (2007) also discuss it in terms of how we, as researchers, affect the process, the decisions and the outcomes of the research. Positivists would critique this position in terms of producing a reliable piece of research (Guba and Lincoln 2004) (see p. 00). Their position holds that **objectivity** is not only essential but possible and indeed that the world and the known exist independently of ourselves.

What Fox et al. (2007) and Silverman (2004) contend is that our values, beliefs and very sense of self impact on and influence the research throughout, and that the research we engage in impacts on and influences us as researchers as well – so positioning research as co-constructed, where the researched and the researcher are interdependent. Sarantakos (1998) positions reflexivity as a dynamic ongoing process that considers all meanings need to be understood within an ongoing flexible reflection on the symbolic and social context.

Reflexivity has a number of interrelated concepts; it can be considered that the 'knowledge that is produced through any qualitative research encounter should be understood as the product of a specific interaction between researcher and informants' (Pink 2004, p. 367). Those being researched are choosing to be part of a piece of research so the knowledge produced is due to the encounter that is framed by the research – thereby challenging any notion of objectivity. However, Snape and Spencer (2003, p. 21) consider that the purpose of reflexivity in qualitative research is the 'striving for objectivity and **neutrality**. We try to reflect upon ways in which **bias** might creep into our qualitative research practice, and acknowledge that our backgrounds and beliefs can be relevant here'.

Reflexivity is also considered to be specific to particular approaches to research as well as processes and aspects of research itself. Reflexivity within **ethnomethodology**, for instance, refers to the process of 'self monitoring by anyone, researcher and researched, which provides the sense of where things are at in the particular situation' (Gomm 2009, p. 290). Reflexivity, according to Garfinkel (1967), is at the core of how we reason out our everyday actions, practical activities and circumstances, 'through which social order is accomplished' (cited in Bryman 2008, p. 494). Bryman (2008) posits reflexivity in this instance as being more about how words and language are not simply representative of the social world but are 'constitutive' of the social world. The

5

practice of reflection and reflexivity can dovetail and indeed merge, being informed by similar critically informed processes.

Useful resource

Etherington, K. (2004) *Becoming a Reflexive Researcher*. London: Jessica Kingsley. A well written text that looks, through the use of real world research (in particular her own journey), at the use of self in research and how reflexive practice can underpin all aspects of the research process.

Evidenced-based practice (EBP)

EBP is about the application of research in practice. Essentially, it is putting into practice evidence (from research) that you have critically evaluated and reflected upon and deemed appropriate to develop best possible practice.

In the context of health, it is concerned with the 'judicious application of current best available evidence when making decisions about the care of individual patients. It integrates clinical expertise with the best available clinical evidence from systematic research and the thoughtful and compassionate consideration of patients' situations in decisions about care' (Sackett et al. 1998, p. 2; cited in Baigis and Hughes 2001, p. 10). Other theorists within this field (e.g. Bowling 2009; Fox et al. 2007; Gomm 2009) see that audit/evaluation, randomised clinical trials and the effectiveness of practice research can all be either encompassed within the umbrella term of EBP (or evidence-based medicine, EBM) or seen as discrete research designs in themselves. Traditionally, though, the reference to 'systematic research' refers to a systematic review of literature (see p. 288), where what is considered the very 'best' of the available research on a particular topic and/or practice has been accessed, analysed and presented in way that brings together the findings of other research in a critical and well considered manner.

The philosophy behind EBP is that all practice is supported by evidence that indicates that this is best practice. In theory, therefore, no practice is undertaken that has not been rigorously researched. The rationales and qualities, and indeed catalysts, for best practice can be multiple and issues of effectiveness can be measured by qualities of cost, time taken, efficiency as well as patient satisfaction, healing and quality of life issues. The government's drive for EBP and a clear link between what professionals do, i.e. their practice, and the research over recent years has resulted in researchers being both encouraged and even 'coerced' (Fox et al. 2007) into carrying out research into their practice. Fox et al. (2007, p. 3) separate EBP into three aspects:

> research should provide the evidence on which professional practice is based;
> service delivery will change based on best available research evidence;
> through evaluation of services, practitioners can monitor the effects of their interventions.

Healthcare rationing (see p. 185) and EBP are often informed by one another. As previously stated, there are a number of drivers that inform EBP, drivers whose meaning in terms of delivering quality care are not straightforwardly situated within 'what is best for the patient'. Clearly finances have considerable impact on how healthcare is planned and delivered. The UK coalition government's 'Big Society' plans to hand over budgetary control to GPs and away from PCTs (to name but one change) are relevant to EBP.

For example, if at present the budget set aside in your health locality for interventions for clinically obese individuals is £50,000 a year, and your budget has been cut overall by 40 per cent, then decisions will be made about how these cuts will be apportioned across all treatments and services, and then within each particular intervention for healthcare. Decisions on treatments and interventions may well, therefore, be informed by what is the most expensive, how many people within the health locality 'need' gastric surgery and which intervention is the most cost effective. The choices of treatment may be framed by cost effectiveness, and EBP would be concerned with assessing the efficacy of those treatments that fall within a particular price bracket.

Ritchie and Vitali (2009), while not disputing the usefulness of and/or necessity for EBP and certainly not denying that it is now a part of health and social care and practitioners' professional lives, question whether some of the more traditional approaches to EBP can capture the complexities of everyday human life. Reducing health to a simple **cause and effect relationship** can neglect the contingent nature of scientific knowledge (Ritchie and Vitali 2009). One of the potential difficulties with quantitative EBP is how to translate the controlled and often experimental conditions of **RCTs** and experimentation to the real world of practice.

The discussions on concepts of health in Chapter 1 (particularly Seedhouse's Foundations of Health), poststructuralism and **social constructivism** are all discourses drawn to develop EBP beyond the narrow remits of RCTs, systematic reviews, experimentation and positivist **epistemologies**.

However, given how funding indisputably prioritises these approaches the debates remain ongoing. Qualitative researchers, as you will see in the rest of this chapter, have endeavoured to challenge the **hegemony** of positivism within healthcare research (Bowling 2009; Ritchie and Vitali 2009). The case study on dementia also explores the limits of EBP, particular in reference to providing quality of life care to people with dementia.

Useful resources

Centre for Evidence Based Medicine (CEBM) guidelines (http://www.cebm.net/index.aspx?o=5653) give overall guidelines for EBM as well as the hierarchy of evidence for systematic reviews (one of the main source of data for EBP).

Greenhalgh, T. (2010) *How to Read a Paper: The Basics of Evidence-Based Medicine*, 4th edn. Oxford: Wiley-Blackwell.

EBP and epidemiology

One area of research considered core in the hierarchy of evidence (i.e. some evidence is seen as more important than other evidence) is epidemiological (or clinical) studies. Epidemiology as a subject covers a vast territory, so this overview is intended to give an insight into its core functions only, to illustrate its significant contribution to the field of health and social care, including health promotion and public health, and to pick out some key points of analysis that can be used when critiquing epidemiological studies.

Formally, epidemiology is defined as:

> the study of the distribution and determinants of health status or events in specified populations, and the application of this study to control health problems. It is concerned with the collective health of people in a community or an area and it provides data for directing public health action. (Bailey et al. 2005, p. 3)

Epidemiology involves the study of populations *not* individuals, and is generally considered to be the science of public health, with its **ontological** and **epistemological** routes very firmly within positivism (see p. 227). Epidemiological study sets out to identify the **incidence** and **prevalence** (or rates) of disease (or risk factors) within populations and detect any changes in this over time (e.g. the rise in HIV or obesity). Epidemiological studies can help to identify who is affected by particular diseases in a population, and to identify the aetiology (causes) of disease.

Its focus is on quantifying this information in the form of generalisable, descriptive or inferential statistics (for more explanation see p. 325). Epidemiological studies also contribute to the assessment of the effectiveness of clinical or prevention initiatives: for example, assessing whether taking statins medication (lipid-lowering medicines) has an effect on death rates from coronary heart disease or if being physically active reduces the likelihood of developing heart disease. Assessing which intervention is 'better' shows the important contribution of epidemiologically based study to EBP.

Probably the most famous British epidemiologist is John Snow (1813–58), who through systematic mapping and logical reasoning identified the source of a cholera epidemic in London in 1853 as the Broad Street water pump, even though at the time there was no knowledge of the bacteriological aetiology of the disease.

Useful resource

See http://www.bbc.co.uk/history/historic_figures/snow_john.shtml to learn more about John Snow and his epidemiological investigation.

Through epidemiological investigation, therefore, it is possible to identify where the burden of disease falls within a population and provide data that contribute to an aetiological (causal/origins) understanding of disease.

Epidemology and health

A variety of data are collected and used for epidemiological monitoring or studies to answer the following:

> Who gets ill?
> Why do they get ill?
> What should the response be?

Some of the key forms of data are noted below.

Rates

These include data on *morbidity* (illness/disease) and *mortality* (death) rates within a specific population or across populations. On one level it might seem nonsensical to assess different rates of death, after all 'The total number of deaths cannot change – one per person' (Marmot and Mustard 1994; cited by Pitts 1996), but what is important is to ascertain the *distribution* of death and illness. For example, are there more deaths than expected among children living in certain areas of the country? Or has the death rate from a particular cause increased or decreased over a period of time? It is important, too, to calculate death *rates* (rather than rely on total numbers of deaths) to enable a comparison over time or between different groups. For example,

Population	Deaths from coronary heart disease (CHD)
A	20
B	200

On face value, there are far more deaths from CHD in population B than population A. However, if they were worked out as a percentage (rate) we might see a very different picture.

Population	Deaths from CHD	Population size	Death rates per 1,000
A	20	4,000	5
B	200	40,000	5

From this table you can see that the death rate is actually the same for both populations. Mortality rates are calculated by taking the number of deaths (numerator), dividing this by the number of people within the population (denominator) and multiplying by 100, 1,000 or another convenient figure (Katz 2000).

Another really important rate is *infant mortality rate (IMR)*. IMRs refer to the number of deaths per 1,000 infants under the age of one year, compared with the number of live births. The IMR is generally considered to be an indicator of the general state of health and deprivation within an area or country (Katz 2000; Bailey et al. 2005).

Another important aspect of rates calculation is to use some form of *standardisation* of rates. Populations differ in terms of key characteristics such as gender and age distributions, so some form of standardising adjusts for these variables. This is important, for instance, because many diseases are more usual in older people. Cancer, for example, is primarily a disease of ageing and so you would 'naturally' expect to see more deaths from cancer in a country or area of the country where there are more elderly residents. Age is in fact the biggest predictor of death.

If differences in death rates persist once they have been 'standardised', this indicates that something other than ageing is likely to be causing this difference in incidence and prevalence of certain diseases. The data can be collated and presented in various forms.

Age standardised

Deaths rates for a particular disease are adjusted to account for different age structures in different populations.

World standardised

Death rates are standardised for a 'classical' population – this allows for comparisons to be made for particular diseases between different countries of the world.

Standardised mortality ratios (SMRs)

This is a very useful measure and is often used in data to compare mortality in different parts of a country. The SMR is a mechanism of compensating for the effect of different age and sex distributions within a population (Katz 2000). The 'baseline' SMR is taken as being 100 (i.e. 100 per cent represents what you would normally expect to see in a population). What is of interest, therefore, in tables presenting SMRs – for instance, across different regions – is to see which areas have SMRs above 100 and which have SMRs below 100. If an area has an SMR above 100, this indicates that *more* people are dying than would be expected (accounting for age distributions etc.). If the SMR for an area is below 100, then *fewer* people are dying than would be expected. It is a common and fairly broad indicator that people's state of health is worse in some areas than others.

It is also important to measure the distribution and frequency of diseases across the population. **Incidence** and **prevalence** data are core to this function. Incidence refers to the number of new cases of disease or disorders over a given period of time, whereas prevalence refers to the total number of people with a disease or disorder over a particular period of time. Prevalence itself constitutes both new and existing or old cases of the disease or disorder, and so reflects new diagnoses as well as those living with a particular condition. Incidence will rise during epidemics and prevalence will fluctuate according to the number of new cases *and* the number recovering, or dying, from the condition.

All the above data are important as they help to identify where particular diseases might be problematic (e.g. rising during an epidemic), changes in disease patterns over time (e.g. mortality and morbidity from coronary heart disease) and who is most affected by a condition (e.g. men or women, or in different areas of the country or a city). Observing patterns of disease – for example, clusters in particular areas, or according to a particular behaviour or exposure (e.g. smoking and lung cancer) – can help to pinpoint the factors that might be contributing to a problem. However, to gain further clarity on this requires further epidemiological investigation and the implementation of particular studies to generate data from which inferences can be made between specific characteristics.

Studies of different types

There are a variety of epidemiological studies that contribute to ascertaining associations between particular diseases and possible causes (Carr et al. 2007) and they broadly constitute a hierarchy of evidence. Systematic reviews and **randomised controlled trials** (RCTs) are at the top of the hierarchy, followed by cohort studies and case–control studies, with expert opinion and anecdotal experience being at the bottom of the hierarchy. As Evans (2003) notes, making blanket decisions about the robustness of sources of evidence is not straightforward, as the effectiveness, appropriateness and quality of the research are important too. However, different studies of different types do manage to ameliorate the impact of various selection and measurement biases, which is why RCTs are generally placed at the top of the hierarchy. This is illustrated by exploring the elements of some of the main types of epidemiological studies from which inferences about the aetiology of diseases can be drawn, namely case–control studies, cohort studies and RCTs.

Case–control studies

In essence this type of investigation involves studying those *with* existing disease and comparing exposures for those *without* existing disease. The first lung cancer study was of this nature. They are useful in the early stages of aetiological investigation as it is possible to check for many factors that might increase the risk of disease or for exploring the possible aetiology of rare diseases, or diseases with a long latency period. They are relatively quick and cheap to undertake. The basic structure of this type of study is given in Figure 5.1.

There are several weaknesses to studies of this type. In particular they are prone to measurement bias as individuals are required to recall exposures (habits, occupational exposures etc., potentially over a lifetime) due to the retrospective nature of the study. The 'cases' and the 'controls' may differ in

5

factors (e.g. age, gender) other than the exposure (e.g. smoking), which could contribute to the development (or absence) of a particular disease and so obscure the true influence(s) on health.

Retrospective: identify what people in the cases (i.e. those with lung cancer) were exposed too, and compare with people in the non-cases (i.e. those with another form of cancer).

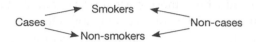

And compare the differences between the two groups. From this, the likelihood (odds) of cases being exposed to a particular risk, e.g. smoking, can be identified and expressed in the form of inferential statistics e.g. odds ratios (ORs).

Figure 5.1 Cases versus controls

Cohort studies

The term 'cohort' comes from the Latin for a group of soldiers who march together in time, and refers to one of the key characteristics of a cohort study. This is that they are prospective or follow-up investigations, which study a group of people over time. They start with a cohort of people (e.g. birth cohort or occupational cohort) who are disease-free, keeping track of their state of health over months or years. It is possible to monitor behaviours or other exposures (e.g. parity or body weight) as well as the development of any diseases, and to look for any correlation (link) between the two. As participants are regularly monitored, some of the problems of recall bias are avoided. They are, however, costly and time-consuming, and attrition rates can be high. It is also never possible to totally account for all the factors that might influence the exposure or outcome of disease, as individuals are not placed in a controlled, experimental environment, and their experiences (and exposures) may differ in ways that are not measured or captured by the study.

Randomised control trials (RCTs)

There are several types of RCTs, but only standard RCTs are referred to here.

Random allocation of participants to:

Intervention group	**OR**	Control group
(change exposure/provide treatment)		('normal' exposure/no treatment)

Compare outcome (death rates, recovery rates) between the two groups.

Data generated from RCTs can provide information about changes in risk, i.e. improvements or increases in the likelihood of a particular event (disease or death) occurring. RCTs can generate inferential statistics such as relative risk (RR) and measures that distinguish real difference (e.g. in outcome) from chance variations (probability measures – p-values).

Figure 5.2 Randomised control trials

It is possible to remove many elements of bias within RCTs. As the participants of the intervention and control group are randomly allocated to each group, they should share the same characteristics, so any measurable differences should be a product of the interventions (Katz 2000). RCTs, particularly **single-blinded**, **double-blided** or **triple-blinded**, can also compensate for the impact of the placebo effect on recovery, i.e. if people think they are on a 'wonder drug' they will get better regardless of any active ingredient. It is also possible to apply statistical tests (inferential statistics) to data generated by RCTs (and other studies) to ascertain if changes and improvements to people's state of health occurred by chance or were the product of the intervention. It is important to have some understanding of these types of statistical tests in order to ascertain the impact or effectiveness of the attributes under investigation, and what follows is a brief overview of some of the main inferential statistics presented in epidemiological papers.

Some basic statistics

It is possible to derive information about particular risks or risk factors from all of the studies noted above. *Risk* is the probability of an event or outcome occurring, usually over a specified time period. In epidemiology it is generally calculated as the number of events divided by the number of people in the population at risk and it is an important measure because the causes of disease do not act in a completely clear-cut way (McConway 1994). For example, smoking does not *inevitably* cause lung cancer. What it does is produce an increased risk of contracting the disease. It is important, therefore, to find a way of making judgements (quantifying) about changes in risk (McConway 1994). Calculations of this nature give you a figure indicating the risk of an event occurring in a given group.

For example, take the case of babies born with neural tube defects (NTD), one group of babies born to women who took vitamin supplements and the other born to women who did not take vitamin supplements. Data from a study by Smithells et al. (1980; cited in McConway 1994) found one case of NTD in the cohort of women (total number of women in this group $n = 178$) given vitamin supplements (these constitute the intervention group) and 13 cases of NTD in the cohort of women (the control group) *not* given vitamin supplements (total number of women in this group $n = 260$).

The risk of NTD in the *intervention group*, therefore, was $1/178 \times 100 = 0.6$ (per cent) and the risk of NTD in the *control group* was $13/260 \times 100 = 5$ (per cent) (McConway 1994).

Relative risk, risk ratio or odds ratio

What is generally more useful is to *compare* the risks of an event occurring between different groups with different characteristics. This is known as the *relative risk or risk ratio* and data of this nature are presented in Manson et al. (1995) (see Case study 5.2).

Taking the example of NTD again, while it seems as if there is a much lower risk of having a baby with NTD if you take vitamins it is sometimes helpful to express this as a single number – the relative risk/risk ratio score (McConway 1994). This is done by dividing the risk score (probability of the event) in the 'active' or intervention group (those taking vitamins) by the risk score (probability of the event) in the 'non-active' or control group (those not taking vitamins). For the figures above the calculation would be as follows:

0.6/5 = 0.12

The risk of occurrence in the supplemented women is about one-eighth of that in the non-supplemented women (0.12/100 [0.12 ÷ 0.12 = 1 and 100 ÷ 12 = 8.33] ∴ 1/8): a lower risk in women who had the supplements.

or 5/0.6 = 8.3: the relative risk/risk ratio = 8.3

The risk of NTD among women who do not receive supplements is about eight times that of those who do receive supplements: a higher risk in those who did not have the supplements.

A relative risk/risk ratio of 1 would indicate no difference, i.e. each had the same, 1:1 risk (Abramson 1984). A relative risk/risk ratio *less* than 1 indicates a change, a lower risk in one group, e.g. a treatment or intervention has benefited (0.12 in the supplemented group noted above) whereas a relative risk/risk ratio greater than 1 indicates a higher risk in one group compared to another (8.3 for women not supplemented). Odds ratios, generated by case–control studies, are interpreted in the same way.

> Is the odds ratio greater than 1? If so, the factor concerned is a possible risk; if less than 1, it's a possible benefit. If the odds ratio equals 1, the factor makes no difference either way. (Bowers et al. 2001, p. 109)

In terms of judging if the risk *is* greater in one group than another a risk ratio of 2 would be considered the minimum indication of a significant change and normally a relative risk/risk ratio of less than 3 would not be seen as significant in observational studies (http://www.numberwatch.co.uk/rr.htm).

The p-value

In the real world things do happen by chance. However, we also might be able to observe that something else, other than chance, is going on, i.e. something (an X-factor) is exerting an impact (either positive or negative) on an event. The *p*-value – '*p*' is for probability – tells us whether an observed difference (i.e. difference in the results) between two (or more) groups or events is likely to have happened by *chance*.

There are a variety of tests that can be done on data, e.g. χ^2 (chi-squared) tests and *t*-tests. The type of test that is chosen depends on the type of data being gathered in the study, e.g. matched versus independent groups. This detail is not explored here, but it is important to know what a *p*-value means if it is presented with data when you are reading a research paper.

The *p*-value is particularly important when trying to identify what might be 'causing' a disease or deaths. Working out the *p*-value for the different rates of death can help us to identify if it was a coincidence that there were more deaths in one group than in another group. For example, if there are more deaths in a group with high blood pressure than in a group with 'normal' blood pressure, did the X-factor (e.g. blood pressure) actually make a difference or not? Was it something else?

Similarly, you might want to know if a particular form of drug treatment for hypertension *lowers* the risk of deaths from cardiovascular disease (CVD). A RCT study could be launched (e.g. with one group taking the medication, one group not taking the medication) to record the rates of CVD deaths in each group. Any observed differences in the rate of deaths between the groups could then be compared and tested (using a *p*-value test of some form) to see if the differences were due to chance or whether they were *statistically significant*. If the results are statistically significant it would *suggest* that the drug treatment was beneficial. Conversely if the *p*-value was not 'significant', the only conclusion that could be drawn is that the *treatment* or *risk-factor* under investigation has *no effect* on the outcome (e.g. recovery or death).

Box 5.2 *P*-Values and Statistical Significance (adapted from Harris and Taylor 2004)

> $p = 0.5$ is *not* statistically significant – it indicates that there was a 50 per cent, 50:50 (0.5 in 1) likelihood of this happening by chance.
> $p = 0.05$ *is* statistically significant – it equates to a 5 per cent (1 in 20) likelihood that it happened by chance.
> $p = 0.01$ *is* statistically significant and is often refered to as being 'highly significant'. It equates to a 1 per cent (1 in 100) likelihood that it happened by chance.
> $p = 0.001$ *is* statistically significant and is often refered to as being 'very highly significant'. It equates to a 0.1 per cent (1 in 1000) likelihood that it happened by chance.

So in epidemiological papers that cite *p*-values you are looking for $p = 0.05$ *or less* for the results to be considered significant and not likely to have happened by chance.

Note: you should also look at the *confidence interval* (CI) if it is cited in a paper. This is an even more important test of the significance of results.

Harris and Taylor (2005) caution us about getting too excited about a *p*-value of 0.05 as they note that if you looked at 20 studies (even if none of the treatments worked), then one study would be likely to have a *p*-value of 0.05 and so appear to be significant.

Confidence intervals

What is being assumed when we undertake an epidemiological study is that the information we elicit (the data we gather), represents that which would be found in the population as a whole (remember here that non-biased, random, sampling is important to ensure representation). In other words, if the values are 'true' they mirror very closely those values which would be found if the data were collected from *everybody* rather than simply a proportion (sample) of the population. However, every sample taken from a population (even when it is done randomly) will differ very slightly from the population as a whole. So some differences (or errors) in the values found in the sample as compared with those that reside within the population as a whole are to be expected. If a particular study was done with another study population (sample), it is likely that we would obtain slightly different results. The confidence interval (CI) is calculated when the aim is to generalise the results of the study sample to the broader population (a 'reference population' that it is believed to represent, e.g. women in the USA) (Abramson 1984). The confidence interval tells us about the preciseness of the statistical estimates computed and whether they reflect the results that would be found from a study of the entire population (a census). They indicate a probable range of true results that would be found within a population.

Risk ratios should therefore be linked to a confidence interval calculation. The CI accounts for 'normal' differences across a population or sample. Risk ratios indicate the degree of risk (none, increased or decreased) between one group and another in relation to a particular 'exposure', as noted earlier. The CI demonstrates whether this risk ratio is statistically significant or not. If the value 1 (for risk ratio or odds ratio) or 0 (for means etc.) is not included in the CI calculated from the relative risk, risk ratio, odds ratio or mean, then the result can be seen as significant. The CI is usually described as a 95 per cent confidence interval. This can be translated as 'being 95 per cent certain that the relationship – i.e. risk – is not simply a coincidence'. Lower than 95 per cent certainty (e.g. 90 per cent) is more dubious.

In addition, depending on what your study is attempting to demonstrate, the width of the CI is also important. A very wide confidence interval (e.g. 1.8 to 65) is not helpful, as the actual 'true' value within a population could be anywhere between these two numbers. A smaller confidence interval (e.g. 10.5 to 20.5) is much more helpful as the true value for the population will reside between these two figures. Larger study samples generally elicit narrower confidence intervals. Results from small studies with large CIs need to be interpreted cautiously.

Means, medians and proportions: the confidence interval

If the CI is given for data citing means, medians or proportions a CI of 0 is deemed *not* to be significant.

With a single population value, such as a population mean score for exam results, the data (score) is not being *compared* with another group, but if a CI is included, its function is to indicate if the study group's mean score is a reasonably precise estimate of the mean score ranges within the population, i.e. a 'plausible range of values for the true (population) value' (Bowers et al. 2001, p. 107).

Drawing conclusions and making recommendations from epidemiological evidence

It has already been identified that the reliability and validity of data coming from different types of studies vary, with some sources being more robust than others. In addition, if any association or risk-factor is identified from a study, this does *not* directly equate to this definitively being the cause of the disease. Instead, it means it is associated with an increased probability (risk) of the disease occurring (Unwin et al. 1997), and is not directly predictable of outcome. Therefore, it is important to give due consideration before any health-related declarations are made. Specifically, Sir Bradford Hill came up with the following criteria:

> The correlation must be biologically plausible. For example, is there a credible mechanism that can explain the association? Knowledge of biological functioning is important here, and it is possible that any existing mechanism has yet to be discovered.

> The correlation must be strong. For example, is the relative risk large? Is the risk so large that we can easily rule out other factors? A relative risk or risk ratio of 1 would indicate no difference, i.e. each had the same, 1:1, risk (Abramson 1984). Weak associations are more likely to be explained by undetected biases and a relative risk even of 2 only indicates a doubling of risk. A relative risk of 4 or more indicates a strong relationship between exposure and the disease. The death rate from lung cancer in cigarette smokers has been identified as being 25 times higher than in non-smokers, i.e. relative risk 25, in some studies.

> The correlation must reflect a biological gradient. Are increasing exposures associated with increasing risks of disease (e.g. the more cigarettes smoked the higher the risk of lung cancer)?

> The correlation must be found consistently. Have the results been replicated by different researchers and under different conditions?

> The correlation must hold over time, e.g. did the exposure precede the disease? For example, as cigarette consumption increased, did the incidence of disease (e.g. lung cancer) increase too?

> The association must preferably be confirmed by experiment (e.g. quitting smoking reduces the risk) (LeFanu 1999; Carr et al. 2007).

5

> **Reflective activity**
>
> If you want to develop your skills of critical analysis go to http://www.sph.nhs.uk/
> what-we-do/public-health-workforce/resource/critical-appraisals-skills-programme.

This has been a very small snapshot of epidemiology, intended to demonstrate the importance of the discipline to Health Studies. As a Health Studies student it is certainly worth familiarising yourself with some of the basic principles of epidemiology, as not only does epidemiological data contribute to the identification and construction of health priorities, and our understanding of what affects our health (see the Obesity case study, for instance), it also informs options for health improvement: for example, stopping, or never starting, smoking. Moreover, understanding epidemiological studies and the data generated is fundamental to developing the skills of critical analysis. With this understanding it is possible to independently interpret and draw conclusions from evidence, which, depending on source, might be skewed, incomplete or false (see the Obesity case study), so the contribution of epidemiology to EBP must never be taken for granted.

It is important too, to remember that other types of evidence and research contribute to our understanding of health matters and it is to this type of research we now turn. In particular we focus on the nature of the research journey you may take in your studies.

5.3 THE RESEARCH PROCESS AND DESIGN

This section explores:

> 'getting started';
> the path to discovering your topic of research;
> searching the literature;
> your purpose and personal location.

Doing your own research

The 'doing' of research is a process; it involves a number of related and interconnected links that move through various stages (Bouma and Ling 2004). Many research textbooks will take you through this process and in far greater depth and detail than we do here. They all, in their own ways, break down the process in fairly similar ways. For instance, Bouma and Ling (2004) look at it in terms of overarching steps; so they consider that your first 'essential' steps involve the process of choosing the research topic and question, as well as selecting a method; the second step involves the collection of the data; and in the third step where the researcher analyses the data and interprets its significance and meaning. Gray (2004, p. 4) adapts a model provided by Gill and Johnson (1997) and describes the research process in the following way:

> exploring and identifying a broad area of interest for research;
> selecting a topic from within this broad area;
> developing a research question, hypothesis or objective;
> deciding on the approach;
> considering and developing a plan;
> collecting the data;
> analysing the data;
> presenting and discussing the findings.

The research design process we will be using here is very much informed by these approaches and what is worth noting in most research textbooks is the recognition that research is a constant, ongoing, interrelated process. That is to say that while there may indeed be steps, stages, phases and aspects to the process, these are all connected with one another and informed by your engagement with the literature, the data and the process in which you are engaged. You may find yourself adjusting, going back to and further developing several of these stages as you progress with your research – the research process is, in other words, cyclical and very often you will find yourself having to go backwards in order to proceed in a way that makes sense.

You will see that the model we provide of the research process is very similar to Gray's (2004, 2009) but with some further detail. Much of our own understanding has been informed by our undergraduate students' engagement with research over the years. Remember that you will often find that you return to aspects as you go along, refining and clarifying:

> choosing a research area or topic;
> engaging with the literature on and around this broad topic;
> considering, reflecting on and identifying your research paradigm, philosophy or approach;
> engaging with the literature;
> developing a more focused research topic;
> engaging with the literature on and around this more focused topic area;
> developing a research question, hypothesis or research objective;
> choosing your methods of data collection and your analytical approach;
> identifying your target population and applying your sampling framework;
> planning and organising issues such as recruitment, access, consent, location, ethics, gatekeepers and stakeholders;
> carrying out a pilot study or trial of methods and method review;
> carrying out the research;
> analysing your data;
> discussing and interpreting meanings and significance;
> reading throughout the whole process.

5

Where do you start?

When embarking on a piece of research you need to start somewhere – and that somewhere is your topic and/or area of interest. This could, in the first instance come from a number of initial sources, but what Booth et al. (1995), Saunders et al. (2000) and Gray (2009) all write is that if possible, it needs to start from a place of interest for you. The reality is that sometimes the reasons you are embarking on a piece of research are because you have been asked to do so by your tutors within a particular course or your employers require it of you, or, indeed, it is a continuous requirement of your practice (and you will find this within health and social industries in particular) that your work is constantly being updated, developed, audited and evaluated.

Other starting points for embarking on a piece of research may be derived from something you have read, heard, a past project that raises more questions than it answered, a topic introduced to you within a different context that grabs your attention and so on. You might have read something in the media, seen something on the Internet, watched something on TV – and want to have more knowledge on and around this topic. Remember, as a beginner researcher you are endeavouring to move beyond anecdotal, personally experienced and media informed beliefs, to ones that are also informed by rigorous and critical research frameworks. This beginning stage is fairly broad, wide-ranging and non-specific – it requires you to engage with the world around you, in its many and varied manifestations, and open your heart and mind with curiosity.

Reflective activity

- What is your topic of interest?
- Who are the people involved in your area of interest?
- What are the events, actions, phenomena that 'make up' your topics of interest?
- What is the context, history, background of your topic?
- What are the multiple meanings, definitions and understandings of the topic
- What are the informing issues and aspects?
- What elements are involved in the topic?

Gray (2004) writes about relevance trees as a potential way of generating ideas. The idea is that you choose a very broad concept, e.g. HIV, and then develop and generate more specific topics, sub-branches and aspects within it. What you will see from the HIV example below is that what ostensibly appears to be a fairly straightforward topic area can suddenly mushroom into something that just seems to keep on going on and on. This in itself is as it should be and Walliman (2001, p. 24) says it well when he stipulates that 'it requires a good deal of thought and knowledge on your chosen topic of study in order to isolate a suitable research problem' – in other words, we need to really explore the topic as widely as possible in order to move on to the next step, which is narrowing ourselves down. We would therefore suggest that you also think about the informing aspects presented in Table 5.1 as a way of contextualising your knowledge base.

Table 5.1 Exploring HIV

Attitudes/beliefs	Meanings/definitions	Services providers
Media Women/men Hetero/homo/bi/trans Government Health providers/services Support providers/services Religion/faith Countries Ethnic groups Children Legal services Policy-makers HIV organisations	Religious Medical/biological Sociological Psychological Critical theory Country Cultural Women/men Heterosexual/homosexual/ bi/trans	HIV voluntary HIV statutory GUM clinics Housing Welfare Legal Primary, secondary and tertiary care Charities Department of Work and Pensions Asylum and refugee charities/ organisations
Who is at risk	**Who is involved**	**Sources of statistics**
Homosexual men Men who have sex with men (MSM) Heterosexual men Heterosexual women Intravenous drug users Babies of HIV+ women/ men Haemophiliacs blood transfusions Health professionals Sub-Saharan peoples National/international	Partners of HIV+ Sex workers People who have sex with HIV+ people Parents of HIV+ children, both adult children and below 18 Siblings of HIV+ Carers and support workers Health professionals HIV support services, voluntary and statutory Immigration officers Schools Communities Friends and neighbours Diagnosed and undiagnosed	Demographics National and global Epidemiology Immigration Home office HIV organisations GUM Police Housing Welfare DWP WHO HPA Advert Aidsmap DOH
Prevention, reduction and treatment	**Sex, gender, sexuality, ethnicity**	**Cultural**
Safe sex – using a condom Abstinence HAART (Highly Active Antiretroviral therapy) Clean needles/not sharing Blood donations tested Caesarean section No breast feeding HIV testing Screening of Infection diseases Religion, faith, cultural traditions and beliefs etc.	Responses Meanings and understandings Service provision Relationships Family Occurrences Demographics Epidemiology Aetiology Family Children	National Global Country Religions Definitions and meanings Responses

5

Historical/context	Policy and law	Demographics
Gender	DDA 2005	Diagnoses
Sexuality	UK Immigration Act 1971	How acquired
Understanding and meanings	Nationality, Immigration and	Who acquires it
Responses	asylum Act 2002	Most at risk
Funding	European Convention on	National
Attitudes and beliefs	Human Rights	International and global
National and global	Home Office Immigration	
Medical and biological	Directorate Instructions 2005	
Sociological	GMC Communicable disease	
	guidance	
	Criminal law and prosecutions	
	DOH	

Clearly this is a wide ranging coverage of an area that is broad and deeply complex – and it is perhaps helpful here to note that this did not all come off the top of our heads but involved making connections, reading, talking with others and engaging in other activities that increased our awareness of possible areas within HIV. You will also see that there are crossovers in terms of areas within areas and repetitions – this is fine as connections are something that you will need to be making when exploring your topic area.

An example of us making connections was the criminal law aspect, which was initially triggered by the media coverage (2001 onwards) of cases in the UK of people being prosecuted and convicted of infecting their sexual partners – what sparked us here was that at least two of them were asylum seekers and one a refugee. We then wondered how the law stood on HIV and immigration or asylum; this then led to issues of healthcare access, which then resulted in a 'discovery' that sub-Saharan populations in this country are considered to be one of the most vulnerable populations for HIV transmissions (Avert 2010).

Reflective activity

Why don't you try something similar with a topic area of your choice and see how you get on. You may need to change some of the **aspect** titles (in bold), add new ones, take these ones away – there is no set way of engaging with this mind mapping process except to be as thorough, ongoing and engaged as you possible can.
Remember to bounce ideas off friends, read around the topic, see what is out there at present in terms of policy, news coverage etc.

Part of the process with which you will be engaging from this point on will be searching out literature, reading, evaluating and exploring. The HIV exploratory map above is one that was informed by an initial exploration of the literature on and around HIV. But this would be the same with any topic area; once you start getting a feel for the topic area itself then areas of focus may start to spring out for you. Or you may already be coming with a fairly narrow and specific focus. Whichever way you come at it you do need to broaden out your knowledge base, in order to provide yourself with a good grounding in the contextual framework of the topic area, before you bring yourself down to a more narrow area (Walliman 2001).

Searching and reading around the topic

Searching and reading, as indicated in our research process model, is an activity that will form part of all stages, and aspects, of your research journey. Some of the reading you will be doing will be around the topic itself, other reading will be on aspects of research design and methods, and still other reading you will be doing will be about the 'how to' approach to developing critical skills in terms of academic thinking. We have already explored some of this with you, so what we focus on here is the topic aspect to your literature search and reading. In section 5.4 we discuss the literature review, a fundamental element of research design.

Literature search

Once a topic area has been chosen then your literature search should be starting in earnest. The purpose of the ongoing literature search and review is: (a) to discover relevant material published in the chosen field of study and to search within this for a suitable 'problem/focus area'; (b) to provide a context and informing background and eventually a rationale for your chosen research 'problem'; and (c) to provide an up-to-date understanding of the subject area, as well as recent and significant research.

Searching the literature needs to be:

> broad and wide ranging;
> concerned with research that has been done in area(s) of interest;
> looking at the background history, policy, law, government, present day influencing factors etc.;
> considering and exploring various disciplines and genres;
> above all a constant search for material that will inform your research throughout.

5

The importance of making a thorough and continuous search of the literature cannot be overemphasised. You will need to be creative, think laterally, explore alternative search terms, visit your librarian at university and ask them about what paper and electronic sources are available to you in your area. Very often your university library will also take you through effective search techniques and engines as a way of maximising your opportunities to access varied literature.

Your second consideration may be to look at sources:

1 Journal articles.
2 Textbooks.
3 The Internet: Google Scholar, Web of Knowledge. (A word of warning about using Internet sites: while we acknowledge that the Internet is a portal to untold wonders, amazing information, useful data and so on we would *strongly* suggest that you apply the same concern about the credibility, reliability, validity, believability, origin, intention and purpose to what has been written as you would to any piece of literature or document.)
4 Databases: Medline, Cinahl, Assia, Psychlit etc.
5 Grey literature sources. ('Grey literature is produced by government agencies, professional organizations, research centers, universities, public institutions, special interest groups, and associations and societies whose goal is to disseminate current information to a wide audience'; Weintraub, http://library. brooklyn.cuny.edu/access/greyliter.htm, accessed 8 July 2010.)

Box 5.3 Examples of some sources of 'grey literature'

http://www.nice.org.uk – National Institute for Health and Clinical Excellence. NICE is an independent organisation responsible for providing national guidance on promoting good health and preventing and treating ill health.

http://www.dh.gov.uk – Department of Health. Provides health and social care policy, guidance and publications, e.g. White papers and Green (consultation) papers.

http://www.dwp.gov.uk – Department of Work and Pensions. Responsible for welfare and pension policy and a key player in tackling child poverty.

It is the biggest public service delivery department in the UK and serves over 20 million customers.

http://www.homeoffice.gov.uk – Home Office – The Home Office is the lead government department for immigration and passports, drugs policy, crime, counter-terrorism and police.

http://www.avert.org – an international HIV and AIDS charity based in the UK, working to 'avert' HIV and AIDS worldwide

http://opensigle.inist.fr/ – a system for grey literature in Europe.

5 Health documents and policy papers.
6 The media. (Be very careful here as to how you use material in both the print and visual media; you will need to consider their sources, the purpose in writing about this and the actual content and message they are endeavouring to convey.)
7 Information leaflets and pamphlets, conference papers, theses.
8 Government publications.
9 Official publications, archives and statistics.

Hart (1998), Sarantakos (1998), Gray (2004, 2009) and Matthews and Ross (2010) are among many research writers who will give you a fairly sound and detailed idea about what potential source materials there are, how to locate them, how to read them and how to use them.

Reflective activity

- Locate three pieces of literature that are related to your research topic (one from the Internet; one from print media; one an empirical research article).
- Read them through and consider the following:
  - What is the writer's point of view?
  - What is the purpose of the article?
  - What do you like about it?
  - What don't you like about it?
  - What do you believe and what don't you believe and why?

5

You the reader and interpreter

Bear in mind that how you read something will be informed by what we have already discussed in terms of your subjective position and motive or personal location (see p. 214). The risk in some ways is that you choose to read and utilise only material that reflects what you already know (think you know), echoes your opinion, supports your belief and/or attitude and deals with the topic area in a way that is very simplistic and lacks depth.

An example of this may be that you believe that it is the parents of obese children who are to blame for their children's condition. As you go through the literature you find research that reiterates this perspective, in terms of overly generalised and basic sources such as the Internet, tabloids and TV documentaries, as well as 'research' that has been carried out by various different bodies, including food companies, advertising and the health industry. Remarkably you end up not only reading material that is supportive of your own point of view, but you also, not surprisingly, produce a review that actually gives a one-sided point of view of a very complex situation.

To engage in a balanced and informative search and review of the literature you need to go back to your mind map and look at the 'players' involved, and you need to ensure that your background reading considers some of these informing aspects. We have tried when presenting our case studies to do just this and get you to move from very fixed narrow positions to ones that are informed and well supported. As a final point this is not to say that parents do not play a role in their children's obesity, nor does it deny that they have responsibility and an active role to play in this health problem, but it does not oversimplify the topic by naming and blaming, but places this in a greater context.

Critical reading and reviewing the literature

The reading for significance, meaning and relevance should always inform how you approach any source material (Hart 1998; Gray 2004, 2009). Hart (1998) consider this aspect to include consideration of:

> The source, i.e. who wrote it and where was/is it located?
> What was the original purpose of the actual study or work that you are reading?
> On what does it focus?
> How was the data collected and managed?
> How did it analyse or deal with the data and material?
> From what perspective does it come?
> Does it do what it said it would do in the introduction/title?
> Are there any ethical issues which need considering?

You will need to consider issues of credibility and believability too when engaging with your literature. More on assessing the credibility and authenticity of your literature is to be found in the documentary research and systematic review sections of this chapter (see pp. 294 and 288). Aspects you need to consider are embedded in the reflective activity below.

Narrowing down

Booth et al. (1995) suggest the following process as a way of focusing on what they call a 'problem area': 'find an interest in a broad subject area, narrow the interest to a plausible topic; question the topic from several points of view; define a rationale for your project/problem' (p. 36). But how do you actually go about narrowing it down to a 'plausible topic' and what steps can you take to help you do this. If we recall the key qualities of research, you can see that one of these is concerned with being reflective, and it is this aspect we want you to engage with throughout (see p. 190).

5

Bouma and Ling (2004, p. 27) posit the process in terms of moving from the 'ordinary everyday question to a researchable question by focusing on one aspect of the issue arousing your interest'. The process of narrowing down is one of engaged activity, requiring you to read on and around the topic area as well as consider some of the informing issues. Partly based on Bouma and Ling's (2004, p. 27) suggestions, we would suggest considering the following steps as a way of bringing down your topic to a reasoned and possible researchable focus.

Reflective activity

- What are the major issues or elements involved?
- What do you know already (or think you know)?
- What is happening to prompt your interest and focus?
- Are you interested in a cause and effect relationship, e.g. obesity is increasing because fast food is more readily available?
- Unpack this relationship further. How and why is this so – and can you be sure you know this?

Purpose

Thinking about your purpose is also a good way of getting you to really consider the reasons for choosing your topic area and the rationale and justification for doing your piece of research. Some thoughts you might like to consider when placing your research topic or focus into a rationale are as follows:

> Do you want to increase your knowledge and/or the knowledge and understanding around a particular phenomenon?
> Is your intention to ascertain the efficacy of a particular intervention or practice?
> Do you want to provide a rationale and/or an explanation for the weaknesses and/or strengths of a particular practice, belief or approach?
> Are you interested in having a greater insight into a particular phenomenon?
> Is your intention to support and/or challenge a particular belief, practice, way of understanding or doing something?
> Is the purpose to highlight a particular aspect of a phenomenon that may need further investigation?
> Do you want to develop your professional or academic profile and acumen?

Again these are merely suggestions but we hope you will be able to see that the process of narrowing down needs to be located within an ongoing critically reflective framework – one that is informed by a clear and reasoned out intention. Going back to Walliman's (2001) and Bryman's (2008) assertions, this process is not one done in a vacuum: a broad knowledge of the area is needed as well as a clear idea about why you, as an individual are doing this, i.e. personal location.

Personal location

Motivation, that which is driving you to do this piece of work, is often informed by your vested interest in exploring and finding out about something. Clearly once you start really unpacking this process you may find that your motivation is almost entirely personally informed, e.g. your grandmother has Alzheimer's disease (AD), has been placed in a home and you are not content with the service she is receiving. Or you are a single mother who has obese children and you want to show people that it is not because you are a bad mother. Our motivation can often be more about ourselves than we think. We often want to 'prove' other people wrong, justify ourselves, blame others, victimise ourselves and others, and so on. We then endeavour to support these personally informed positions by locating them with what we think is a piece of research, e.g. we do an Internet search and find lots of websites reiterating what we already believe or potentially oversimplifying the complex issues we want to research; or we read a paper that we already know to reflect our beliefs and values.

Reflective activity: an example

Go onto the Internet and do a search: 'single mothers and their obese children, UK'.
- What kind of data does it come up with?
- What do you believe and why?
- What don't you believe and why?
- What questions do you have from this data?

We need to be very reflexive here (see above, p. 191), as this will facilitate you to catch yourself in one-sided perspectives and ill-informed and selective viewpoints. For instance, you may well feel, based on what you have witnessed with your grandmother, that the care received by older people in homes in substandard, i.e. you theorise that the individually specific (your grandmother) is applicable to a *generalised* population (clearly an unsupported but very common approach taken by students when first embarking on a piece of research). In order to support and explore this view further you will need to be able to rationalise the need to actually do a piece of research in this area. This means locating yourself, and the research, within a contextualised framework that is about increasing knowledge, providing insight and clarifying and/or supporting, developing or challenging present day practice. The element of self-reflection needed may include the following:

> Why are you interested in this area – what are your personal motivations?
> What professional or knowledge motivations are there within this?
> What do you want to get out of this piece of research? Often asking yourself what you want at the end is a good way of clarifying your actual focus. What can happen here is that when we reflect on our hoped for outcome we realise that often we want to 'change the world'; or 'we want to somehow

"prove" what we already believe is so'; or even we want to lay blame for children being obese, or care in homes for people with dementia being substandard, with a particular group, individual etc.

> Whose position or point of view do you already support and why? Here really consider what you believe already – again this may well be simply based on reading the tabloids, having a personal experience, having watched something on the TV or heard a friend speak about something. This requires honest reflection on your part. You don't necessarily need to share this with others but you do need to consider how your own invested interests can impact on how you do a piece of research. An example of this may be that, based on personal experience, you believe that standards of care for people with Dementia are poor. Without acknowledging this attitude you may well end up designing a piece of research which (unintentionally) supports that opinion – i.e. looking at the standard of care within a Dementia care home from the perspective of the relatives who have moved their relatives from at least one home already.

> What is your role and place within the topic? Are you someone who is impacted upon by the topic area? Do you work in the area? Have you witnessed people being affected? Have you have been told to focus on this area and so on?

> What are your intentions regarding what you want to do with it? Is it a piece of work you need to hand in to demonstrate your understanding and application of research? Is it something you want to actually do eventually and so on?

> Who and what is it for?

> Who is it going to be about? This may sound like a fairly obvious question but clarity here can be so helpful. If you want children's stories of their eating behaviours then make sure your focus is on them; if it is about children but from the perspective of the parents or health workers then make sure you make it clear that it is the stories of parents and health workers on whom you are focusing. Very often pieces of research that can come our way purport to be about one population but are in fact about another population telling stories, giving opinions or talking about experiences of another population.

Critically unpacking motivation, personal location, purpose and context

Below we have a 'worked' example of what might have been the informing motivations and drivers for MacRae's article on the experiences of people with early-stage Alzheimer's. Clearly all we can ascertain is from the article itself and what she has written, so it is our interpretation based on the information she has provided.

Case study 5.1 A critical interpretation of purpose

Source: MacRae, H. (2008) '"Making the Best You Can of It": Living with Early-Stage Alzheimer's Disease', *Sociology of Health and Illness*, 30(3), 396–412.

Why would this area be of interest/context? MacRae (2008) seems to be interested in how the individuals who are given an early diagnosis make sense of the illness itself and their lives. She gives background to this area and some of the research that has gone before. Her research could be partly prompted by the way in which Alzheimer's disease is negatively constructed in terms of medical definitions but also in terms of the media and society. Much of the research within this area has focused on the acute stages of AD and/or the carers' perspective, often rendering the individual with AD as invisible and negating the notion of AD as a progressive illness, i.e. one that has stages. Her background considers the dehumanising understanding of AD, where the individual is seen as a burden to the families, caregivers and society as a whole. But what MacRae (2008) is pulling on here is that recent research (e.g. Kitwood 1997; Phinney 2002; Young 2002) would indicate that how the individual makes sense of their experience and the illness and how they respond and cope with it challenges the idea that the individual loses self-identity – this discourse extends to how labels around illness can locate people in particular ways – so rather than it simply being individuals with AD losing their identity it is more about how others treat them so that this process happens. MacRae is interested in looking at developing the recent research to explore early stage AD individuals' own perspectives around meanings and how they create meaningfulness for themselves.

Relevance/so what factor. If society, the media and indeed medical meanings couch Alzheimer's in terms of loss of individuality, social burden and victimhood then the way we treat someone with AD will be implicitly and explicitly informed by these beliefs. Therefore, when we treat someone as if they are no longer fully human and, as soon as we hear the label AD, we locate them in terms of acute stages we might lessen their ability to function, engage with society, create meaningful lives. This can inevitably lead to disenfranchisement, depression, loss of motivation and self worth. If we gain insight into how individuals actually make sense and develop meaning than perhaps practice can be impacted upon in terms of actively supporting individuals with AD.

Personal location. To give individuals with early stages of AD an opportunity to voice their experience. To challenge popular discourses about AD and to extend meanings of AD beyond a simple homogeneous population given the definition of having a disastrous affliction that is greeted, and treated, with stigma, abhorrence and fear. MacRae is very keen to highlight this misconception and its impact on people with early stages of AD, and to enable the individual to be supported in living a more meaningful life.

Purpose. For both health care workers and those individuals who are newly diagnosed to understand that 'given the opportunity persons with AD can create meaningful lives' (p. 409), so removing some of the negative stigma and fear responses.

Who is involved? People with early stage AD. The gatekeepers (often people we need to have contact with in order to gain access to the actual population), in this case the geriatricians at a particular hospital.

Who are the intended audience? Healthcare workers and personnel in particular but also, because it is challenging popular discourses, just about everyone else too!

5

The 'so what factor'

It is worth noting here what we mean by 'the so what factor'. In research the 'so what factor' is a fairly crucial consideration when exploring your topic and engaging in the narrowing down and focusing process. You may find your tutors asking you this very question when you present your ideas for your research. Essentially what it is asking of you, as a reflective/reflexive researcher, is to consider the purpose, personal location and meaning, relevance and/or significance of your chosen research question. It is asking you to move into a research position, rather than simply presenting a question or topic area that has very little usefulness or contextual meaning.

Reflective activity

To explore the 'so what factor' further, let's look at a question that you might want to address that is linked with the topic of dementia: 'family responses to a relative with dementia'.

Using (a) the McRae (2008) example in Case study 5.1 and (b) the dementia case study (Case study 4.4), consider the following:

- What might be the purpose of 'doing' a piece of research like this?
- Who might be interested in doing this research and why?
- What is the context or background that might inform this piece of research?
- What would its significance or 'so what factor' be in terms of knowledge or practice?
- Why might it be useful to do a piece of research like this?

Risks of focusing without reflection/reflexivity

Walliman (2001), Gray (2004) and Bryman (2008)all consider processes of narrowing down and focusing in the initial stages and emphasise the importance of reading literature on and round the topic area, but also consider similar ways of being systematic and reflective in how you engage with the topic itself, Walliman (2001) and Gray (2004) also consider what to avoid when narrowing down.

Your own personal agenda regarding your own lack of knowledge base

The purpose of your research is for your own personal information rather than located within wider debates about increasing, informing, clarifying or exploring knowledge bases within wider contexts and contributing to public knowledge and interests, e.g. you are thinking of going through IVF and you want to find out what the DoH policy is about how many implantations you can have – this is not research but merely ascertaining certain information. If, however, your subjectivity was located within the framework of considering lesbian couples' experience of going through IVF then there may be more veracity for this piece of research.

Simply considering a research problem or focus that is only concerned with comparing one set of data against another

> Merely comparing HIV positive white, gay, male populations with white, male, heterosexual populations doesn't tell us anything new or informative about the meanings and relevance of this data. The research problem would need to be clearly situated within a framework of rationale, purpose, context and relevance – e.g. using the two data sets as a way of exploring the potential implications for developing future health promotion prevention strategies.

Setting up your question to find a correlation between two sets of data without a context or purpose

> You could be looking for data on poverty and the apparent link with obesity without actually revealing the causal link and its significance in terms of the 'how, why, when, where and what'. So you need to move beyond generalisations that are simplistically presented and look at the actual meaning of the relationship (if indeed there is one). Let's say you are seeking to isolate variables like poverty (however you define that) and obesity (again how will you define this) in a causal relationship. What would the significance and meaning of this be? What is the purpose of this and the context? How might these be related and when and why … and so on.

Devising a problem that requires a simple yes or no answer

> The temptation is often to seek absolute answers to your questions and pursuit of knowledge but actually, in research, this needs to be formed within an informing context of how and why things may be the way they are, their history and background, how they work, the implications and relevance. Again let's go back to the case studies we have looked at and consider HIV – you may be keen to find out if people with HIV are prevented from working in the health industry. Why would you want to know that, what might come before, what is the significance of you even asking this question and so on?

What this all means for you

> Overall what seems to be the message is that you need to ensure you do not engage in research within a vacuum – that is, without considering what has gone before, what the background and context of the topic under investigation is. The key here is to avoid oversimplifying your topic and only looking at it from one angle and/or source. By critically reflecting on your own points of view you can learn to differentiate between a well considered research topic and one that is situated in rather uninformed and unsubstantiated claims. As you develop your skills of searching the literature, and thinking through your ideas in systematic ways, your curiosity will take flight in ways that go far beyond media-derived headlines and Internet chat rooms.

Concluding comments

Within this section we have introduced you to some of the initial steps you will need to undertake within research. Issues such as purpose and motivation, as well as your initial exploration of the topic, are framed in reflective activities that enable you to 'give it a go'. The discussion on EBP centralises the importance of research within health and its impact on practice, while the worked through example of McRae's (2008) research illustrates how these positionings can frame research. All research is informed by your purpose and intention, and where you are positioned within the phenomenon itself. Thus, who you are, why you are doing the research, what you have read around this topic and how you know what you know are all fundamental to the explorations you need to undertake.

In the next section our understandings of knowledge, and your purpose in undertaking the research, are explored in much greater detail. While this is separated into a distinct part this does not mean that you won't already have thought about these aspects already, it is just a way to organise the material you need to learn about when embarking on your research journey.

5.4 CORE PRINCIPLES INFORMING THE RESEARCH PROCESS

This section explores:

> research paradigms;
> deductive and inductive reasoning;
> variables, reliability, validity, generalisability and credibility;
> types of research design;
> the literature review;
> research question;
> ethics;
> sampling;
> access.

The previous sections explore the meanings of research, its purpose and ways of choosing and developing your topic area. This section takes this process further by looking at the essential framing aspects of research in terms of its fundamental informing principles. In order to produce a rigorous and well designed piece of research these elements cannot be missed out or superficially addressed. While we acknowledge that the application can be challenging, particularly when considering the language used around these aspects, we hope that you will find the discussion below helpful in developing your ideas. Within the research texts we have suggested to you at the beginning of this research section (see p. 187) you will find discussions on these aspects and it is advisable to utilise a broad range of sources to really get to grips with some of the more complex elements within research principles.

Your research paradigm

Your approach to research and indeed your understanding of the world is informed by a set of beliefs – a set of beliefs that organises and makes sense of how you understand the nature of the world in particular ways. The questions you ask, they ways you ask them, the focus you take and the way you engage with the literature are all informed by this set of beliefs – what is known in research as your *paradigm*. You will also find that writers use a slew of terms to describe this essential concept and these can include research philosophy, theoretical approaches, qualitative and quantitative approaches, inductive and deductive reasoning and so on. As with many other issues concerning approaches, while the words may differ the fundamental concern will be very similar – and that is how your research is going to be shaped and driven by your theoretical positioning.

Bryman (2008, pp. 696–7) considers a paradigm to be 'a cluster of beliefs and dictates that for scientist [*sic*] in a particular discipline influence what should be studied, how research should be done, and how results should be interpreted'. Walliman (2001) also considers the influence of a paradigm and positions it in terms of how a belief in a particular theoretical approach may influence the researcher's view of the world and, therefore, the topic or phenomenon itself. Creswell (1998, p. 74) provides us with an even clearer definition and considers paradigms to be 'a basic set of beliefs or assumptions that guide [our] inquiries. These are assumptions related to the nature of reality (the ontology), the relationships the researcher has to that being researched (the epistemological issue) … and the process of the research (the methodological issue).' What all these theorists are saying is that we all have a particular belief and/or theoretical position that impacts not only on how we view the world around us but also how we relate and see ourselves positioned within that; and as a consequence how we undertake research.

Once you start reflecting on your research topic, the literature you engage with, the questions you ask, what you believe and what you feel more challenged by and why, the idea that we come to our research topics from a rather personal and particular point of view begins to make sense.

A research paradigm involves three aspects and/or parts and Creswell (1998) alludes to them in his summation of how he defines a research paradigm. Below we offer further explanation of these particular terms so that you can begin to become familiar with them.

Ontology

'What is the nature of the "knowable"? What is the nature of "reality"?' (Guba 1990, p. 18). Gray's (2004, p. 16) definition refers directly to issues concerning research and describes ontology as 'the study of being, that is, the nature of existence … [it] embodies understanding what is'.

Fox et al. (2007) considers the understanding of ontology in three particular ways, while Guba and Lincoln (1998) break it down into four.

1 Ontological meanings can be situated within the 'existence' of an objective world (positivism); a world that exists independently of human belief and culture. This truth/known is observable and can be measured and verified as existing. Matthews and Ross (2010, p. 25) emphasise the essential nature of objectivism in positivism, which 'asserts that the social phenomena that make up our social world have an existence of their own … apart from and independent of social actors (humans) who are involved'. Examples of positivistic informed frameworks include RCTs; epidemiology; quantitative systematic reviews; experimental designs; cause and effect statements of truth; validity, reliability and generalisability; deductive reasoning.

Reflective activity

Think about the term 'the elderly', often used to define a particular group of people. To hold an ontological view that is informed by positivist beliefs you would have to absolutely 'know' that this group existed independently and outside of human influence. Thus, for you the 'elderly' will have a particular unitary and universal meaning.

- Now think of the phenomenon of 'dementia'; what do you absolutely 'know' (knowledge that exists independently of outside influences) about this term?
- How does this knowledge impact on how you might 'treat' this group?

2 Fox et al. (2007) then consider the socially constructed world/reality, positing that realities are constructed by groups of people with shared meanings. Thus, realities are multiple and groups of people continuously create, respond to and interact with these realities to make sense of their world (social construction/constructivism is an example of this). Matthews and Ross (2010, p. 25) define this as follows: the 'social phenomena making up our social world are only real in the sense that they are constructed ideas which are continually being reviewed and reworked by those involved in them (the social actors) through social interactions and reflection'.

Useful resources

Go to the case study on dementia (Chapter 4, Case study 4) and read the section on alternative views to biomedicine. This gives you some idea of how we can construct, and then create, particular understandings of dementia that impact on how people with dementia understand dementia, but also on how those of us without dementia understand it.

3 Fox et al. (2007) talk about the individually constructed world/reality (interpretivism) where the individual experiences and then constructs, interprets and makes sense of their own world; so in effect individuals

construct and interpret their own world (e.g. phenomenology). This form of ontology considers the experiencing and the living of, and within, a phenomenon as that which is known – this, like social construction, is an ongoing and dynamic process where meanings and experiences intertwine and inform one another.

4 Gray (2009) and Matthews and Ross (2010) add to this range of ontological understandings the term realist. What this ontological position holds is that there is such a thing as an external reality that exists independently of social actors but that there is more to reality then meets the eye (or the senses), a dimension, according to Matthews and Ross (2010, p. 26), 'which is hidden from the senses, which cannot be directly observed … but their impact can be observed in the way people behave'. Very often critical research theories are located within this ontology – believing that the powerful structures and mechanisms that are invisible, taken for granted 'truths' are hugely influential on the way we behave, feel and interact with one another.

Reflective activity

Go to the examples provided for you in the section on generalisability (p. 255), and consider the one that states 'Boys like cars'.

- Why do boys like cars?
- What are we saying about the nature of boys?

Epistemology

The second related strand of paradigms is epistemologies, how we know or understand what we know. Guba (1990) defines this in terms of the nature of the relationship between us (the researcher/the knower) and that which we 'know' and/or understand. Gray's definition (2004, p. 16) states that 'epistemology tries to understand what it means to know. Epistemology provides a philosophical background for deciding what kinds of knowledge are legitimate and adequate.'

Fox et al. (2007, pp. 10–12) again break this down, as they did with ontology, and divide them into particular understandings.

1 For positivistic approaches the relationship of the researcher to the objective world is free of values, the researcher does not influence or impact on this world and can be detached from this reality – asking it questions and getting answers back.

2 The socially constructed world is one where the researcher is part of what emerges in terms of multiple realities, so the researcher here interacts with, interprets and relates to that which they are researching. Matthews and Ross (2010) also see the subjectivity of the researcher within this

5

view, the interactive nature and co-construction of multiple realities being an integral aspect of how we understand and relate to the world.

3 In the individually constructed world, the individual gains insight into their own and other people's worlds, they believe they impact and bring their own individually constructed view to the research and work with that in order to gain insight into other people's worlds. As with socially constructed views, this is a subjective position that is worked with in terms of interpretation and inclusion (Matthews and Ross 2010).

4 Realism's epistemological position is very often located within critical realist debates (Bryman 2008; Matthews and Ross 2010) and epistemologically locates the researcher as the 'discoverer' or identifier of the hidden structures and mechanisms that result in 'structural mechanisms' of inequality and injustice. This offers us the epistemological role of being able to challenge, change and even negate these mechanisms through the process of identification and empowerment (Matthew and Ross 2010). The case studies on dementia, HIV and obesity in particular all engage with this framework when trying to unpack some of the powerful stigmatisations and discriminatory practices that function in all three areas of practice.

Schools of paradigms or methodolologies

You will find, as previously said, that writers will often divide different schools of paradigms and/or approaches into particular broad umbrella terms that encompass particular ontological and epistemological positions. For instance, Sarantakos (1998, p. 33) divides them into three groups, which, he feels, best reflect these varied positions.

1 Positivistic/quantitative: positivism, neopositivism, methodological positivism, logical positivism.
2 Interpretative/qualitative: symbolic interaction, phenomenology, ethnomethodology, hermeneutics, psychoanalysis, ethnology, ethnography, social linguistics [social construction, narrative enquiry].
3 Critical: critical sociology, conflict school of thought of Marxism, feminism [critical disability, queer theory, postcolonialism, Marxist approaches, critical cultural/race studies, poststructuralism, critical citizenship studies].

There are two aspects you need to consider when reading around these informing frameworks. First, paradigms act as a map or framework for the questions you ask, the kind of problems or issues you explore, the angles and perspectives you take, and the way in which you ask questions. Second, you will see terms like 'qualitative', 'interpretative', 'naturalist', 'anti- or non-positivist' etc. used interchangeably and synonymously to denote similar meanings. The key here is to consider that the language used can vary and it is up to you to develop the skills to identify the key characteristics embraced within each approach.

Language and methodologies (a brief word)

Methodology, in reference to paradigms, refers to how and what method you use to collect your data. Clearly your choice of method is absolutely informed by your ontological and epistemological position, as these elements frame the very nature of the data you want to investigate and your role in that investigation. Thus, coming from a positivist paradigm you will want to measure the independent existence of particular phenomena using methods that are designed to be structured, objective and distanced.

However, the term methodology can also be used in other ways, which while clearly connected, have particular meanings of their own. Thus, you may find the term 'methodology' being used synonymously with paradigms and indeed methods, as well as being understood and written about in the following ways:

1 Used to describe the research model that a project has used to frame, contextualise and carry out the research, so one could infer from this that each project has its own unique methodology, i.e. combination of aspects.
2 Used more commonly as distinctive, mutually exclusive theoretical or research principles that guide the research, i.e. very much similar to the way in which principles of research are determined in a paradigm and taken to a framework of engagement, such as ethnography – the study of cultures, mores, norms and rituals through emersion within the natural setting etc.

Approaches included in this text

You will observe that this text does not cover all the possible paradigms mentioned. What we have chosen to do instead is discuss a number of them, focusing on their characteristics and applications. Bryman (2008), Bowling (2009), Gray (2009) and Ross and Matthews (2010) are a few of the texts that explore a greater range of approaches within all of the three broad paradigmatic schools.

We deliberately address the various approaches in different ways, to reflect their clear, often oppositional, way of engaging with knowledge and its 'creation'. We start with positivism, as this is still the most powerful paradigm within health and social care research. It is as a result of the considerable limitations of this paradigm that interpretative and critical research theories emerged. You will see that we have unpacked positivism's meanings, significance and applications in ways that reflect its ontological and epistemological positioning.

We then look at interpretative approaches (including phenomenology, ethnography, social construction and symbolic interactionism) and endeavour to unpack a number of approaches that can fall into paradigmatic, as well as methodological, frameworks. Finally, we address critical approaches to research (feminist, critical disability, queer theory, postcolonial/critical race studies etc.). We look at only one of the possible critical approaches available to us and we do so deliberately. First, we feel that feminist methodologies are

5

one of the main critical theoretical research approaches; second, they have had a profound influence on the development of other critical approaches, particularly in their political positioning and epistemologies. Third, feminist methodologies have particular characteristics that are specific to them, and these are explored further.

While the style taken within these sections attempts to explain, or even describe at times, the meanings of interpretative and critical approaches, embedded within you will find a critically analytical approach as well. Within each section we consider some of the limitations and/or areas to address should you decide to engage with any of these approaches.

Reflective activities

Within the sections that follow we have embedded empirical research articles in each of the discussions. These are used to give you 'living examples' of how the particular paradigm or methodology informs the design, method and research process as a whole. Thus, the reflective activity for these sections is the reading of the research article itself. The engagement with these is part of your research journey, applying your learning to your own research topic and the literature that you access.

In some ways all of the case studies have been heavily influenced by critical theory, as well as interpretism and positivism. What we hope is evident is how these three approaches inform the way in which the topics under investigation are discussed and developed. Thus, these case studies are intended to be working examples of the complexities of how knowledge can be understood.

Box 5.4 Interpretative Research

Key qualities of interpretative research

> In-depth and interpreted understandings of social world.
> Small-scale samples purposively selected.
> Data collection in close contact with participants.
> Detailed, information-rich and extensive data.
> Emergent analysis – description and patterns.
> Represents the social world.
> 'Perceives the researcher and the researched as equally important elements of the same situation' (Sarantakos 1998, p. 46).
> Inductive, i.e. through collecting the data, and analysing its meanings etc., one develops a theory, beliefs etc.

Aspects of interpretative research that are challenged

> Non-consensus over methods and/or meanings and approaches.
> Often lack of clarity and vagueness in terms of the rationale for utilising a particular method and/or analytic approach.
> Endeavours to make generalisations from a very small sample.

> Sampling can often be based on a convenience approach and produce results and a population that therefore represent a 'biased' position.
> The impact of the researcher on in-depth and responsive approaches to interviews and focus groups, i.e. how our own interpretations and responses can inform and impact on others (see social construction).
> Descriptive and 'unscientific'.
> Interpretative and not based on measured outcomes.
> Subjective.
> Lack of reliability and validity (according to positivist criteria).
> Can't be generalised.

Box 5.5 Critical Research Theory

Key qualities of critical research theory

> Research leads to action and change.
> Research is engaged with the respondents.
> The researcher is part of the hidden structures so research is very reflective and reflexive so that the ways in which these structures impact on the researcher are also made visible.
> Often uses mixed methods.
> In-depth and rich, as well as measured.
> Interpretative and objective.
> Theoretically inductive and deductive.
> Politically situated.
> Exposes the power and 'false consciousness' structures that are embedded in our ideas of reality.
> Empowering and enfranchising.

Aspects of this approach that are challenged

> Idealistic.
> Politically partial.
> See too the challenges to both qualitative and at times positivist research, as this approach can utilise mixed methods.
> Can essentialise concepts.

Positivism

Positivism is sometimes referred to as the scientific paradigm. Positivism originates from the work of the French philosopher and founder of the academic discipline of sociology, Auguste Comte (1798–1857). Comte postulated that there were three epochs of human thought and knowledge:

> theological, where knowledge and thought was based on belief systems (supernatural, religious);
> metaphysical, where knowledge was based on, and informed by, philosophical and theoretical thinking (dominated by lawyers and theologians);
> positive, where knowledge was based on, and informed by, scientific thinking (dominated by scientists and engineers).

Comte's philosophy and ideas were informed by his experiences of revolution in France during the first part of the nineteenth century, and is reflective of the significant shifts in thinking occurring during the Enlightenment (Bilton et al. 2002). He determined that what was necessary to improve social order and facilitate effective social change was to develop a scientific understanding of society. Comte thought that the 'positive' stage of thinking encapsulated benevolence and welfare for all (Noble 2000).

> The basic theme of positivism is that only science, firmly grounded in non-metaphysical fact and the discovery of the laws of causes and effect which explain the observable universe, can finally liberate the world from ignorance or disorder. (Noble 2000, p. 43)

The main principles of positivism reflect an objective ontology and that it is possible to identify 'facts' about the social and physical world (Crichton and Mulhall 2008). It is asserted that all knowledge is scientific and science is often regarded as the highest form of genuine knowledge (Benton and Craib 2001).

Empirical study (observation and experimentation) is the key component of positivist investigation, with the main focus on the collection of quantifiable data (Crichton and Mulhall 2008) as it is deemed essential to verify knowledge (Davey 1994b; Quinton 1997). It is claimed that through such investigation, universal laws can also be identified that predict and explain phenomena, as positivism is broadly descriptive and normative (Lacey 1995).

> The philosophy of positivism was the view that science could tell us the final truth about the world … [it] was thought that science could replace prejudice, superstition, blind tradition and the intolerant conservatism of the *ancien regimes* everywhere, and … the blind utopianism and mindless savagery of the revolutionary masses. (Nobel 2000, p. 46)

Box 5.6 Positivism

Key qualities of positivist research

> Measured.
> Structured.
> Generalisable.
> Valid and reliable.
> Replicable.

> Large scale.
> Deductive, i.e. one applies a general principle to the researched and research.
> Researcher is objective/distanced.
> Controlled.
> Experimental.
> There is an objective truth, known, independent of social actors.

Aspects of the positivistic paradigm that are challenged

> The belief that there is an independently existing known.
> Knowledge is positioned as being value free.
> The objectivity of researchers.
> Reductionism throughout.
> Essentialised conceptualisation of variables.
> Decontextualisation of phenomena.
> Fixed research designs unresponsive to contextual realities.
> Accepts that populations can be fully 'known' and then generalised.
> Limitations of cause and effect reasoning.
> Results obtained in controlled experimental conditions do not apply to the messiness of the real world.

Positivism and health-related research

The positivist paradigm informs much of the knowledge base gathered from the natural world, including the biological functioning of the body and scientific and medical study such as epidemiology (Crichton and Mulhall 2008) (see p. 194). A particular influence of positivism, in research and epidemiology, is the development of the *hypothetico-deductive* method. Essentially, this refers to the structured process of reasoning and investigation to put ideas, 'facts' and 'truth' to the test. A theory or hypothesis emerges from observations or logical reasoning with regard to a particular phenomenon, although Karl Popper, a philosopher (1902–94), asserted that scientific investigation was a speculative and creative activity too. From the formulation of a hypothesis, i.e. provisional explanations about a phenomenon, the proper way to proceed with scientific discovery is to put theories (hypotheses), (e.g. that obesity contributes to mortality) to the test (i.e. undertake some form of empirical study, experiment or observation) (Davey 1994b). A hypothesis is a supposition that is tested by collecting facts that lead to its acceptance or rejection.

For example, in 1947 the Medical Research Council asked Bradford-Hill et al. to investigate the (possible/proposed) link between smoking and lung cancer, based on observations that increases in the incidence of lung cancer had proceeded increases in rates of smoking (Sir Richard Doll, at the time, also thought that lung cancer might be linked to increasing urban pollution with the growth in the use of motor vehicles).

5

Testing a theory or hypothesis requires the formulation of specific outcomes or predictions. In the case of smoking and lung cancer this could be expressed along the lines of:

H (Hypothesis) = People who smoke cigarettes are more likely to die of lung cancer than non-smokers

However, according to Popper it is impossible to conclusively *prove* that a hypothesis is correct, as no one is able to undertake all lines of investigation and collect *all* the evidence that might be available in the world on any particular matter (Davey 1994b). This means that, at least in theory, it is possible that evidence contrary to the hypothesis does exist – it simply has not be collected or observed. Take, for example, the hypothesis below:

H = all swans are white

A survey of swans could be undertaken in a random selection of counties in the UK and only white swans are found. This, however, does not prove the hypothesis beyond all doubt as evidence has not been collected from *all* possible sources, i.e. every country. It would take the discovery of just one black swan (as do exist in Australia) for this statement to be shown to not be true or not proven (Gambrill 1999).

This also demonstrates the contingent nature of discovery. Prior to 'finding' Australia all the *available* evidence might support the above hypothesis (i.e. all UK swans are white), but as mechanisms for discovery advance and other research is undertaken, the potential for new evidence to emerge that refutes old 'truths' is obvious. This is why Bradford-Hill, for example, proposed that before any claims about a relationship between X and Y (smoking and lung cancer) can be made, the correlation must be found consistently. Any study that found contrary evidence (e.g. the one black swan) should be a cause to doubt the 'truth' of the hypothesis.

Box 5.7 Good versus bad studies

Please note: evidence emanating from some studies is better than others, simply due to the fact that some have a more robust study design. For example, evidence drawn from a survey in your local park of a group of 20 swans (all white), is not as substantial as that drawn from a UK-wide survey of 200,000 swans (also all white) – numbers do count when making inferences from sample groups to the population as a whole.

In general, therefore, the only safe conclusion that can be drawn from research evidence regarding a hypothesis is that it *might* be true – we cannot conclusively state that it *is* true.

Karl Popper reasoned that instead of trying to *prove* a hypothesis to be true, scientists and researchers should in fact try to find out if a claim is *not true* (disprove their hypothesis/falsify a claim) (Davey 1994b). The purpose is to set out to investigate the antithesis of a theory, hypothesis or claim. This is called the *null hypothesis*. For inferences (and claims) to be made, 'Statistical testing of an association requires the formulation of a null hypothesis' (Abramson 1984, p. 31). Researchers can then examine the evidence for and against the null hypothesis. If the evidence against the null hypothesis is sufficiently strong they can reject the null hypothesis and if the null hypothesis is *not* true then the hypothesis is likely to be true (Davey 1994b).

Take the smoking and lung cancer example again – the null hypothesis would be:

> Null Hypothesis = People who smoke cigarettes are *not* more likely to die of lung cancer than non-smokers.

(We know that this is not true – so the opposite, people who smoke, are more likely to die of lung cancer – is likely to be true.) The purpose of a scientific or, in this case, epidemiological study is, therefore, to test the null hypothesis. If the null hypothesis is shown to be false (i.e. the data shows that those who smoke are actually *more* likely to die from lung cancer than non-smokers), the hypothesis that 'people who smoke cigarettes are more likely to die of lung cancer than non-smokers' is given some credibility.

It is this pattern of reasoning that is fundamental to epidemiological study, which informs a great deal of EBP. This sort of study process is also essential when attempting to determine such matters as the therapeutic effectiveness of new medication or surgical interventions (e.g. as opposed to no treatment or existing therapies) but this approach has attracted criticism when it comes to the more holistic study of humans or societies.

Criticism of positivism

Bilton et al. (2002) note that the positivist perspective is criticised for asserting the existence of social 'facts' about the world that exist separately from human interactions and subjective experiences and for ignoring the 'socially constructed' nature of ideas and influences about the way human society should and does function. Positivist study also requires close, objective, scrutiny of matters that can be tested, which is difficult to achieve within complex human societies (Davey 1994b). Many subjective states, such as anxiety, love and 'goodness', are difficult, if not impossible, to measure, and the claim that scientific explanation discovers *the* truth (reductionism – a single explanation) is rejected when it comes to human society. Reductionism in scientific investigation also involves in practice the exploration of a phenomenon at its 'lowest' level, e.g. at the level of the chemical, cell or atom, to explain why a particular event occurs (e.g. how the heart beats), but this is criticised for disconnecting individual parts from the totality of functioning. Social scientists assert the need for a much more holistic approach whereby phenomena can only be comprehended through the exploration of interactions and relationships at all

5

levels (Davey 1994b). Moreover it is increasingly recognised that social inter-actions and subjective matters influence the 'facts' too (see the case studies in Chapter 4) and as Davey (1994b, p. 19) writes:

> the claim that scientific research is about the objective discovery of 'facts' and to conceal from the public gaze the reality that it is conducted by human beings who make mistakes, follow hunches, complete with each other for fame and funding, get bored and occasionally fake their results. In other words, scientific research is a social activity which is often 'dressed up' to look as though it isn't.

None of this is intended to imply that scientifically focused research is essentially corrupt or unnecessary. Instead it emphasises the necessary caution that should be placed on any claims of ultimate, indisputable truth, and the need to recognise the social context within which knowledge operates.

Case study 5.2 An example of positivism

Context and purpose: The Manson et al. (1995) study set out to investigate the relationship between weight and health. Specifically, they 'examined the relation between body-mass index and both overall mortality and mortality from specific causes in a large cohort of middle-aged women enrolled in the prospective Nurses' Health Study ... also assessed the role of weight gain since the age of 18 and the ratio of waist circumference to hip circumference in predicting mortality in the cohort' (Manson et al. 1995, p. 679). They were concerned too about the increasing prevalence of obesity and permissiveness in recommended weight standards across the USA and, additionally, wanted to assess the validity of the link between leanness (being thin) and mortality.

Approach: This epidemiological study is a prospective cohort-study of 115,195 US nurses. It started in 1976 when study participants filled in a questionnaire giving details of age, current weight and height, current and past cigarette smoking, other risk factors and medical history. These questionnaires were repeated every two years and information about weight at 18, food frequency and physical activity was requested in 1980. All information was self-reported (and therefore subject to error through measurement bias) and in recognition of this, some validity checks were made.

Findings: The data collected from the questionnaires was used to calculate relative risk of death between women grouped into different weight categories based on body mass index (BMI). Over the 16 years follow-up included in this study there were 4,726 deaths, 881 from CHD, 2,586 from cancer and 1,259 from other causes. The conclusions drawn from this study and highlighted in the abstract reads as follows:

> We examined the association between body-mass index ... and both overall mortality and mortality from specific causes in a cohort of 115,195 US women enrolled in the prospective Nurses' Health Study. ... Body weight and mortality from all causes were directly related among these middle-aged women. Lean women did not have excess mortality. The lowest mortality rate was observed

among women who weighed at least 15 percent less than the US average for women of similar age and among those whose weight had been stable since early adulthood. (Manson et al. 1995, p. 677)

The conclusions are based upon statistical associations between BMI and mortality – in other words a *risk* of death linked to specific weight categories (BMI). The study presents data on the risk of death in one group compared with another (those with a higher BMI compared to a lower BMI) – the *relative risk*. The risk ratios (RR) for mortality between groups of women with different BMIs are all very small. The largest RR (adjusted for age and other variables) was 1.5 for those with a BMI ≤ 19 compared with those with a BMI ≥ 32. This equates to a *possible*, 1.5 more people having a bad outcome (death) or 15 per 1,000. None of the RR were suggestive of a *strong* correlation. Some of the relative risks calculated were also less than 1: BMI ≤ 19 compared to BMI 19–21.9, 22–24.9, 25–26.9 = 0.8. This indicates a benefit from being heavier. In addition, the relative risk for BMI 27–28.9 compared to BMI ≤ 19 was 1, i.e. there was no difference in the risk of mortality between these two groups. For women who were former smokers the RR was below 1 (i.e. indicating a beneficial effect of weight, although not statistically significant) *except* for women with a BMI ≥ 32, and this was below 2.

Risk shifts in favour of the hypothesis (that obesity is bad for health) *only* when smoking is taken out of the equation (43.8 per cent of thin women smoked), early deaths are excluded and reported stable weight is taken into account. These tabulations relate to small numbers (1,168 and 531 respectively) and the small increase in risk (2 at its maximum) is only statistically significant for BMIs ≥ 27. When CHD, cancer rates and 'other causes' are worked out for women who never smoked the RR does increase and is statistically significant for BMIs ≥ 27 again (CHD and cancers) and is at its maximum of 4 for CHD deaths. This only includes 184 deaths. For 'other causes' the increase in risk (which is marginal, being less than 2) is only statistically significant for women in the BMI category 29–31.9.

Evidence-based conclusions?

This is not a comprehensive critique of the Manson et al. (1995) study, but it is worth drawing your attention to the validity of this conclusion given the nature of the study and evidence presented in the paper. According to Campos (2004),

> What this study actually demonstrated was that the odds that a mildly 'obese' middle-age middle-class non smoking white woman would die of cardio-vascular disease (or anything else) over the sixteen-year course of the study were extremely low. (Campos 2004, p. 16)

Source: Manson et al. (1995) 'Body Weight and Mortality among Women', *New England Journal of Medicine*, 333(11), 677–85.

5

Ethnography

Ethnography is a particular tradition and/or approach to research that can be of great use to health studies. You will find, particularly in dementia research, for instance, that there is a great deal of research that relies on the ethnographic approach to gain insight into a particular setting. Ethnography is largely rooted in anthropology, which considers (Smith 2002; Bryman 2008; Matthews and Ross 2010) that the only way we can truly gain insight into a particular group, setting, culture etc. is by living with and becoming immersed within the setting. Realities are therefore creations within groups and settings, within the context with all its contributing aspects.

Ethnography, like many qualitative and/or interpretative approaches is concerned with naturalistic settings, i.e. within the actual environment of the phenomenon. It is also very much embedded in what Smith (2002) calls 'finding the social' and inductive in its reasoning, i.e. research is discovery. It relies primarily on engaged observation as its main method of data collection. Sarantakos (1998, p. 196) describes it as 'the science of "ethnos", that is, nations, people or cultures ... interested in relationships between people and the physical, socio-political, personal, cultural and historical aspects of their life'.

According to Fox et al. (2007, p. 14) its purpose it to analyse how 'cultures' (and the term culture in this instance can mean organisations, events, communities and groups) organise and behave in their natural setting. Harper and La Fontaine (2009, p. 238) understand the purpose of ethnography to be 'the study of people within their living and/or working environments, the goal of which is to achieve a rich and detailed understanding of actions, beliefs, constructions and meanings associated with that group'. For Matthews and Ross (2010) one of the key qualities of ethnography is the researcher's total immersion and involvement in the research context, so that they 'witness' and are part of what is said and done first hand rather than it being a retrospective account of action and speech.

Usually ethnography does not only use observation as its method of data gathering; the research can involve the utilisation of interviews, focus groups and even surveys (Tritter 2007) as a way of supplementing the observational data. Interviews may be in response to what emerges in the field, so the researcher seeks to understand and clarify that which they have observed. Sometimes interviews will be in the form of informant interviews, again embedded in the emergent design but often concerned with having explanations.

Mixed method approaches, which include observation, are often designed as case studies where there is an in-depth focus on a particular culture using multiple methods as a way of endeavouring to fully 'understand' the emergent realities. Bowling (2009, p. 386) understands that ethnography centralises the use of observation as its main source of data, but that it 'involves a *triangulated* approach to research: for example, using a combination of unstructured interviews and record research to supplement and validate the observations'.

Box 5.8 Ethnography

Key qualities of ethnography

> In-depth and engaged.
> Over a long period of time in order for full immersion to take place, which in turn allows the realities of the group or context being observed to emerge in their natural setting.
> Inductive.
> Naturalistic.
> Can be used with groups or settings with which it may be difficult to engage.
> Largely relies on in-depth observation.
> Concerned with gaining insight into and providing a picture of peoples, groups or organisations through involved fieldwork.
> Interested in how people interact and events take place (Matthews and Ross 2010) as they take place.
> 'Allows the factors influencing professional and clinical practice' (Harper and La Fontaine 2009, p. 240) to emerge, be seen and 'understood'.
> Allows the implicit taken-for-granted practices in which we engage to be rendered visible; therefore it acknowledges that realities emerge through our everyday actions, behaviours and responses as they occur.

Aspects of ethnography that are challenging and challenged

> The potential for role conflict of the researcher/observer role and the involved participant role.
> Being an ethnographer in a 'strange and new place' (Robson 2007) requires an enormous amount of skills and experiences, including what to observe, who to speak to in terms of informant interviews and so on, while, as Robson (2007) says, those doing research in their own practice or a familiar setting need to be able to 'set aside their own preconceptions', i.e. render the familiar unfamiliar.
> Ethics in terms of how long you have known the other participants and developing a relationship: (a) what you do with disclosures and witnessing inappropriate practice; and (b) how you deal with the relationships when you leave the field.
> How to work with covert and overt ethnography – do you tell everyone or only certain informants? Providing a well based rationale for covert observation requires a great deal of thought and rigorous justification located within sound ethical frameworks.
> Matthews and Ross (2010) also consider that issues such as gaining access can be challenging and long drawn out.
> The challenge of decisions about how to record, when and with what.

5

> How do you ensure credibility of design, i.e. that you are exploring what you intended in the most feasible and rigorous manner?

> Harper and La Fontaine (2009, p. 243) problematise 'its subjectivity and reliance on interpretation ... The use of small samples or groups of people which mean that findings cannot be considered generalisable.' A counter challenge to this is that: (a) ethnographic research does not set out to generalise, seeing that an in-depth engagement with a small population will allow the quality of interaction, behaviours and relationships to emerge in real world situations; and (b) all research is subjectively located and ethnography works with subjectivity in ways that are designed to reduce its impact.

> Being time-consuming and thus costly to undertake (Matthews and Ross 2010).

Case study 5.3 An example of ethnography

Context. Globally HIV is on the increase and the design of interventions to prevent or reduce this are multiple. When working with populations, such as female sex workers who are particularly marginalised and disenfranchised, research has shown that interventions need to be designed to be community based, with the intention of engaging and empowering the disempowered populations. According to the findings many of these fail to succeed in reducing the prevalence and spread of HIV but a particular community-based project in India, The Sonagachi STD/HIV Prevention Project (SHIP) in Kolkata, achieved significant changes in safe sex behaviour, reductions in STI prevalence and low rates of HIV, at the same time bringing about a process of collectivism and participation among sex workers.

Purpose. They were interested in looking at what it was in this particular project and/or community that facilitated the success, so rather than evaluating success based on measurements and outcomes it was concerned with exploring the context and environment – as it considered issues of power, context, agency and organisation culture as an often unacknowledged influence on what 'makes an intervention work in one place and not in another'.

Approach. The researchers rationalised that in order to fully engage and gain insight into the culture of the context of implementation, an ethnographic take was needed – particularly given their stance on 'naturally occurring events and influences in the setting and environment of the intervention that might act to contribute to or impede intervention success' (Hawe et al. 2004, p. 788; cited in Evans and Lambert 2008).

Method. Their design was multiple and included interviews, both individual and group, as well as participant observations. Their interest was in recognising the messiness of intervention and placing it within the context of relationships, power, history, politics and influences. For them, projects are implemented through a range of everyday formal and informal practices that are imbued with cultural meanings and values. They also recognise that projects are implemented with and through 'agents' who are embedded within broader social relationships (of which a project is just one). Finally, they stress that ethnographies must engage with the concept of 'power', paying attention to whose voices, interests and ideas come to dominate within projects at different times and why.

There were two periods of ethnographic research (fairly early on in the life of the project and then a few years later), with the original focus of the research, i.e. women's sexual health and vulnerability to HIV, mushrooming and responding to the context, to particularly focus on SHIP. Very often a key to critical ethnographic research is the response to the environment and culture, the unexpected often becoming visible and researchers then engage with that context's culture (Silverman 2004; Bryman 2009; Gray 2009). The two researchers (again very often an element of acknowledging the interpretative nature of ethnography may well be to have more than one researcher; moreover, from a practical point, given the complex and multilayered nature of cultures and the non-sequential nature of implementation and management of interventions, having two researchers would enable – if necessary – researchers to be in more than one place at one time) were immersed in the day to day running of the process, organisation and management, engaging with the project on lots of different levels. They went to meetings, were involved in the everyday project work, training sessions and field work of the trainers, spent time with the trainers and in the sex workers' club room and so on. In other words they observed not only the interventions themselves but the informing organisation context as well. It was only through this in-depth participant observation and ethnography that some of the informing elements that enabled this project to be so successful emerged.

Findings. First, the project, and its multiple participants and layers, openly engaged with the inevitable power and political manoeuvring and debate that occurs in organisations, across different groups, managing and implementing change and individual roles and agendas. While it was uncomfortable, this enabled the 'private/hidden stories' that ethnography is so interested in to emerge and the realities of these contexts to be worked with rather than glossed over in what the researchers termed the 'warmly persuasive rhetoric of participation'. Second, there was a commitment to the mobilisation and empowerment of the sex workers by SHIP and other participants. So the political ideology of community and the mobilisation of workers' rights were embedded in how the project was run and worked with the participants. Peer educators were recruited from within the sex worker communities and the commitment of the project to workers' rights enabled the peer educators to become 'agents of change' – despite working within the rather formal and didactic nature of the intervention itself.

Limitations of ethnography

There are a number of weaknesses or potential criticisms of ethnography and this project, not least that the researchers were invested in the project itself – so their commitment to it was informed by their role as both researcher and participant observer within the project itself – so the likelihood of them impacting on the very practices they were there to observe was high. If acknowledged explicitly and worked with then this does not necessarily mean that it is a weakness; instead their own role is simply part of the micro picture (see also participant observations).

Source: Evans, C. and Lambert, H. (2008) 'Implementing Community Interventions for HIV Prevention: Insights from Project Ethnography', *Social Science and Medicine*, 66, 467–78.

5

This philosophical positioning has already been explored and critiqued, in some depth, in Chapter 3, so what is presented here is brief, with the unpacking of the article being the main focus. Social constructivism, another interpretative approach, considers 'the existing social reality, which we take for granted, as a "social construction" of members of a given society' (Flick et al. 2004, p. 65). Thus, what and how we create meaning and understanding is something that as group(s) of people we do together, but in ways that are often implicit rather than explicitly intended. Fox et al. (2007) emphasise the shared nature of the meanings, constructions and interactions, defining reality in terms of its multiple constructions, which can shift and constantly develop within the contexts, involving particular people.

Engaging in a piece of research that is informed by constructivism would have the purpose of gaining insight into how people make sense of their world with others. Speedy (2008) explains this as a collaborative creative and meaning-making activity that makes up the 'space' between and among people. The implication here is that the constructions themselves are active agents as well a result of this interactive engagement. Gergen and Gergen (2003, p. 15) explain it as being 'principally concerned with explicating the processes by which people come to describe, explain, or otherwise account for the world (including themselves) in which they live. It attempts to articulate common forms of understanding as they now exist, as they have existed in prior historical periods, and as they might exist should creative attention be so directed.'

Case study 5.4 An example of social constructivism

Context, purpose and approach. This piece of research was part of a larger study, but was interested in looking at how groups of people make sense of and construct meanings around STIs and in particular HIV/AIDS. The concern here was looking at what do people draw on to make sense of HIV/AIDS. Previous research had clearly indicated that how people understood and constructed HIV/AIDS and how they behaved were related, so the researchers were interested in looking at these multiple constructions of reality. The researchers acknowledged the importance of the legacy of apartheid as well as the conservatism of both white and black South African populations, where sexual matters are positioned as fairly taboo and unspoken. So the social context, history and arena in which people live are seen as informants to how people may understand and construct their worlds.

Method. The methods used were as open and qualitative as possible in order to allow people to fully explore their meanings and the unspoken, and to allow what the researchers constitute as misconceptions and misunderstandings to emerge. They used ten focus groups and tried to focus on recruiting groups that were particularly considered 'at risk', i.e. miners, prisoners, sex workers, young people, as well as community workers. They very often worked with pre-existing groups as well. They had two all-male groups, five all-female groups and three groups with both genders.

5

The format of the group was informed by a semi-structured guide and a number of vignettes that were introduced to the groups to engender discussion.

Findings. What became apparent was that HIV/AIDS was socially constructed as promiscuity, prostitution, dirtiness, immorality, women/gender blamed, shameful and so on. Discourses of 'othering' people with HIV/AIDS also emerged, as did the process of 'exceptionalism' when individuals who had HIV/AIDS wanted to locate themselves outside of the above social construction. Thus, there was separation in terms of both 'I'm not like them' and 'the victim/I didn't know' discourses. By engaging in these discourses the powerful nature of stigmatisation was revealed, and its implications for their lives and how they live and treat others.

Source: Shefer, T., Strebel, A., Wilson, T., Shabalala, N., Simbayi, L., Ratele, K., Potgieter, C. and Andipatin, M. (2002) 'The Social Construction of Sexually Transmitted Infections (STIs) in South African Communities', *Qualitative Health Research*, 12(10), 1373–90.

Phenomenology

Phenomenology is an interpretative approach that is particularly concerned with gaining insight into and exploring the lived experience of individuals in relation to a particular phenomenon from their own point of view (Robson 2007). It is what both Bryman (2008) and Gray (2009) would assert to be the antithesis of positivism. That is, it says that the world is a social and subjective construction and the researcher is part of that world (having experiences and views of their own) and the phenomenon under exploration. So here again you will find that this approach can be used a great deal in the health industry (Fox et al. 2007; Bowling 2009), including EBP. Very often the focus will be on 'what is it like and what does it mean to have dementia/be infertile/be obese/have HIV'. The interest here is on the perspective and experience of the individual who has had the experience. Thus, realities are individually mediated by a repertoire of constructs that each individual draws on to make sense of their experience of the world.

This requires a great deal of reflection on your part in terms of what you think and believe already. Phenomenology acknowledges the subjective position of the researcher (Snape and Spencer 2003; Gray 2009) and that your relationship to the individual(s) and the phenomenon under investigation will have a considerable bearing on what emerges throughout the research. What phenomenology asks the researcher to consider is 'bracketing', which is the process of clearly acknowledging your own beliefs, meanings and experiential constructs and then setting them aside during the process of research (this can be a contentious practice; Edmund Husserl, the 'father' of phenomenology, and Martin Heidegger, a student of Husserl, are two philosophers whose work has informed this discourse).

The focus for phenomenology is therefore the belief that 'each individual holds a unique story about what has happened in the past … there is nothing more fundamental than experiences. Reality is what a person experiences ... how the individual makes sense of and constructs his or her own world' (Fox et al. 2007, p. 11). Sarantakos (1998, p. 48), referring to Husserl, 'suggests that people are active creators of their world, and have a consciousness that communicates to them everyday experiences and knowledge'.

Box 5.9 Phenomenology

Key qualities of phenomenology

> In-depth and engaged.
> Behaviour is a product of how people experience and interpret the world (Bryman 2008).
> Inductive in that it endeavours to construct theories and identify patterns and meanings from the data itself (Gray 2009).
> Interpretative.
> Largely relies on in-depth (unstructured) interviews and engagement with participants.
> Often collaborative in terms of sharing meanings and outcomes (Speedy 2008).
> Works with small samples (Bowling 2009; Gray 2009).
> Concerned with the lived experience of individuals and their meanings, understandings and responses from their perspective (Fox et al. 2007; Bryman 2008; Gray 2009).
> Research is ongoing and often meanings that are interpreted from the data are taken back to the respondents to be further developed and confirmed; thus there is a sense of collaborative meaning making driven by the respondents' own points of view (Gray 2009).
> Very often, for instance, more than one interview will be carried out with each respondent in order to enable the respondent to confirm the 'accuracy of representation'.

Aspects of phenomenology that are challenging and challenged

> Questioning the possibility of bracketing off your self in order not to influence the respondent with your own perspectives. How will this be achieved?
> The challenge of trying to understand what is happening, e.g how an individual says things happened or occurred and what 'actually' happened may differ; this is only a problem if you situate your findings as trying to explain what happened rather then positioning them as how people understand and experience what happens.
> Trying to make sense of how other people make sense of their world is complex.
> Given that behaviour is understood to be a product of how people

interpret the world, there are elements within this paradigm of almost causal relationships, e.g. people overeat because … or doctors when 'treating' dementia patients often see them as problems due to their …

> 'Common sense' 'assumptions about the validity of individuals' accounts of experiences are uncritically accepted' (Bowling 2009, p. 139); though other phenomenologists would endeavour to analyse these assumptions and accounts rather than simply uncritically accepting them.

Case study 5.5   An example of phenomenology

Context. Since the advent of ART (antiretroviral therapy) people have been living longer with HIV, which has resulted in an increased morbidity and long-term health needs and HIV-related disabilities. As a result, and given that the poor, disenfranchised and marginalised populations in the USA are more vulnerable to HIV, there is an increased need to provide care for people in nursing homes. There is little research on the experiences and needs of people living with HIV (PLWH) who are in the advanced stages of the disease and receiving long-term care in homes. Research with people living with cancer and with older people in residential settings has indicated that the concept, understanding and experience of dignity can inform the quality of end of life experiences and their experience of care. Historically many nursing homes didn't accept PLWH and research has focused on the reasons for and meanings of this. There is little insight into what the experience of receiving care may be for such a marginalised population, as well as little research on the actually meaning and understanding of dignity.

Purpose. This research is interested in gaining insight into what it is like to be poor and living and receiving care in HIV/AIDS care settings and the experience of and meaning of dignity to the people there.

Approach. The study is interpretative phenomenological and seeks to 'understand rather than explain or predict participants' worlds. Participants' concerns, habits, and practices reveal what matters most to them as they live their everyday lives.' The researchers are interested in gathering the respondents' stories in as non-intrusive manner possible, within a particular culture or setting – i.e. the care home. It is only through an in-depth understanding of participants' concerns, experiences and understandings that their realities can emerge.

Method. It is part of a larger multi-method research project but this paper focuses on unstructured group interviews – these groups were seen as being an arena in which stories and narratives were able to emerge, while allowing for openness in exploring their experience of institutionalism, as well as facilitating individuals to compare and contrast their stories with one another. The researchers only interviewed the respondents once, which from a phenomenological perspective could be challenged, as this reduces the ability to fully explore interpretations of the researcher and ongoing experiences of the researched, and restricts further opportunities to explore that lived experience. The researchers therefore limited the respondents' opportunity to clarify and develop their understanding in ways that best reflect their reality.

Findings. Dignity for the participants is defined as being respected by the carers

5

and themselves – respect here was defined as having choices and being asked and spoken to with respect. Given their vulnerability already in terms of their health, the stigma of HIV and their own disempowered and marginalised position, the respondents expressed how lack of 'respect' contributed further to their sense of marginalisation. The offset of being treated with respect and being offered choice often enabled individuals to feel able to 'get back on track', take ARV and develop skills and knowledge outside their experiences.

Limitations of this type of phenomenological study

The rationale for a group interview was around previous research, which indicated that focus groups enabled story telling and swapping of experiences as well as being 'safer for informants whose voices have not been heard or are marginalised' (Hughes et al. 2008, p. 345). However, the weakness of this approach in phenomenology is that it reduces the ability of an individual to explore their own meanings without feeling impacted upon by other's own stories and responses. A way of addressing this might have been to take back the transcripts and the analysis to the groups for them to respond further. There are strengths and weaknesses in the focus group method and at some level the implication of the focus group, i.e. looking at shared meanings and experiences, would move this more to a social constructivist piece of work. It can also be challenged for introducing the notion of dignity as a concept in and of itself. The residents knew each other and again, as with much of the writing on and around focus groups, this can be a strength and/or a weakness. Finally, the participants were paid, and this can create a particular dynamic within research that emphasises even more the potentially privileged position of the researcher compared to the respondents.

Source: Hughes, A., Davies, B. and Gudmundsdottir, M. (2008) '"Can You Give Me Respect?" Experiences of the Urban Poor on a Dedicated AIDS Nursing Home Unit', *Journal of the Association of Nurses in AIDS Care*, 19(5), 342–56.

Symbolic interactionism

This is an approach that is again used within health professions as a way of acknowledging and working with how people interact with one another and the symbolic meaning we give to interpersonal relations and how language forms part of that process. It is seen as relatively similar to phenomenology but with the emphasis being on the meaning-making (Gray 2009) process of inter-action. Bowling (2009) defines it as being concerned with how we give symbolic meaning to our social interactions and experiences and then create (continue to create/confirm) a sense of self and, therefore, identity. For Bowling (2009) and Gray (2009) words and objects (including actions) are loaded with meanings, what Bowling calls 'cultural meanings' (p. 140). It is the interpretations of these on which we act. So the uniform of a 'police officer' is given the symbolic meaning of power; we then interact with that symbolic meaning based on our interpretations of that symbol.

Sarantakos (1998, p. 49) considers that 'social life is formed, maintained and changed by the basic meaning attached to it by interacting people, who interact on the basis of meanings they assign to their world: social life and objects become significant when they are assigned meanings ... social life is expressed through symbols. Language is the most important symbolic system.'

The focus here is on interaction and communication, and how people develop their sense of identity through that (Gray 2009); within this identity is not something that is a given, nor is it fixed, but it is in constant construction as we respond to social situations, experiences and people.

Useful resources: symbolic interactionism

A 5 minute podcast by Michael Buhn (http://www.youtube.com/watch?v=rNWhBq1HQ5g).

A short paper on some of the elements within symbolic interactionism (http://www.colorado.edu/communication/meta-discourses/Papers/App_Papers/Nelson.htm).

Blumer, H. (1969) *Symbolic Interactionism: Perspective and Method*. Englewood Cliffs, NJ: Prentice Hall. Herbert Blumer is considered to be one of the central thinkers to this area of theory. This seminal text provides an introduction to some of the elements within symbolic interactionism. (access to the first 20 pages is available via *Google Books*)

Box 5.10 Symbolic interactionism

Key qualities of symbolic interactionism

> Our sense of self is a result of the symbolic meanings we give to our interactions and experiences (Bowling 2009; Gray 2009).
> In-depth and engaged.
> Interpretative.
> 'Interaction takes place in such a way that the individual is continually interpreting the symbolic meaning of his or her environment ... and acts on the basis of this imputed meaning' (Bryman 2008, p. 17).
> The meanings we make of the world, and of ourselves, come from social interaction (Gray 2009).
> These meanings are not fixed or concrete but are constantly being amended in response to experience.
> Our sense of self, and identity, is equally responsive to our experiences (Gray 2009).
> Can be used in multiple ways within various approaches and designs.
> Often used within ethnography (Gomm 2009; Gray 2009).

5

Case study 5.6 An example of symbolic interactionism

Context and purpose. The researchers here are interested to see how women survive and live with HIV/AIDS in their communities. They are particularly interested in seeing ⊾

how the women, through interactions with the community, are given meaning and ascribe meaning to their status and how this impacts on their behaviour and ways of being. The researchers believe that these meanings are 'social products that are created through the defining activities of people as they interact. The meaning of objects to a particular person arise fundamentally out of the way the objects are defined by those with whom he or she interacts' (Klunklin and Greenwood 2006, p. 34).

Approach. These meanings are fluid, rather than fixed, and can be informed by the knowledge and understanding people may have of HIV/AIDS, so as knowledge develops so will meanings attached to HIV change.

Method. Women were interviewed a number of times and their behaviour within these interviews closely observed. The focus of the research was to see how, through the interaction with the community and their own internalised processes, these women function and act.

Findings. What emerges from this research is the joint action between those with HIV/AIDS and those in the community who do not have the disease. Findings indicated that people adjust their ways of being to fit in with how HIV/AIDs is seen within communities. They then internalise this, and are part of the process by which HIV/AIDS and therefore the women are 'designated' as dirty and lethal. There was an expectation of this happening and the women, and the rest of the community, developed strategies of managing it and keeping separate from each other. The women with HIV were able to reduce the impact of this, first, by somehow separating their selves from the disease and, second, by making proactive decisions and taking actions that they initiated by hiding themselves from the rest of the community. What emerged was that both the the actions of distancing from and hiding were almost the same.

Source: Klunklin, A. and Greenwood, J. (2006) 'Symbolic Interactionism in Grounded Theory Studies: Women Surviving with HIV/AIDS in Rural Northern Thailand', *Journal of the Association of Nurses in AIDS Care,* 17(5), 32–41.

Feminist methodologies

This is a critical research theory and, therefore holds particular ontological and epistemological meanings. Grundy (1987, p. 19; cited by Fox et al. 2007, p. 55) uses the term emancipatory research to identify critical approaches, considering the main objective of emancipatory research to be 'fundamental interest in emancipation and empowerment to engage in autonomous action arising out of authentic, critical insights into the social construction of human society'.

Having said that, there is within this approach a huge range of extent, quality, perspectives and meanings and we would strongly suggest you explore this more fully. Below we have suggested a few sources that you might find useful. Given that feminist methodologies can be so diverse, we have given here a brief overview and chosen not to provide, as we have with some of the other sections, a list of key characteristics of and some of the challenges to feminist research. Instead, we reiterate our previous suggestion about further reading as well as reading the rest of this section and the feminist theory discussed in Chapter 3 as a way of starting you on the road.

Useful resources: feminist methodologies

Haney, L. (2002) 'Negotiating Power and Expertise in the Field', Chapter 13. London: Sage.

Kitzinger, C. (2004) 'Feminist Approaches', in C. Seale, G. Gobo, J. F. Gubrium and D. Silverman (eds), *Qualitative Research Practice*. London: Sage.

Jarviluoma, H., Moisala, P. and Vilkko, A. (2003) *Gender and Qualitative Methods*. London: Sage.

Letherby, G. (2003) *Feminist Research in Theory and Practice*. Buckingham: Open University Press.

Given this proviso what we discuss here are some of the overarching qualities and aspects that make up feminist methodologies. Jarviluoma et al. (2003, p. 1) centralise the importance of acknowledging that values, informed by patriarchal norms and male dominance, inform the nature of reality (ontology). Thus, given that all research and knowledge is informed by these often invisible taken for granted structures, to truly engage in research that enables truths to emerge,

> the cultural construction of femininity and masculinity, cannot be avoided in any research activity. It is present in all human action and its products, including researchers and their research ... gender is central to the way we perceive and structure the world and events in which we participate. It influences all aspects of our being, of our relationships and of the society and culture around us. Gendered conceptualisations, norms (what is considered to be proper behaviour), values (the personal characteristics that are highly valued), and attitudes (the kinds of prejudices that come into play when we meet a person of a different gender), have a profound effect on both the person and social, the micro and macro levels of our lives.

Thus, the purpose of feminist methodologies is to give voice to the groups, largely women but increasingly other disempowered groups, who have been marginalised through patriarchal society (Devine and Heath 1999). Feminist methodologists argue that research reality is determined by male interests, legitimising their experiences and views of reality (Kitzinger 2004) as 'normalised and universally applicable'. Thus women's experiences were rendered invisible, elided with patriarchally determined universal norms or problematised as being different, and therefore rendered invisible or dismissed as meaningless and irrelevant (Kitzinger 2004; Speedy 2008; Matthews and Ross 2010).

Following this line of reasoning, all research that does not acknowledge and work to challenge these powerful patriarchal structures is, therefore, only partial

(Devine and Heath 1999; Jarviluoma et al. 2003) at best. Therefore, the role of the feminist researcher is to explore, reveal and reflect on this 'false consciousness' and expose a fuller picture of reality or realities that is not simply filtered through patriarchal discourses. Like all critical approaches it sees power as endemic to all knowledge construction, and focuses on gender as the main way in which knowledge and power are organised (Bryman 2008; Gray 2009).

Given the unequal power dynamic that forms part of epistemological frameworks of research, most feminist research endeavours not to engage in research that simply replicates these power differentiations (Kitzinger 2004; Speedy 2008). Speedy (2008) discusses this power dynamic in research as being between 'the perceived' and 'the perceivers', and being imbued with any number of social and political inequalities. Thus the endeavour is to carry out non-exploitative research by rendering these rather complex but invidious power structures as transparent as possible (Speedy 2008; Matthews and Ross 2010). It is therefore highly reflective, acknowledging the role of the researcher in the construction of knowledge and as being part of the process. Speedy (2008) writes about this in terms of researchers being consciously committed to exposing the structural inequalities and power dynamics that exist between them and the researched. Hence, there is often a commitment to collaborative and shared ownership of the research process: 'the most distinctive feature of feminist qualitative research is the emphasis placed on reflexivity or engaging in reflection about the research process ... the researcher is expected not simply to produce emancipatory knowledge, but to demonstrate that she has come to view her own life differently through conducting empirical research' (Travers 2001, pp. 137, 138).

Thus, part of the objective throughout the research as well as in the analysis, and dissemination, of results is to implement change and raise consciousness or awareness through the sharing of knowledge. It is through active commitment to emancipation that change can be brought about (or at least women can be equipped with knowledge that they might otherwise not have had) and hegemonic forces embedded in social structures can be challenged. For feminists this can happen on both micro and macro levels, as well as in 'inter' and 'intra' personal ways.

Finally, 'feminist researchers are concerned to do research which reveals what is going on in women's lives (and men's too, because to fully understand women's lives we need to also understand what men are thinking and experiencing), and to undertake research in a way that is non-exploitative ... the concern for feminists is not just with what we do but how and why we do it and the relevance of the techniques and approaches we choose. Feminist research accounts acknowledge the 'messiness' of the research process and consider the details of doing research and the relationship between this and the knowledge produced' (Letherby 2003, p. 6). Ultimately the aim of feminist methodologies is to empower and transform, challenge and equip both the researcher and the researched with alternative views and perspectives.

Case study 5.7   An example of feminist research

Context and purpose. The aim of this piece of work was to look at how mothers of obese children were engaging with practices. Previous research clearly shows the importance of parents' own behaviours and norms on children's eating behaviours but also on their role in helping to change the children's eating behaviours and physical activity. Research also clearly indicates that women continue to be situated as the main parent to blame in terms of children being obese.

Approach. The researchers clearly indicate that they are coming from a feminist approach as they recognise 'the need for continuous recognition of gender as basic to all social life, recognition of consciousness-raising as an integral aspect of research methodology, acceptance of inter-subjectivity and person knowing a legitimate sources of knowledge, acknowledging the ethical responsibilities in research, and understanding of the transformative and empowering aspects of feminist research' (Jackson et al. 2005, pp. 7–8; see also Cook and Fonow 1986)

Method. By acknowledging and working within the belief system of gender being a main contributor to organising meanings and social life, they endeavoured to work with women in ways that did not situate them as 'to blame' but acknowledged the impact of this discourse on how women made sense of their experience with the children. They undertook in-depth interviews with these women, situating them as proactive beings and situating them within a family environment and context rather than as separate from this context.

Findings. The approach enabled findings to emerge that emphasised the importance of the role of partners in enabling change strategies to take place. Rather than only focusing on the overweight child for change strategies, the women endeavoured to integrate approaches within the whole family context. By engaging in feminist approaches, women's realities of being part of a family and influenced and informed by this context were allowed to emerge, thereby potentially informing future intervention strategies that emphasised the importance of these contextual realities. This approach enabled the power structures within families, male partner's roles in influencing behaviour, food choices and engaging with change, to be rendered visible.

Source: Jackson, D., Mannix, J., Faga, P. and McDonald, G. (2005) 'Overweight and Obese Children: Mothers' Strategies', *Journal of Advanced Nursing*, 52(1), 6–13.

5

Concluding comments on paradigms

The five paradigms that have been unpacked, in a variety of ways, have, we hope, given you some insight into the ways in which a paradigm informs the research question and focus, its design, the methods and analysis used and the significance of the findings and how that is positioned. However, paradigms are informed by a number of aspects that help to frame your research even further.

What follows is a discussion of the way you reason out what you 'know' and what you think you 'know'. These two 'thinking' styles are clearly part of how you engage with meanings and will also have a profound impact on the methods you use and where you position yourself in this.

Deductive and inductive reasoning

It is worth exploring, when considering your purpose and approach to knowledge, as well as the focus of your research question, how you actually make sense of knowledge. Deductive and inductive reasoning are two key characteristics that will inform your research topic and question, as well as how you engage in the field and 'doing' of research, and even how you analyse it (see also Chapter 1 and the Enlightenment section in Chapter 2, p. 37).

Bowling (2009, p. 131) defines deductive reasoning as being when 'the investigator starts with [a] general idea and develops a theory and testable hypothesis from it', while inductive reasoning begins 'with the observations and builds up ideas and more general statements and testable hypotheses from them for further testing on the basis of further observations'. You can see from her meanings that her focus is on the testing of a theory and that ultimately all research should lead to engaging with more 'scientific inquiry'. However, Bryman (2008) doesn't see their purpose in quite the same way. He posits that the way we reason reflects our subjective stances and our belief systems in relation to knowledge. So he sees deductive theory as being informed by a 'known' field of knowledge and its theoretical underpinnings; then the role of the researcher is to deduce a hypothesis from that field of knowledge and make it operational, i.e. workable and doable. The problem with deductive reasoning is that very often it can be rooted in fairly flimsy and limited reasoning and then drive the gathering of the data.

If your notion of validity and reliability is located within positivist frameworks, and you therefore only access theory and literature that also frames knowledge in the same way, then you may negate understandings and approaches that, while giving insight into a particular concept, do not do so utilising what is positioned as 'scientific inquiry'.

For instance, you may well believe, and the field of knowledge you have accessed reflects this, that dementia care is substandard. Your method of collecting data to test this theory will position and use as measurements concepts that measure the characteristic of substandard in particular ways, as well as what you term 'dementia care'. Deductive reasoning is often supported by a theoretical stance. In this instance your 'stance' may be biomedicine, which is constructed on finding cure and reducing effects through experimental identification of the epidemiology and aetiology of a particular disease. Thus, for you dementia care is about the use of particular types of interventions and EBP, supported and informed by biomedical evidence. Your hypothesis will be constructed within this paradigm and through testing its validity; your hypothesis will then be rejected or accepted depending on the results you collect.

But what if the care protocols within nursing homes, which are based on EBP, reduce interventions to merely a cause and effect relationship, without reflecting that interventions are impacted on by a whole host of contextual issues, such as the relationships, personalities and approaches of the carers and the recipients? In this case, deductive reasoning could be potentially inflexible and limiting, and indeed, particularly with reference to dementia, frequently is. Deductive reasoning can and does, according to critical research theorists, serve the interests of hegemonic forces of conformity, control, invested power interests and the unacknowledged, but pervasive, influence of discrimination and stigmatisation (Parker 2005; Bartlett and O'Connor 2007; Milne 2010).

But according to Bryman (2008) inductive reasoning can and does form a part of deductive reasoning, particularly when you are trying to make sense of the results or end product. In other words, when analysing results, going over the research design, questioning the validity and reliability of a piece of research and trying to reason out what went wrong, why it went wrong and how to 'fix it', the researcher engages with inductive reasoning.

Inductive reasoning, according to Gray (2009), is about engaging with the data and developing theories, suggesting patterns and analysing relationships from the data itself – a more emergent process. Bryman (2008) talks about how the relationship between theory and research is informed by understandings and theories being the *outcome* of the research. This does not mean that inductive 'reasoners' do not have theories or ways of understanding their research topic and questions – clearly to produce a credible piece of research you will need to be rooted in what is already believed or believed to be known – but what inductive reasoning asks of the researcher is to ground their understandings in the data that is being gathered. Thus it is what emerges from this process that informs our understandings and the potential to develop embryonic theories.

Clearly there are problems with this form of reasoning. Gomm (2009) believes that the difficulty with inductivism is that, given that we develop theories and understandings from the data, in order to truly claim findings from the data to have the potential of developing a theory, you would have to do this many times and the responses would have to be consistent. However, this could be further challenged as drawing on the positivist values of replicability, but inductive reasoning can by its in-depth and authentic engagement with the field provide deeply informed insight into phenomena that can develop our understanding further. The philosophical challenges of this position are fairly complex and if you want to explore this further we would suggest you access some of the suggested reading as well as looking at the sections on Enlightenment and social construction in Chapter 2.

Further principles that inform your research

Often embedded within the paradigms and certainly within the overall design and purpose of your research are various elements that provide further parameters to your paradigm. These items have a profound impact on the choices you make regarding your overall aims and how you will attempt to achieve these aims. They are concerned with the quality of knowledge and hierarchical notions of what constitute valuable and worthwhile research approaches and findings.

Variables

The term variable is utilised and operationalised in research in a number of ways. Bowling (2009) defines a variable as an 'indicator' that represents a particular concept. Bryman (2008, p. 33) develops this definition further as 'an attribute in which cases vary' – his emphasis is on when these attributes or characteristics vary (e.g. gender, age, class, health); if they are the same then he defines them as a constant. Matthews and Ross (2010, p. 31) encapsulate understanding of a variable as 'an attribute or characteristic of cases (for example, individuals, organisations, objects or situations) which can vary from case to case'.

Variables can be problematic to define, as they can be seen to oversimplify, in often very descriptive terms, characteristics and their meanings. So, for instance, if you are wanting to test the theory that 'private fertility clinics allocate more IVF treatments to heterosexual women than lesbians' you will need to absolutely define your two variables and be able to rationalise the conceptualisation of these two variables as being representative of differing attributes, and establish that this 'difference' is the causal link to the outcome. An oft-levelled criticism of this process is the essentialising of characteristics in distinct and separate identities. A second challenge is levelled more at the level of relationship, questioning whether it is a causal one or more of an association.

Variables come in many different forms and again we would recommend you to access your research texts for a far more broad and explanatory discussion. For the purpose of this chapter we briefly attempt to define two particularly pertinent characteristics that are of relevance to the development of a hypothesis.

The independent variable and dependent variable concern the cause and the subsequent effect of differing conditions and their relationships. Bowling (2009) explains this further by explaining that the dependent variable is that which the researcher/scientist wants to explain, and the independent variable is that which is the explanation for, or precedes, the dependent variable. An example of this may be:

Obesity is on the increase in children under the age of seven – effect (dependent variable).

Fast food consumption in children under the age of seven has increased by 58 per cent since 2005 – cause (independent variable).

Your hypothesis might therefore look something like this:

Fast food consumption in children under the age of seven causes an increase in obesity within this population.

As you can see, the complexities of being able to test this require a great deal of planning and designing. As a final note Gomm (2009) provides an easy and helpful reference table that defines and differentiates these two associated variables.

Reliability

Walliman (2001) locates the practice of reliability within what he and Cohen and Manion (1994; cited in Walliman 2001) identify as scientific approaches, often elided with positivism. Reasoning and our senses can be, if utilised 'correctly', dependable tools for the measurement and recording of data and ideas. Interpretists would absolutely refute this as an unrealistic possibility, and would instead contend that reflexivity, rigour and transparency are ways of working with our subjectivities – subjectivities that inform our engagement with every stage of research (Sarantakos 1998; Silverman 2004; Bryman 2008). Critical theoretical (e.g. feminist) researchers would challenge the notion of 'correct', as the implication that there is a 'right' way and a 'wrong' way is located within powerful taken for granted 'beliefs' built on invested hierarchical interests that aim at maintaining a status quo located in patriarchal, racial, 'ableist' inequalities.

Robson (2002) unpacks the term reliability, specifically referring to research design, by considering reliability as meaning that the method of data collection, if used within the same conditions elsewhere, will elicit the same outcomes as the previous research. Clearly this could be construed again as somewhat unrealistic and naive, particularly if your ontological and epistemological beliefs are that people, contexts, meanings and situations are not absolute and are in constant flux.

Positivists work very hard at producing what they position as reliable tools of measurement and will militate against possible researcher and participant error and bias by, for instance, piloting their methods, having more than one observer (for instance) when engaging in structured observations and having

5

ongoing up-to-date knowledge of the field they are researching. They may also test out the methods more than once, carry out tests or experiments that are 'blind' and engage with sampling frameworks that are as representatively random as possible (see **RCT**, systematic reviews, structured interviews, questionnaires, epidemiology and structured observations for examples of 'reliability in action'). It is worth noting here that positivists also acknowledge the contested nature of reliability and instead work to maximise reliability rather than seeing it as an absolute attainable quality. Good examples of this can be located within research articles that endeavour to establish reliability but acknowledge the limitations of this too.

Fox et al. (2007) see reliability, along with validity and generalisability, as working to achieve the main goal of positivist research, which is replicability – defined here as the consistency and stability of a measurement over time and place, meaning that it could be repeated elsewhere in almost exactly the same way (Gomm 2009). Being able to produce a reliable piece of work requires the research to be 'without bias or error' and the participants to be 'representative of the population under investigation and in no way distorted or skewed'. Bryman (2009, pp. 149–50) considers reliability to be about the consistency of the measure itself. He unpacks this as having three key qualities: (a) stability, referring to the stability of the measure itself, i.e. whether it produces results that have little variation over time; (b) internal reliability, which refers to how consistent the relationships of some 'indicators' to other 'indicators' are within the measurement scale; (c) inter-observer consistency, which refers to how consistent, between researchers, are the data and methods that researchers are gathering, measuring and analysing (Gomm 2009).

Reflective activity

Go to the obesity case study in Chapter 4 and look at the discussion on the reliability and validity of BMI as a measurement for obesity.

5

Validity

There are a number of different forms of validity (Bryman 2008; Bowling 2009; Gomm 2009; Gray 2009) in quantitative research, and its most fundamental application refers to whether the measurement tool or instrument designed to test and/or measure a particular concept actually measures that concept (Bryman 2008; Bowling 2009) – in other words, does it do what it says on the label? David Gray (2009) explains it rather clearly by relating 'the operationally defined subject area', i.e. what you clearly defined and set out to research in your aims, to 'the research instrument subject area' – what the method you have chosen actually measures. So for Gray (2009) these two elements must exactly match in order to achieve validity. Fox et al. (2007) and Bryman (2008), as previously noted in the discussion on reliability, see validity as one of three of the core interrelated concepts needed to establish the replicability of a piece of research. Interestingly, Robson (2002) claims that a measurement tool can be reliable and not valid. When an instrument is devised that measures the efficacy of an intervention, such as an extreme diet programme for obese men, the results may be the same when applied to other populations: for example, the average weight loss is five stones during the programme, but it is not possible to predict the long-term weight loss when the programme ends.

Validity is a contested area, in which social constructionists and realists counter the claim that any instrument can absolutely claim validity. When reading through empirical research articles you will see that very few researchers will make an out and out claim for validity (Gomm 2009); most will instead claim that they endeavoured to 'counter threats to validity' (Bryman 2008; Gomm 2009). Lewis and Ritchie (2004) clearly differentiate between quantitative and qualitative validity and claim that qualitative validity is more concerned with 'representation, understanding and interpretation' (p. 272). They go on to quote Hammersley (1992, p. 69; cited in Lewis and Ritchie 2004, p. 272): 'an account is valid or true if it represents accurately those features of the phenomena that it is intended to describe, explain or theorise'.

As previously stated, validity has a number of differing but interlinked forms within quantitative research – all with the intention of establishing the validity of the research. Some of these include internal validity, which means that the causal conclusions that are drawn between two or more variables, like the impact of an intervention on a control group and an experimental group, are sound; some include external validity – whether the results can be generalised to a larger population (Bryman 2008; Gray 2009). Gomm (2009) differentiates this in terms of, first, the research instrument itself – whether the tool produces results with the same degree of accuracy over a wide range of subjects and settings – and, second, the findings: whether what was found within this piece of research is also 'true' of other people, in other settings and times.

Face and content validity

Face validity is also another aspect of establishing a research instrument's validity and, interestingly (given that objectivity is considered an essential criterion for positivist and valid 'scientific research'), at some level requires the researcher to subjectively decide whether the elements within the tool are actually relevant, appropriate, clear and straightforward (Bowling 2009). Gomm (2009) agrees with Bowling (2009) as to the superficiality of face validity and positions it as not only being the most commonly engaged with aspect, but also being concerned with 'whether according to appropriate judges an instrument looks as if it measures what it is supposed to measure' (p. 379). Instead of face validity theorists encourage the rigorous researcher to engage with content validity – which is 'whether an instrument deals with all the relevant aspects of the construct an instrument is supposed to measure'

(Gomm 2009, p. 379). Bowling (2009) positions content validity as more systematic, and therefore more rigorous, than face validity and defines it as 'the extent to which the content of the instrument appears logically to examine and comprehensively include, in a balanced way, the full scope of the characteristic or domain it is intended to measure' (p. 167).

Qualitative approaches to validity

While these writers are positioning validity largely in terms of quantitative research, qualitative theorists also discuss the nature of, and need for validity. Lewis and Ritchie (2004), for instance, while questioning the nature of quantitative understandings of validity, at the same time suggest that validity is and can be still a concern of qualitative researchers. Perhaps at the core of the difficulties is the degree to which qualitative researchers challenge the notion that there is a truth and this truth can be validated (Lewis and Ritchie 2004; Sarantakos 2005; Robson 2007). So instead the emphasis within the qualitative research is more concerned with asking questions such as:

> ❯ Has the phenomena, as understood or seen through the eyes of the respondents, been represented as rigorously as possible (Lewis and Ritchie 2004)?
> ❯ Has the method chosen been the most effective way of gathering data that will best represent the phenomena being explored (Fox et al. 2007)?
> ❯ How is the data affected by the researcher's personal location and interpretations? Is there enough 'internal evidence for the explanatory accounts that have been developed' (Lewis and Ritchie 2004, p. 274)?
> ❯ How might the researcher's framework (paradigm) impact on the data (and indeed the field); has the analysis emerged from the data (Fox et al. 2007)?
> ❯ Fox et al. (2007, p. 18) provide a further validity criterion of 'theory validity – are the data explained by appropriate theory?'

As a final comment on validity (often referred to as credibility, which is discussed further a few pages on in this text), within qualitative research it is useful to consider the notion of content validity as defined by quantitative researchers. The relevance of 'knowing your field' is just as pertinent to qualitative researchers as it is to quantitative researchers. While the definitions of 'knowing' may differ – positivists can and do believe there is a known while qualitative researchers believe that realities are subjectively constructed and can, therefore, be multiple and individual according the paradigm engaged with – it is just as important for qualitative researchers to have an in-depth knowledge about the field they are researching. While emergent data and flexible responsive research design are inherent to a rigorous piece of qualitative research, this does not preclude qualitative researchers from wanting to ensure that they have awareness and knowledge of the complexities that may exist in and around a phenomenon. Unlike positivists, qualitative researchers are not looking to produce conclusive evidence to support the supposed existence of 'a fixed and measurable phenomenon' but are instead looking to explore, expand, investigate, clarify and expound on it. Validity or credibility for a qualitative researcher means that how we choose to engage in research, the questions we ask and the methods we choose are informed by an in-depth knowledge of what may, or may not, be relevant to the area under investigation.

Reflective activity

- What do you want to measure for your hypothesis?
- How does what you want to measure 'answer' your hypothesis?
- What tool of measurement would be most appropriate to use?

Generalisability

Again, as with reliability and validity, this is more of a concern for positivist quantitative researchers then qualitative researchers, though a number of theorists (e.g. Gobo 2004; Perakyla 2004; Fox et al. 2007; Gray 2009) explore the possibilities and applicability to qualitative research.

If you are intending to make generalisations from the data, this in essence means that you are making claims that what is ascertained in one place, with one group of people, at a certain time will also be true of other places, people and times (Gomm 2009). To make such generalisations your research must be valid and reliable; hence Fox et al.'s (2007) and Bryman's (2009) claim that these three elements work together to produce a piece of work that is 'true' and replicable. Gomm (2009) extrapolates on the efficacy of making generalisations by emphasising the need to be absolutely specific about what it is you are making claims for and for whom (Bowling 2009; Gray 2009). This relates as well to your sampling framework and how 'representative' the sample you have selected is of the whole target population (explored further on in the text).

We are often tempted by what Gray (2009) calls a typical human trait, to make generalisation with very limited information and, even further, informed by personal experience and opinion. A generalisation in this guise is often utilised by media sources as a way of giving more impact (validity/truth) to their opinions – and it is, after all, largely opinions and attitudes that inform how the media represent the news. As a critical and reasoned thinker you need to move beyond this position and start substantiating claims you make with robust evidence and clear sources for your data. In our experience popular generalisations made by students can look like this:

> Poor people eat convenience food because it is cheap.
> All young women like reading glamour/celebrity magazines.
> Boys like cars.
> All Muslims practice their faith in the same way.
> Children who are sexually abused go on to abuse as adults.

When generalisations such as these are made, we are endeavouring to position our assumptions, perspectives, beliefs, values and attitudes as generalised 'fact'. Embedded in these statements are on the whole un-researched, reactionary belief systems, which, in order to justify themselves, are positioned as generalisations. Very often the source of your generalised beliefs is informed by personal experience, your own norms and values, the media you read or don't read, the people with whom you associate and so on. For a student, researcher and critical thinker this is clearly unacceptable and needs to challenged at all levels of thinking.

Box 5.11 Reasoning through a Generalised Opinion

All young women like reading glamour/celebrity magazines

1. You read celebrity magazines a lot.
2. You read them because you like the pictures; the ease of the writing style; the celebrity 'gossip'; the information on clothes and makeup; the 'stories' about celebrity lives; shock/horror revelations about celebrities and 'normal people'.
3. You also feel reassured reading them because: (a) the magazines routinely point out, using both unflattering photos and captions, the 'faults' in female celebrity bodies; (b) they 'reveal' that celebrities suffer heart break, humiliation, loss and insecurities about their bodies and lives; and (c) they routinely humiliate, shame and expose celebrities by showing them in less than flattering lights. By 'making them like you', your own experiences and feelings are 'normalised' and you are reassured that these 'perfect people' who you hold up as ideals to strive for are 'human' too.
4. You and your social circle all read similar magazines and talk about the content.
5. At some level you feel uncomfortable about some of the content and even your liking of these magazines, as they represent or stereotype you in ways you are embarrassed by and don't want to be associated with, i.e. superficial, obsessed with your looks, enjoying other people's 'suffering' and 'unhappiness' etc. etc.
6. In order to justify, rationalise and explain your reading, and liking, of these magazines you make the above generalisation.
7. Generalisations such as these can be a source of comfort and certainty; you can feel that you are merely conforming to what you have positioned as a very **essentialised** idea of young women or girls of your age.

> Instead of it being a choice, influenced by a number of differing contexts, and representative of your norms, values and decisions, you have reduced it to being 'what all young women do'.

Reflective activity

Choose another one of the five generalised opinion statements above. As we have done in Box 5.11, try to reason out the process that may take place in making a personal opinion become a generalisation.

Generalisations in quantitative research

In quantitative research the efficacy and power of generalisations are strengthened by a valid, reliable and very well designed piece of research. Gomm (2009) considers that the main aspect of generalisation within quantitative research concerns its **representativeness**: the people, units or cases you have 'done' the research on statistically represent the whole population you are making claims about (Bryman 2008; Bowling 2009; Gray 2009). As many researchers will admit, it is an incredibly difficult absolute claim to make. Qualitative researchers would question the ability to make claims of representativeness given how social context, the social world and individual characteristics cannot be absolutely defined and measured.

To make a claim for representativeness you really need to 'know' (and have access to) your population and the variables and characteristics that are meaningful in terms of how you design your **sampling framework**. Practicalities such as gaining access to the full complement of the target population from which to select your representative **sample** can be hugely complicated. For instance, if you are doing a piece of research titled 'Comparing the effectiveness of gastric bands to gastric bypasses in long-term weight loss in the clinically obese', how will you get hold of everyone who has had both interventions? These interventions are carried out in the NHS and private clinics in the UK and also abroad – their record keeping may vary as well as their access-to-data policies.

The second aspect of generalisation is that of the theoretical claims you are making and whether these claims can be more widely applied. Again, as with representativeness, theoretical generalisations are heavily contingent on the validity and reliability of your design and method – and what Gomm (2009) identifies as the specificity of the claim (Gray 2009) and the matching of that with the method.

Credibility in qualitative research

Credibility is sometimes identified as trustworthiness, transparency, dependability, plausibility, authenticity or transferability. These terms are concerned with processes, utilised within qualitative research, to substantiate and strengthen the research. Interestingly it is not just an 'end' product but an ongoing process that qualitative researchers engage with throughout the research. As more often than not qualitative researchers are concerned not with what they consider **reductionist** definitions of validity, reliability and generalisability, but with the rigour of their research. Terms used to establish this can be interchangeable. Bryman (2008) provides an extensive discussion of the various aspects and meanings applied to establishing and working with qualitative research. He, like Gray (2009), Silverman (2004) and Matthews and Ross (2010), posit that there is a need to establish different criteria for assessing qualitative research rather than simply endeavouring to map qualitative research into validity and reliability characteristics.

Among some of the aspects and meanings to consider are:

> Credibility. This has a number of strands, including ensuring that the approach and method used to collect data is, for want of another word, above board and reflective of good practice. Second, the research findings are given to the respondents to ensure that their 'social world' has been represented (Bryman 2008). Third, more than one researcher analyses the data and then it is cross-checked for consistency (Gray 2009). Matthews and Ross (2010) consider that the checking of findings alongside existing theory is another way of establishing the credibility of the findings.

> Transferability. Qualitative researchers are not looking to generalise or make statements of applicability to other contexts and populations in their research. Instead what they do is provide very rich and detailed contextual descriptions so that 'others' can make judgements themselves as to the findings' relevance to other contexts (Bryman 2008; Gray 2009).

> Dependability. This is often concerned with the **transparency** of the research, which Matthews and Ross (2010) define in terms of transparency of practice. Thus researchers keep very clear and open records of the procedures and steps they took throughout the research, as well as their findings and ultimate analysis. This enables other researchers to access and potentially 'audit' the trail (Bryman 2008). Matthews and Ross (2010) further add to this concept by stipulating that the data set must be complete, that nothing is lost, inaccurate or misplaced.

> Confirmability. This concerns what Bryman (2008, p. 379) describes as 'acting in good faith', which is about the researcher, while acknowledging subjectivities, beliefs and values, endeavouring to minimise their impact on the design, direction and analysis of the research.

> Rigour. Bowling (2009) writes about the maintenance of rigour within qualitative research, the characteristics of which are very similar to Bryman's (2009, pp. 381–2) model and include being systematic, transparent and explicit throughout the research; acknowledging the theoretical stance and values of the researcher from the beginning; and endeavouring, where possible, to have more than one investigator involved in the research at some stage, enabling separate reports to be constructed and then cross-checked for added depth and consistency.

> Authenticity. This 'relates analysis and interpretation to the meanings and experiences that are lived and perceived by the subjects of the research. This means the research being aware of the multiple voices contained with the data, and the subtle, sometimes conflicting realities within it. Do the interpretations ring true? Have rival explanations been considered?' (Gray 2009, p. 174). Clearly this has similarities to credibility, but with added emphasis on the explicit acknowledgement that working within qualitative research involves working with the messy, multiple and complex meanings that individuals give to their lives and experiences need to be represented – rather than simply eliding them into convenient categories.

Useful resources

May, T. (2002) *Qualitative Research in Action*. London: Sage.

Williams, M. (2002) Generalizations in Interpretative Research, pp 125–43 , in T. May (ed.) *Qualitative Research in Action*. London: Sage.

Designing your research

As you continue to unpack the issues framing your approaches to research you will be getting a clear idea that everything within research has a purpose. To engage with research without considering your paradigm will often result in a piece of work that lacks substance and consistency. To consider what you intend to measure and/or investigate without analysing how you will define your remit and hoped for outcomes can result in a piece of work that is both unreliable and unworkable. Very often these elements are encompassed within particular designs, designs that are intended to best reflect your overall research intentions. The discussion below briefly looks at some of these designs, designs that are clearly linked to your paradigm.

Research design

The overarching design of the research relates, as previously noted, to your overall purpose. Gray (2009) considers that there are four different forms that your research may take, while Matthews and Ross (2010) initially describe three possible designs dependent on what you actually want to do with the data you collect. Interestingly, Matthews and Ross (2010) consider this stage to be particularly informed by your research question or hypothesis, and further in their discussions also include an evaluative design or purpose, while Gray (2009) also links design with purpose. However this is understood, what is of relevance to you is to consider which descriptor best fits your purpose.

Exploratory

An exploratory study is often considered when there may be little known about your particular phenomenon (Gray 2009), and you want to investigate what is occurring and then ask questions of it. Bear in mind that an exploratory study still requires a wide ranging reading of the available literature and 'expert' insight; as Gray (2009) so aptly posits, having done some reading you may well find that the study is not so much exploratory as explanatory or interpretative. A criticism of exploratory studies can be that they are so open and wide ranging that they have no particular purpose or focus.

Descriptive

Matthews and Ross (2010, p. 111) consider a descriptive study as one that is concerned with describing 'the current (or past) situation', while Gray (2009, pp. 35–6) understands the purpose of descriptive study as being to 'provide a picture of a phenomenon as it naturally occurs ... [seeking] to "draw a picture" of a situation, person or event or show how things are related to each other'. Studies of this type, while insightful, are criticised for reducing data to mere items with no explanation about them.

Explanatory

These are studies that intend to 'explain and account for' (Gray 2009) descriptive data, so moving beyond the 'whats' and into the 'hows' and 'whys' (Gray 2009; Matthews and Ross 2010); they can often be concerned with looking at the correlation and/or relationship between variables and endeavouring to explain them. A weakness of this is, as with descriptive studies, reducing concepts to variables and presupposing that a phenomenon can be explained and accounted for.

Interpretative

These are studies that seek to explore people's experiences and their interpretations, views, understandings and perspectives (Gray 2009). So the key here is that you are interested in other people's, and potentially your own, interpretations of their worlds and life events. To make this purposeful and fulfil the 'so what factor' that we have previously discussed you need to be able to frame these sorts of studies in discourses of, for instance, humanism and interpretist or critical theory. The weakness of research like this can be that it is so interpretative and individualistic that it renders your findings potentially 'without value to health studies' unless you can locate them within ongoing theoretical discussions and inductive reasoning.

Evaluative

An evaluative study or design is essentially interested in assessing the value or efficacy of something, usually an intervention, in relation to its impact on the situation and phenomenon it was intended to address (Matthews and Ross 2010). Evaluation has its historical roots, according to Gray (2009), in the 1970s and the evaluation of the accuracy of various measuring techniques, and, therefore, is very positivistically informed. The range and meanings of evaluation have developed since then and while it is still often concerned with evaluating efficacy, it can also look at evaluating the outcomes and at what contextual issues might have impacted on and informed that intervention (Bryman 2008).

Bowling (2009) would absolutely dispute this as she sees evaluative studies as located within what she defines as 'scientific methods', which look to measure outcomes, as well as the ongoing changes that occur as the project or intervention continues. Bowling (2009) is particularly interested in the use of evaluation in health research and understands evaluation to be either formative (collecting data as the project runs and then using that data to either develop or improve the intervention) or summative (collecting data about the project with the aim of deciding whether it should be continued or not). David Gray (2009) discusses in great depth the differing types and purposes of evaluation. From a purpose point of view it is worth noting that the methods and approaches vary widely and you would be well advised to read further on this topic.

Experimental

Briefly, your purpose or design may well have the characteristics of an experimental approach. Bryman (2008) considers true experimental design in social science research as not only unusual but also almost impossible to design. Given that the characteristics are concerned with manipulating the independent variable in order to see its impact and influence on the dependent variable, and this usually requires controlled, replicable, reliable and valid conditions, it is no wonder that social scientists struggle to design such a piece of research.

Gray (2009) acknowledges this difficulty but considers the possibility of designing quasi-experimental research, which bears many of the characteristics of experimental design (which is often considered to be the most reliable, and therefore of the highest standard), but rather than manipulating the independent variable they would observe the differences between the two groups. So it may still consider utilising control groups, but these would be ones that already exist rather than being randomly selected. Experimental design and purpose is contested and has to be rigorously and very clearly delineated – it also has various 'types' – and a fuller discussion can be found in both Bowling (2009) and Bryman (2008).

5

Action research

'Action research is a participative method of research that both seeks to gain more knowledge and aims to change people's circumstances for the better by engaging them in the research process' (Waterman 2007, p. 133). Thus your purpose or design may well be with this intention in mind. Action research, EBP and evaluations can be linked in terms of looking to improve and/or assess practice and then develop ways forward. Purpose, in this design, may be not only to evaluate the outcomes of a particular intervention but also, based on the results and outcomes of that, to look at working with all the 'players' within the implementation of the tool and pooling knowledge and experiences as a way of developing research that can facilitate change.

Action research uses mixed methods; an example is questionnaires to measure an outcome for an intervention, then focus groups to work with the data collected from this research and develop a new intervention. The focus groups may be made up of service users, service providers, workers and carers, families, managers of services and so on. These focus groups may be ongoing, working at developing and implementing change, looking at new measures and evaluating ongoing efficacy and management. There may be interviews with workers and service providers to get a more in-depth view on the experiences of these interventions and what works and what doesn't. Documentary data may be accessed in terms of case and medical records to look at some of the processes and outcomes. Given that action research is largely designed to facilitate and implement change it is used in EBP as a way of auditing and evaluating practice. Given its focus on implementing change, through empowerment and co-ownership, it is not surprising that (participatory) action research can often be informed by critical theoretical approaches, e.g. feminism, critical disability or critical race approaches. Waterman (2007) provides a well discussed outline and application of action research in health.

Useful resources

Coghlan, D. and Brannick, T. (2009) *Doing Action Research in Your Own Organization*, 3rd edn. London: Sage.

Gray, D. (2009) 'Action Research and Change', in *Doing Research in the Real World*, 2nd edn. London: Sage, pp. 312–34.

Ladkin, D. (2004) 'Action Research', in C. Seale, G. Gobo, J. F. Gubrium and D. Silverman (eds), *Qualitative Research Practice.* London: Sage, pp. 478–90.

Waterman, H. (2007) 'Action Research and Health', in M. Saks and J. Allsop (eds), *Researching Health: Qualitative, Quantitative and Mixed Methods*. London: Sage, pp. 133–51.

Case study

Case study research is about collecting various forms of data as a way to get more 'rounded and arguably more valid findings' (Tritter 2007, p. 303) on a particular phenomenon. Yin (1991, p. 23) defines a case study as 'an empirical inquiry that investigates a contemporary phenomenon within its real-life context when the boundaries between phenomenon and context are not clearly evident; and in which multiple sources of evidence are used'. Typically a case study design is over a long period of time, and the term itself can refer to the study of individual cases; though cases can mean an organisation, a particular individual, ailment or treatment or a case study of an event. Clearly it is a focused design that endeavours to work within the real life context or natural environment (Sarantakos 1998) of the phenomenon under investigation. Its intention is to study 'whole units' as opposed to partial pictures of a unit, and it is often used in terms of considering the whole process, structure and implications of a unit or case. A case study might be concerned with exploring 'schools' responses to obesity in teenagers' – thus it would access policy data and policy-makers, interview school nurses, work with students identified as obese in terms of eliciting their experiences of services and responses, potentially work with the parents of obese teenagers, look at the teaching models available around health and so on – all within one school. Thus, it is not just about mixed methods of data collection; it also attempts to engage with all the people involved as representative of the 'totality' of the case under investigation (Sarantakos 1998). As a design it is often flexible, responsive and communicative, engaging with the case as fully as possible. Case study research often works alongside action research, triangulation and mixed methods approaches.

Useful resources

Case studies

Yin, R. (2009) *Case Study Research: Design and Methods,* 4th edn. London: Sage.

Gray, D. (2009) 'Designing Case Studies' in *Doing Research in the Real World*, 2nd edn. London: Sage, pp. 246–77.

Research design overall

Bryman, A. (2008) 'Research Designs', in *Social Research Methods*, 3rd edn. Oxford: Oxford University Press.

Lewis, J. (2003) 'Design Issues', in J. Ritchie and J. Lewis (eds), *Qualitative Research Practice: A Guide for Social Science Students and Researchers*. London: Sage, pp. 47–76.

The literature review

Various research writers have discussed and considered the vital purpose of a literature search (discussed in section 5.3) and review within the design of your research. Gray (2004, p. 54) writes that 'it is *not* sufficient to simply read around the topic, the purpose of the literature review is to provide an increasingly focused argument or set of concerns based on a synthesis of subjects or related subjects'. Frankel and Devers (2000) wrote that there is a balance to be had with a literature review, which considers the need to ensure that the research problem is set within a solid review of the literature, to ensure contextual breadth, while at the same time seeing the risks of limiting your literature review in ways that disable creativity and ongoing development. Miller and Crabtree (1999, p. 94) state that the 'initial literature review is used to identify the existing descriptive, theoretical, and analytical categories for the research topic … the initial goal is to search out the literature's assumptions and expectations and then to identify key conceptual domains'. Thus, your literature review is intended to develop your topic focus and ultimately your research question.

The function of searching and reading

One of the fundamental purposes of a literature review is to provide background, context and a broad view of the topic in which you are interested.

While you engage with this aspect you are rather like a detective, following leads, gathering background clues and information, looking at what information is out there, where you might need to locate this material and who or what may be connected with the topic.

As you increasingly become familiar with what is out there you will find yourself narrowing yourself down, finding a focus embedded from within the literature. This is where many students become unstuck and it refers back to what Frankel and Devers (2000) describes as the 'premature review' – that is, your focus is so narrow and specific that you miss out on looking at vital material that would give you background and context. As with everything in research the literature search and review process is not to be done in a vacuum, as you also need to consider your subjective position and your invested interests.

An example of this might be that you start off from a very specific location of wanting to look at all research that is connected with HIV prevention in sub-Saharan populations in the UK – you therefore only look for, and at, material that is directly linked and refers to this area. You don't look at the overall picture, the local, national and global discourses and approaches around HIV, you don't think about the implications of gender and/or class, you neglect recent policies within the UK around HIV, you don't explore the legal and immigration policies and approaches. In effect you produce a piece of work that is partial, leading and uninformed; rather like poorly researched media reports, you have simply skimmed the surface and done yourself and the topic no favours in your oversimplification of a complex area.

Reflective activity

Using the topic area that you have been working on throughout your research journey so far, consider the following when reading and making informed decisions about your literature:

- What is the relevance of the material to my area of study?
- How does this inform the 'bigger picture' and add to the informing context?
- What is the source and how credible is it?
- What does this tell me about what beliefs, concepts and issues are connected with my chosen topic?
- What is the purpose of me utilising this?

Your process of sifting through the potentially enormous amount of published material is one that needs to be fairly systematic and thought out. Your decisions regarding the literature that you may include or exclude for your topic will be informed by ascertaining its use, relevance, credibility and reliability.

Always remember that the purpose of an ongoing engagement with the literature search and review are, according to Gray (2004, p. 52):

> up-to-date understanding of the subject and its significance and structure;
> identifies the kinds of research methods that have been used;
> is informed by the views and research of experts in the field;
> assists in the formulation of research topics, questions and directions;

> provides a basis on which the subsequent research findings can be compared.

Gray (2004) goes on to say that the literature search is not simply something that you do at one isolated stage in the research process and then never engage with again. It is something that is continuous, ongoing and always exploratory.

Box 5.12 Skills Involved in Writing a Relevant Literature Review

> Your inclusion/exclusion criteria: deciding what to include and what not to include. This will be informed by your research question, design and purpose, but deciding which articles to include and which not can be daunting (Matthews and Ross 2010).
> Structuring the review so it makes sense in terms of the purpose and context of the research you are undertaking.
> Ensuring that the material you include in the review is relevant and meaningful in terms of the research question and design (Hart 1998; Bryman 2008).
> Establishing the credibility, authenticity, reliability and believability of the material you are utilising.

The review

A great source of insight into what a literature review looks like is to explore research dissertations in the library as well as research articles from within journals. As these materials are usually written about research that has been done they will have read around and explored available material on their chosen topic. What may confuse you is that more often than not within research articles, you will find not a clear subheading of 'literature review' but instead 'Introduction', 'background' or 'context'; it might not even be given a subheading but simply form the first part of the article before the methods section. Finally, you may find that research articles subhead it by the particular aspect within the topic they are discussing. Alternatively, if you look at research dissertations and/or theses then you will find often extensive literature reviews.

Reflective activity

Locate the following two articles and read their literature reviews:

MacRae, H. (2008) '"Making the Best You Can of It": Living with Early-Stage Alzheimer's Disease', *Sociology of Health and Illness*, 30(3), 396–412. Read the following sections, which form part of the literature review/background/context: Introduction; The cultural meaning of Alzheimer's disease; Alzheimer's disease and academic research.

Bond, V., Chase, E. and Aggleton, P. (2002) 'Stigma, HIV/AIDS and Prevention of Mother-to-Child Transmission in Zambia', *Evaluation and Program Planning*, 25, 347–56. Read the following sections, which form part of the literature review/background/context: Introduction; Stigma, stigmatisation, discrimination and denial; The situation in Zambia; Children's and women's rights.

You will see from these articles that how they construct their literature reviews is informed by their purpose, paradigm and topic area focus. However, despite the variability in how we may write a review, Gray (2004, 2009) and Hart (1998) both consider that there are various core or basic elements that need to inform the structure of the review. These include:

> 'An introduction that lets the reader know how the review is to be organised and structured' (Gray 2004, p. 53).
> The main body, which will cover various constituted aspects of the data, knowledge, theory and previous research that informs the topic.
> The conclusion or summary, which draws together the meaning, significance and key themes within the literature and leads to your research question.

The role of a literature review

When you are producing a critical review, Hart (1998, p. 180) suggests, the following are useful to develop a sound argument:

> Structure: use a reliable structure that is explicit.
> Definition: define the terms you will use carefully using clear examples.
> Reasons: provide the reason for anything you have included as support.
> Assumptions: substantiate your assumptions; do not leave them as implicit. Use only reliable assumptions that are free from value judgements or are based on valid reasoning.
> Fallacies: avoid fallacies, such as generalisations, abstraction and misplaced concreteness.
> Evidence: use only reliable documented evidence in the public domain that is legitimate and relevant, and not trivial.
> Avoid appeals to authority, convention and tradition.

Remember, the role of the review is to provide an increasingly focused argument for the topic you have chosen and the eventual focus that you are taking. Gray (2004, p. 54) adds to Hart's (1998) advice by noting that the critical reviewing involves:

> an assessment of the strengths and weaknesses of some of the theories;
> a clear understanding of the topic;
> a citing of key studies in the subject territory;
> a clear indication of how the review links to your research question;
> a definition of the boundaries of your research;
> a selection and synthesis of existing arguments to form a new perspective;
> through gradual refinement, a clear demarcation of the research problem.

We often describe the literature review as being like an inverted equilateral triangle (see Figure 5.3).

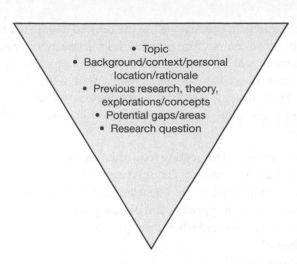

Figure 5.3 Literature review triangle

The idea is that in the literature search and initial reading you start off broad and eventually, by dint of critical and systematic reading, you eventually reach your research question – the focus of your research. The reader needs to be able to see how you got to your research question and that what you are asking is based on the literature you have worked with and written about. Again look at other pieces of work that have a literature review and see if you can almost plot the path towards their research question. Have they substantiated their research area, and have they provided the relevant background and rationale and dealt with up-to-date research and theories informing their ultimate research question?

Useful resources: writing a literature review

Aveyard, H. (2010) *Doing a Literature Review in Health and Social Care: A Practical Guide*, 2nd edn: Maidenhead: McGraw-Hill/Open University Press.

Fink, A. (2005) Conducting Research Literature Reviews: From the Internet to Paper, 2nd edn. Thousand Oaks, CA: Sage.

Hart, C. (1998) *Doing a Literature Review: Releasing the Social Science Research Imagination*. London: Sage.

Jones, K. (2007) 'Doing a Literature Review in Health', in M. Saks and J. Allsop (eds), *Researching Health: Qualitative, Quantitative and Mixed Methods*. London: Sage, pp. 32–54.

The research question

Refining your topic area to a research question is often one of the most challenging and time consuming aspects of research design (Gray 2009; Matthews and Ross 2010). The term research question can be used interchangeably with hypothesis, statement of intent and/or aims and objectives. When reading through your research textbooks you may note that there is a disparity in how these terms are used, but overall what they are all concerned with is the focus and direction of your research. In this text we use the term to denote the focus of the research in terms of your aims. The possibilities for research questions, informed by the rigorous and systematic developmental process, can be endless – as you will see in the research material that is used in the rest of this chapter concerning HIV, obesity, artificial reproductive techniques and dementia. The overall purpose of your research question needs to clearly consider the following:

> What area in particular are you subjecting to further investigation?
> Can you rationalise and justify your question, statement etc.?
> Is it located within and informed by the literature search and review?
> Is it informed by your research approach and philosophy?
> Is it 'do-able' – what is possible and what is not possible?
> Are there ethical issues?
> Is it clear and concisely stated?
> Is it based on and informed by research literature, practice and emerging issues?
> What is its significance or importance and relevance to the field of knowledge?
> Continue searching and reviewing the literature, now focusing on this particular area or question.

Hypothesis

(For a more detailed reading on this see the sections on positivism and health, and epidemiology.) According to Matthews and Ross (2010, p. 58) a hypothesis is 'a testable assertion about a relationship or relationships between two or more concepts'. Bryman (2008) specifies that the process of deduction is central to the development of a hypothesis, and that it is intended to test a theory. Bowling (2009) emphasises the ongoing nature of hypothesis testing, in that if a hypothesis is rejected then it is refined and developed further and then tested again. Bowling (2009) notes that hypotheses have a number of different forms, including causal (when we predict that due to one or more particular phenomenon another phenomenon will occur) and substantive (more tentatively located within theoretical assumptions of the conceptual relationship between dependent and independent variables). To be able to position anything as a hypothesis you will need to have done a great deal of reading and research on and around the topic of choice and be able to clearly demonstrate your theoretical position and belief.

For instance, if you decide, informed by the substantial research findings you have read, that you want to focus on the role of parents and child obesity, than your hypothesis may look something like this:

Parents who have obese children engage 50 per cent less in planned physical activity than parents who don't have obese children.

Within this you would clearly need to ensure you define your terms and variables.

This is a fairly exact exercise where there needs to be no ambiguity or blurred meanings. In order to locate the hypothesis firmly in a strong theoretical position you will need to ensure that it is deeply embedded in the literature you have read and presented in your review. You are testing a theory or a number of theories and either falsifying or supporting them. Fox et al. (2007, p. 115) emphasise the rigorous nature of your role within this, as 'Hypotheses are usually based on previous research and theory and are predictions the research has about the connection between two or more variables.'

There are variations within hypotheses and we would suggest that you again refer to various research texts to get a much broader and more detailed account of the design and process of development. A final comment on a hypothesis is that it largely, though not exclusively by any means, utilises quantitative methods in order to measure the phenomenon or phenomena being tested.

Challenges to hypothesis testing

There are a number of criticisms of this process of testing theory and the causal relationships within social sciences in particular. To truly produce the conditions needed to test the effect of one phenomenon on another you would engage with an experiment (Bryman 2008; Bowling 2009), and to design an experiment to test the effect of planned physical activity on obesity and non-obesity in children would be extremely complex and problematic. Thus, in social research 'quasi' experimental designs may be implemented, although given the complexity not all positivist research is looking to test a hypothesis, and will instead look to exploring relationships and 'answering' questions.

Research questions, statements of intent and aims and objectives

The first thing to note about these terms is that they are used by different theories in a variety of ways. You will find that research textbooks consider them to be either explicitly concerned with looking at possible relationships between variables or connected to a theoretical position and/or framework (Gray 2004). Gray (2004) even goes as far as to stipulate that they more often than not end with a question mark. 'Why is HIV on the increase in gay male populations in the UK?' Now clearly here you are looking for an explanation of something you know to be true. You would also have to believe it was possible to find this out – that there was a truth out there and it is possible to ascertain that truth. The question also clearly indicates that you believe there is a cause for the increase in HIV in the gay male population. Going even further, you would also have to believe that there is a concept 'gay male' that can be reduced to a variable. All of this connotes positivist positioning and tools that could seek measurable outcomes.

Fox et al. (2007, p. 115) provide an interesting outline of definitions and meanings of research questions, emphasising the role of methodology and theoretical framework in the development of the research question. They consider that it is the 'aims and objectives' that develop the research questions and define these as follows: 'The research "Aim" should state clearly what the study is intended to find out. The research objectives are specific issues to be looked at by the work, which are related to the overall aim. Objectives are generally related to specific empirical outcomes and form the basis for the "research questions".' Bouma and Ling (2004) consider this in terms of the research objective, positing that this approach is largely descriptive and concerned with looking at what is happening within a phenomenon.

The idea, then, is to develop a statement of an objective that clearly and succinctly states what it is you are exploring, describing or investigating without looking to test a set of beliefs or measure relationships between variables and/or situate your research in terms of causal relationships. If we develop this in terms of the case studies then your research objective may look something like this:

> The experience of sub-Saharan women living with HIV in the UK.
> Investigating the role of family in the care of a relative with dementia.

While clearly this contrasts with a hypotheses, you still need to refer back to the list of qualities needed in the development and positioning of a research question – how did you get to these questions, what has come before and what informs your particular perspective or focus? Bouma and Ling (2004) stipulate the importance of clarifying our concepts and being absolutely clear what we mean by our descriptive terminologies. The importance of being clear cannot be overemphasised; asking yourself questions around your meaning can help you to be absolutely clear. Let's take a question from above and do this now:

Investigating the role of family in the care of a relative with dementia.

> What do we mean by family? Are we considering all blood relatives? Are we considering siblings, parents, children, aunts, uncles etc.?
> Will they need to live with the person with dementia or are you interested in all the family?
> Are we only considering people living at home or in a home?
> Are they family members who are 'officially' considered to be the carer of the relative or simply relatives who take an active role in the relatives care?
> What do you mean by care – physical input?
> What do you mean by role – active or passive?

Finally, Bryman (2008) and many other theorists consider the development of research questions in relation to the chosen and intended methodologies. For Bryman a research question is located within qualitative research and is inductive in nature, i.e. it is through the collection of data and engagement within the field that potential theories or insights can be developed. Thus while research questions still need to be succinct and clear they may have 'varying degrees of explicitness' (Bryman 2008, p. 371). Researchers still need to be clear what it is they want to explore and at the same time leave it fairly open; this enables you to see what emerges from the field rather than limiting it too much by providing a restrictive definition. Clearly, there are strengths and weaknesses to both approaches but you, as a researcher, need to explore what is most suited for you.

Let's go back to the question: 'Investigating the role of the family in the care of a relative with dementia.'

> You don't want to limit your definition to those family members who are actively involved because you want to see the overall picture and what emerges.
> Your focus is on the family involvement, irrespective of whether the relative is in a care home or living at home.
> Given that you want to explore family responses, you realise that terming it as a 'role' may be too prescriptive, so you widen the term to be more encompassing, allowing for a wider range of experiences.
> The term 'investigating' implies a more specific 'finding out what is happening' focus; you are are clear that you want it to be an emergent process that allows all aspects of all involvement to be considered.
> You realise that the term 'care' may be restrictive, so you change it to 'involvement' and reposition your statement as follows: 'Exploring family involvement with a relative with dementia.'

Reflective activity

- Using your own topic area, devise a research question or statement of intent.
- Then, using the example worked already as guidance, refine your statement to one that you feel best communicates your intention.

This process of refining and defining your research question, hypothesis, objective etc. can take time and very often may even involve a readjustment of the question, more particularly in the case of qualitative as opposed to quantitative research, as you progress. It also requires you to think about what you want from the research and what objectives and/or outcomes you are looking for. You may often see a research question written as below, with aims attached:

The experience of sub-Saharan women living with HIV in the UK
Aims:

> Women's stories of what it is like for them living in the UK.
> The impact of HIV on their lived experience.
> How women respond to their life conditions.

Reflective activity

Go back to the research you have refined and see if you can devise two or three aims that further focus your research.

What this process does is make it even clearer what it is you intend to explore within the piece of research you are doing. It also gives fairly clear hints, if you don't know already, on your theoretical perspective and framework.

Useful resource

White, P. (2008) *Developing Research Questions: A Guide for Social Scientists*. Basingstoke: Palgrave. This is a very good step-by-step approach to developing viable research questions.

Ethics in research

Ethics in health studies research need to be embedded in all the aspects of your design. You will find that most research writers will provide varying degrees of discussions and materials on ethical codes of conduct, ethical behaviour and attitudes, design and procedures, and as ever we would strongly advise you to explore this much further than we are able to do in this section.

A good place to start is with Silverman (2006, p. 315), who suggests that before we even embark on doing research we should ask ourselves two reflective questions:

1 Why are we researching this topic? Will our findings contribute in some way to what we value as the common good? Or are we just interested in furthering our educational or research career?
2 Do we want to help and, at the very least, protect the people we study? Or are we using them simply as research fodder?

Gray (2004, p. 61) provides a fairly long and detailed checklist of ethical issues that need to be considered and established when carrying our research:

Privacy – the right not to participate. The right to be contacted at reasonable times and to withdraw at any time.

Promises and reciprocity – what do participants gain from cooperating with the research? If promises are made (such as a copy of the final report) keep them.

Risk assessment – in what ways will the research put people under psychological stress, legal liabilities, ostracism by peers or others? Will there be political repercussions? How will you plan to deal with these risks?

Confidentiality – what constitutes the kinds of reasonable promises of confidentiality that can be honoured in practice? Do not make promises that cannot be kept.

Informed consent – what kind of formal consent is necessary and how will it be obtained?

Data access and ownership – who will have access to the data and who owns it? Make sure that this is specified in any research contract.

Researcher mental health – how will the researcher be affected by conducting the research? What will they see or hear that may require debriefing or counselling?

Advice – who will the researcher use as a confidante or counsellor on issues of ethics during the research.

As you can see this goes well beyond the often simplistic understanding of ethics as being only in relation to confidentiality. What needs to be considered within the researcher's personal ethical code are implicit, and indeed explicit, considerations of researchers' power, motivation, openness, moral code and own set of values and norms. It is not enough, therefore, to choose a research topic on obesity and decide to interview three friends of yours who have been given this medical label simply because they are conveniently there. You will need to think beyond the convenience, and what also may be considered exploitation, of these 'sitting ducks' and really engage with an ethical reflective exercise that asks you to consider your respondents as human beings rather than simply cannon fodder to do with what you will.

One of the challenges for many students and all researchers is the engagement with their own moral and ethical codes. The discomfort may come when you realise that what you think is acceptable behaviour might actually be located outside Grey's (2004) ethical code. There is, unfortunately, a great deal of research that does not thoroughly consider the ethics of the research topic, how the research is managed, how the researcher behaves and treats the respondents or the well-being of the researched. Feminist researchers in particular have drawn attention to this often exploitative and dismissive approach to research and have done much to improve the exploration of research ethics beyond fairly baseline meanings.

Embedded within much of the discussion regarding the research articles we have used are issues of ethics. Ethical considerations are apparent in Briggs et al.'s (2007) work, where they started off intending to be observers but, due to the field and the needs and discomfort of the carers, they spoke with the carers and became to a 'lesser extent' involved. The ethics here were about responding to a human condition, and having compassion as well as an ethical commitment to the well-being of all. Briggs et al. (2007) also discuss the ethics of, once having developed a relationship, how to exit the field well – an area that is often the concern of ethnographers and feminists in terms of engaged approaches to research.

Brotsky and Giles's (2007) covert participant observation of 'ana' communities contrasts with this concern for the respondents and seems to give little consideration to the impact of the researcher on the respondents. For Brotsky and Giles (2007) their justification of 'going undercover' is framed in terms of the ends justifying the means – i.e. the benefits that might be gained by engaging with the field. This is not to say they have not attempted to frame their research in ethical commitments. Thus they explore issues of 'informed consent', which they don't seek even retrospectively because the respondents 'would be extremely unlikely to give retrospective consent' (p. 96). Deception was acknowledged and justified because 'it was felt highly unlikely that access would be granted to a researcher openly disclosing the purpose of her study' (p. 96). Their third concern was about the well-being of the researcher and her exposure to the material, and they therefore provided support and help to her in order for her to be able to retain a sense of herself.

Doyal and Anderson's (2005) ethical concern, particularly in a feminist piece of work, was about the respondents and the impact of discussing and opening up the areas under discussion. Their commitment was rooted in non-exploitation of the respondents, so they provided psychological support for women who were distressed.

Getting rubber stamped

Research will have to be approved by organisational bodies dedicated to ensuring that ethical codes are followed. Within Jackson et al.'s (2005) research on mothers' strategies for working with their obese children they note that their research was approved by an ethical committee and they abided by institutional codes of practice in gaining informed consent from all participants. In some ways it is surprising that in an ostensibly feminist piece of work the attention paid to issues of power, influence, impact and collaboration is fairly minimal. What is even more intriguing is that they acknowledge the sensitivity of the research but did not return the transcripts to the respondents – instead focusing on reflexivity within the research team.

Bryman (2008) has written an entire chapter on the political nature of ethics in social research, in terms of accessing, gaining permission and what types of research are more likely to receive permission than others. Issues of who is funding the research and what is the purpose of the research can also frame ways in which research is permitted. Ethical permission can often be associated with research that is considered to be more 'scientifically' informed – i.e. engaging with the gold standard of RCTs and experimentally designed research (Bowling 2009). Here it is interesting to explore some of the hoops that need to be jumped through in order to gain access to particular populations and research. Bowling's (2009) chapter discusses these issues within the context of healthcare research.

Considerations such as access, who the population is and how 'vulnerable' they may be can all make a big difference to whether your research receives the go ahead. The Declaration of Helsinki (recently updated – see http://www.wma.net for further details) has particular codes and definitions regarding vulnerable populations, largely associated with clinical and medical research, and it is worth noting the implicit, and explicit, engagement with notions of power, choice and justification that is core to this framework.

What is defined as vulnerable, and how do we as researchers take this into account when planning our research? What qualities identify someone as vulnerable, and are people always vulnerable or can it be contextually impacted upon depending on the phenomenon under investigation? One of the core facets to vulnerability is the impact of power differentiations on relationships, treatments, responses and even access to levels of care and respect. It is a complex discourse and one that you will need to engage in to produce a piece of research that has taken into account these issues. Clearly, given understandings of vulnerability, issues of informed consent, choice and freedom to engage and withdraw are also implicated within ethical frameworks. Your rationale for wanting to access particular populations needs to include your role within this, and how you will work with issues of vulnerability. It is not unusual at all for research bids and proposals to be knocked back because these issues have not been addressed sufficiently.

Useful resource

Rogers, W. A. (2004) 'Evidence Based Medicine and Justice: A Framework for Looking at the Impact of EBM upon Vulnerable or Disadvantaged Groups', *British Medical Journal*, 30, 141–5. (http://jme.bmj.com/content/30/2/141.full).

The notion of vulnerability, while largely associated with respondents, can also be used in reference to researchers and their own well-being in undertaking research. This can be as straightforward as physical safety but also refer to the emotional and mental impact of working within your research field. While in some ways this tends to be more associated with the immersed nature of qualitative research, it also has resonance for positivist research, where the impact of treatment may mean the difference between life or death, or certainly affect quality of life issues.

Permission is therefore an important element in terms of gaining access to your research area and participants. All EBP and research that goes through any organisation will need to go through this process and this can take various lengths of time; the frameworks can be more or less rigorous and the aspects that need to be abided by may vary. Very often a period of adjustment will need to be structured into your research plan, as it is very common not to have immediate ethical approval: many committees will require you to further tweak your work to ensure that all aspects can be justified and are considered safe practice. This process will be more, or less, explored in research articles and dissertations. Zwakhalen at al. (2007) and Clare et al. (2008) both simply indicate that they gained permission from appropriate channels involved in the research – what went on behind the scenes is not shared.

5

As a final note we rather liked Sarantakos (2005, p. 23) presentation of ethical guidelines in terms of the 'ten commandments on ethics'.

Thou shalt not …

> Include in the study or continue working with a person who demonstrates resistance or discomfort relating to the study or the research topic.
> Attempt to convince a person to take part in the study, when this person is not in a position to respond adequately to the research question.
> Fail to explain all relevant aspects of the study to the respondents before they agree to participate.
> Promise anonymity and confidentiality if it is likely that this promise will not be honoured.
> Fail to respect the respondent's privacy.
> Deceive the respondents in any way.
> Subject respondents to procedures that may entail physical or mental stress.
> Include in the study techniques whose degree of safety is questionable.
> Violate professional research standards, for example by fabricating, falsifying, or concealing data.
> Accept a contracted research project that violates ethical and/or professional standards.

Useful resources

Ethical guidelines: association websites

British Association of Counselling and Psychotherapy (http://www.bacp.co.uk).

British Psychological Society (http://www.bps.org.uk).

Economic and Social research Council (http://www.esrc.ac.uk).

National Research Ethics Service (http://www.nres.npsa.nhs.uk/).

Research Governance Framework for Health and Social Care (http://www.dh.gov.uk).

Social Care Research Ethics Committee (http://www.screc.org.uk/).

The World Medical Association has produced a 2009 Medical Ethics Manual that can be downloaded (http://www.wma.net).

Resources for further reading

Alderson, P. (2007) 'Governance and Ethics in Health Research', in M. Saks and J. Allsop (eds), *Researching Health: Qualitative, Quantitative and Mixed Methods.* London: Sage, pp. 283–300.

Bryman, A. (2008) 'Ethics and Politics in Socal Research', in *Social Research Methods*, 3rd edn. Oxford: Oxford University Press.

Fox, M., Martin, P. and Green, G. (2007) 'Undertaking Ethical Research', in *Doing Practitioner Research*. London: Sage, pp. 95–111.

Matthews, B. and Ross, L. (2010) 'Research as an Ethical and Cultural Issue', in *Research Methods: A Practical Guide for the Social Sciences*. Harlow: Longman.

Sampling in research

Once you have identified the research question and your purpose then a decision needs to be made as to who (or what in the case of documentary research) are best placed to provide you with the data you are seeking. This is known as your 'target population'. The target population represents the overall population you want to research; within this you will also be able to present the variables and characteristics that make up this population.

So, for instance, in Doyal and Anderson's (2005) research they stipulated that their target population involved the following characteristics:

> over 18 years of age;
> had to have been diagnosed with HIV for at least 6 months;
> had to have lived in the UK for at least 6 months;
> needed to identify themselves as black African;
> accessing specialist HIV clinics in London between July and December 2001.

In addition they ensured that their sampling framework (how you are going to choose the actual respondents from this population) reflected the various nationalities in the overall population.

Jackson et al.'s (2005) target population was fairly broad and included the following requirements:

> mothers of at least one overweight or obese child;
> the child must be living with them;
> be able to speak and understand English;
> willing to participate in the study.

They recruited their participants from Sydney, Australia, in 2003–4. The location itself was seemingly more informed by convenience in terms of where the researchers were based than a random selection of urban populations.

Haas's (2002) research on social support within gay male relationships

5

used the following criteria to decide on the target population most able to provide insight into the aims of the research:

> in an ongoing intimate romantic relationship;
> one or both partners were HIV+ or had AIDS;
> both partners agreed to participate in the study.

The choice of your population is directly informed by your research question and in addition you will need to support how you have defined the population and how you understand this criterion as having relevance to the research aims. Clearly the target population can mean a very large number of people and depending on the type of research you are doing you will more often than not decide to narrow down your population by using a sampling framework, i.e. the process by which you will select your actual respondents.

Before we briefly provide you with the two main ways in which sampling takes place it is worth noting that there are occasions when your target population and your sample are one and the same thing. For instance, you want to research 'How members of the Stratford Over Eaters Support Group experienced the interventions of an eating disorder re-education tool'. Clearly your target population will be all the members of this group and instead of selecting only a few (because, after all, there are only eight of them, and they are all members of an active group) you consider that to get as full a picture as possible you will need to interview all the members of this group. The narrower and more specific your research question in terms of location, arena or phenomenon the more possible it is for your target and sample population to elide.

There are often very practical reasons for using a sampling framework, including:

> it is unlikely that you will be able to reach the whole target population;
> responses can come back more quickly when you rely on a smaller number of people;
> it is more possible in terms of finance, time, resources and so on;
> you are interested not in generalising but in engaging with a few people or cases in-depth.

There are essentially two very broad approaches to sampling in research and these are probability or random sampling and non-probability or purposive sampling. Within each of these approaches there are a variety of ways that can be engaged with that are not covered here.

Probability or random sampling (usually associated with quantitative research)

A *probability sampling* method is any method of sampling that utilizes some form of random selection. In order to have a random selection method, you must set up some process or procedure that assures that the different units in your population have equal probabilities of being chosen. Humans have long practiced various forms of random selection, such as picking a name out of a hat, or choosing the short straw. These days, we tend to use computers as the mechanism for generating random numbers as the basis for random selection. (http://www.socialresearchmethods. net/kb/sampprob.php)

Sarantakos (1998) describes the random sampling framework as employing rigid and strict rules of probability by which every unit within the population has an equal and known probability of being selected; moreover, a large sample is needed in order for a high degree of representativeness to be established.

So the overall intention of random sampling is to represent the whole population as accurately as possible in order to make generalisations and form conclusions (Bouma and Ling 2004) from the sample to the larger population. There are various ways in which we can go about randomly selecting populations and their utilisation will again depend on our research question, the population, what is practically possible and, finally, which is the most reliable method. Research literature talks about simple random sampling, stratified sampling, systematic sampling and cluster sampling to name some of the main sampling methods (Bouma and Ling 2004).

Non-probability or purposive sampling (usually associated with qualitative research)

Non-probability sampling is often more concerned and informed by in-depth engagement with a select number of people. Very often these can also be 'hard to find' or access populations from a particular 'walk of life' etc., which makes them hard to access through a random sample frame. Non-probability sampling 'is less strict and makes no claims to representativeness. It is generally left up to the researcher or the interviewer to decide which sample units should be chosen, and is employed in exploratory research, observational research and qualitative research' (Sarantakos 1998, p. 141).

As with probability sampling there are a number of ways in which you can go about selecting your non-probability sample and these include convenience, snowball sampling, quota sampling, accidental sampling and so on. Very often the researchers using these methods are not even attempting to claim generalisability or indeed representativeness: the purpose of their research is such that it is the in-depth engagement with the chosen population's experience and understanding that is of interest. Their philosophical position is such that perhaps they also do not believe that there is such a thing as a representative population, there is merely an interpretation of one.

Box 5.13 Issues to Consider when Selecting Your Sample

> How will you access your population/sample?
> How will you approach this population?
> Where will they come from?
> What practical arrangements do you need to consider in order to access your population?
> What are your inclusion and exclusion criteria, what is the justification for these criteria, how do they relate to my aims and objectives, and what relevance do they have?
> Where will the research take place and in what form?
> How will you contact the sample and when?

Sarantakos (1998, p. 154) provides this final advice regarding the selection of your sampling framework and suggests that 'you use sampling frameworks which relate/reflect the philosophy of the type of research, so that it is informed therefore by the underlying qualitative framework'.

Useful resources: sampling

Bowling, A. (2009) 'Sample Size and Sampling for Quantitative Research', in *Research Methods in Health: Investigating Health and Health Services*, 3rd edn. Maidenhead : Open University Press, pp. 183–212.

Gobo, G. (2004) 'Sampling, Representativeness and Generalizability', in C. Seale, G. Gobo, J. Gubrium and D. Silverman (eds), *Qualitative Research Practice*. London: Sage, pp. 405–26.

Ritchie, J., Lewis, J. and Elam, G. (2003) 'Designing and Selecting Samples', in J. Ritchie and J. Lewis (eds), *Qualitative Research Practice: A Guide for Social Science Students and Researchers*. London: Sage, pp. 77–108.

Gaining access to your field

The process of accessing the field that you intend to research is, as with all aspects of research planning, an aspect that you will need to consider in your design. The ability to access, or indeed not access, your intended population can inform your research question and should you encounter any difficulties in accessing your population you may even find that your research question needs to be amended. This issue of access isn't just about 'how' you will find the population or locate them (although both of these are clearly significant) but also about how you will get hold of them. Very often this is where the roles of gatekeepers and stakeholders, particularly in healthcare research, come into play. Very often it is only through the gatekeeper that you will be able to access your population and gatekeepers are usually powerfully located in the healthcare hierarchy in terms of being managers and/or in the case of privately run care homes the owners of the organisation.

Gatekeepers can be concerned with protecting the interests of the potential group or setting you want to research; this protection may be about ethical rights to privacy, data protection, vulnerability and issues of non-exploitation. However, it can also be about power and ownership of data, and an invested interest in the research itself. Thus gatekeepers can, and do, become stakeholders and your access to the field may be contingent on certain conditions that are set by stakeholders. The difficulty with this, within your research, may be that in order to access the dementia care home the gatekeeper or stakeholder requires to have access to the data you collect and/or know who you interviewed and what they said. It might involve them stipulating the form your research takes and what measures are to be researched.

Within the research articles discussed in the next section various processes of access have been adopted by the researchers – some of them rather random (e.g. sticking up posters in public places), others informed by where (and with whom) the researchers work and still other access processes informed by knowing someone who knows someone etc. The key here, when considering issues of access, is fourfold. First, you need to be as clear and transparent as possible in the steps you take to gain access. Second, you need to give yourself time to gain access and to know your field and possible avenues to pursue. Third, if your access is dependent on other people then you need to consider how this might have impacted on your sample, and your sample's freedom to participate. Finally you need to be prepared to have doors closed to you, resulting in a reconfiguring of your research question and aims.

Useful resource

Lee, P. (2005) 'The Process of Gatekeeping in Health Care Research', *Nursing Times*, 101(32), 36 (http://www.nursingtimes.net/nursing-practice-clinical-research/the-process-of-gatekeeping-in-health-care-research/203728.article).

The fundamentals of research

The foundational underpinnings and informing aspects of your research design are clearly fundamental to producing a solid piece of research. Without an exploration of these elements the tendency is to produce research that lacks substance and the necessary vigour required to make sound decisions about the next stage of your research journey – which is choosing the methods and methodologies.

5.5 METHODS, ANALYSIS AND WRITING UP

This section explores:

> pilot trial studies;
> different methods, including questionnaires, systematic reviews, interviews (structured, semi-structured and unstructured), documentary research, observations (structured, participant and non participant) and focus groups;

5

> qualitative analysis;
> quantitative analysis;
> writing up your work.

Methods (methodologies)

The choice of what method or methods are best situated to collect the data you need in order to 'answer' your research question is one that is framed by a number of interlinked issues. Thus, your decision will be based on discourses of *validity*, *reliability*, *credibility* and *generalisability*, as well as your research *paradigm*, the design itself and mediating issues of *ethics*, *sampling* and *deductive* and *inductive* reasoning (all items introduced in the previous section). The rationale for your choice of method must be located within these interweaving elements. This is not to say that time, cost, accessing your population and your skill base will not also form part of this consideration, but what we would encourage you to do is to be transparent to yourself, as well as within the research, about how these aspects also informed your decision.

Below we unpack a number of methods, which broadly fall into qualitative and quantitative categories.

Quantitative methods	Qualitative methods
Structured interviews	Semi structured interviews
Structured observations	Unstructured interviews
Surveys/questionnaires	Participant/non-participant
RCT/experiments/quasi	observations
experiments	Focus groups
Systematic review	Documentary/media analysis
Meta analysis	Systematic review

Useful resource

A podcast by Alan Bryman on methodologies and engaging with research and methods (http://www.youtube.com/watch?v=bHzM9RIO6j0).

Piloting quantitative methods

A key process in establishing the validity and reliability of your research tool is to 'test' it first. This, in quantitative research, is what piloting is concerned with and is considered an absolutely vital stage of the research design. By trying out the method on a small sample of the population and testing out its validity measures, the researcher can then adjust, amend and even redesign the method itself to ensure maximum efficiency. They may do this a number of times until the pilot demonstrates validity as far as possible. They, as with qualitative researchers, may work with other researchers to try to reduce the potential impact of personal influence on the design and implementation of their research method.

Research pilots like Zwakhalen et al.'s (2007) work on pain scales are often used as a way of further developing an intervention measurement or tool – thus in their research they found that while the amended tool did indeed measure levels of pain within populations living with dementia, they also saw this pilot as a way of taking the data to develop a reduced item pain scale for clinicians.

Trialling qualitative methods

In qualitative research, given the more flexible and responsive methods used, researchers often work in a number of ways to ensure that their method is as credible as possible. So they try out their interview/focus group guide on colleagues and other individuals who are involved in the research phenomenon they are exploring. They may construct a guide with a number of people, pooling knowledge, and they may practise their interviewing and observation techniques. Thus they are concerned not only with the actual credibility of the method in terms of effectively exploring the phenomenon under investigation but also with the process of 'doing' the method. In other words they are interested in the 'how' as well as the 'what' of their method. For instance, with observation, given that they engage with the field for a long time, their trialling may be planned into the introductory stages of their research field. They would be considering and reflecting on what they were observing, how they were observing, their potential to impact on the field, their interpretation and partiality and so on – acknowledging a time of adjustment and response to the field as a way of trialling the method.

Mixed methods and triangulation

We have not in this text looked at the use of mixed methods in great detail, though the articles we have unpacked have often used more than one method. The rationale for using mixed methods may be the desire to 'triangulate', i.e. cross check consistency and meanings using different methods. It may also be that you recognise that the quality of data that emerges from a focus group needs to be developed further through in-depth interviewing. Or you may be using a case study, ethnography or action research design, where the methods needed are multiple in order to get a 'full picture' of the phenomenon being investigated.

Useful resources

Bowling, A. (2009) 'Mixed Research', in *Research Methods in Health: Investigating Health and Health Services*, 3rd edn. Maidenhead : Open University Press, pp. 432–61.

Bryman, A. (2008) 'Mixed Methods Research: Combining Quantitative and Qualitative Research', in *Social Research Methods*, 3rd edn. Oxford: Oxford University Press.

Creswell, J. W. and Plano Clark, V. L. (2007) *Designing and Conducting Mixed Methods Research*. Thousand Oaks, CA: Sage.

Teddlie, C. and Tashakkori, A. (2009) *Foundations of Mixed Methods Research: Integrating Quantitative and Qualitative Approaches in the Social and Behavioral Sciences*. London: Sage.

Tritter, J. (2007) 'Mixed Methods and Multidisciplinary Research in Health Care', in M. Saks and J. Allsop (eds), *Researching Health: Qualitative, Quantitative and Mixed Methods.* London: Sage, pp. 301–18.

Types of method

Questionnaires

This is largely designed to be used as a quantitative/positivist method of data collection, and can be used in research that is triangulated, as well as being of a case study or action research design. At a fundamental level a questionnaire involves posing a number of questions, in an organised and structured manner; it is often referred to as a survey (Bryman 2008; Gray 2009). It is located within a deductive reasoning framework as the questions are predetermined measurements (constructed on valid concepts) informed by a predetermined theory. Thus the purpose of a questionnaire is to measure the predetermined indicators that make up the phenomenon to be quantified and analysed (Calnan 2007).

The concepts (see variables, p. 250) that are to be measured then need to be defined into indicators (Fox et al. 2007; Gray 2009). Designing questions so that they measure what they are intended to measure (see validity, p. 252) requires a great deal of skill and theoretical conceptualisation. This is in order to ensure that the wording, the order in which you 'ask the questions' and the structure of the questionnaire as a whole, as well as each construct, are absolutely clear, unambiguous and representative. Clearly here the ontological position of positivism is in evidence, as to reduce concepts into clearly predetermined items you have to 'know' not only that this is possible, but also that what you have developed exists independently of any 'outside influence'. By this we mean that you 'know' that concepts such as attitude, stress, eating behaviours, dementia, safe sex practices and so on can be defined and measured. As a method they are extremely popular, as once designed and disseminated, they can produce large amounts of data that can be analysed to produce what are believed to be quantifiable answers to particular questions (Bryman 2008).

It is an inflexible method, in that the structure and predetermined questions are fixed, with no room to be responsive to what interpretivists see as the messiness of life (Silverman 2004). Interestingly enough, the tools and measurements used in questionnaires are used to test what is believed to exist already. Questionnaires can be used in a number of ways: postal, 'randomly' handed out, face-to-face structured interviews, over the phone and even on the Internet via various websites.

A face-to-face questionnaire (see structured interviews, p. 305) requires you to personally ask each respondent the questions; bearing in mind the necessary qualities of reliability, replicability, validity and generalisability to ensure that your research produces 'true' results, this means asking questions of people in exactly the same order, with the same tone of voice, the same probes and prompts, and the same wording (and if you need to repeat the question then this too is set beforehand and not deviated from). Given these conditions, you can see why face-to-face questionnaires are rife with challenges of validity, as well as why they are a popular form of data collection. Whether you carry out questionnaires face-to-face or 'from afar' the quality of objective researcher remains the same – that is, the distance between the researcher and the researched is maintained so that the results are not 'invalidated'.

Questionnaires allow you to ask a large number of people the same questions – so your sample size can and indeed needs to be large and certainly representative of your population as a whole (Bowling 2009; Gray 2009). As with any method you need to rationalise your reasons for selecting the method. Your rationale must be informed by the 'type' of data you are looking to collect and not simply based on practical considerations of 'it's quick' (debatable given the length of time it takes to design a questionnaire, pilot it and endeavour to improve the response rate), 'it can be sent out to lots of people at the same time' (clearly a large sample to make useful claims from the data is necessary, but it also needs to be informed by positivistic values and beliefs) and/or 'it's cheap' (while money clearly informs many of the choices made in health research about what method is used, this does not mean that the questionnaire is actually the most effective method of data collection for your research). Thus your reasoning must be based on the purpose of your research, your paradigm and how the method is the most appropriate method to collect the data your research requires.

One of the main weaknesses of questionnaire design can be largely due to the researchers themselves, and their lack of theoretic rigour, limited knowledge base and the complexities of the phenomena under investigation. A good example of this is Forder's (2008) research on age discrimination, in which she found that satisfaction measures and questions used with the 'elderly' to 'ascertain' the quality of services provided were inappropriate, given this population's tendency to minimise their condition and their (understandable) fear of stigmatisation.

Another example of a researcher not engaging in wide enough reading could be: 'School nurses' (SNs) role in the promotion of health eating and physical activity for preteens'. You 'know' that SNs have a defined role and this has an effect on promoting healthy eating and physical activity in preteens. Your questionnaire is therefore designed to measure these concepts. You decide that your theoretical position means that all concepts can be defined and then measured. You set about designing a questionnaire but have not read through the NICE (2006) 'Guidelines on Obesity: The Prevention, Identification, Assessment and Management of Overweight and Obesity in Adults and Children'. This provides guidelines to local authorities and schools – so clearly it will have implications for the SN role. But because you have not read widely enough your questionnaire will have enormous gaps in it and you will miss some crucial information.

5

The variation in questionnaires is vast and we would again strongly advise you to read around this but below are some of the characteristics of a questionnaire.

Key qualities of questionnaires

> They are impersonal – contact between respondent and questioner is either remote or very distanced.
> They are fixed – questions can't change depending on how the respondent answers the question.
> They can be anonymous.
> There is no limitation to geography and location (as long as language etc. is appropriate).
> They can be relatively economical in terms of time and cost in targeting a large number of people (Walliman 2001).
> They can be postal or personal, i.e. asked face-to-face with the respondent.
> They need to be piloted at least once to ascertain the validity of the method.
> They must be clear. Gray (2004, p. 187) emphasises the difficulty in designing a questionnaire that is 'valid, reliable and objective'.
> They are standardised and predetermined.
> They can be relatively straightforward to analyse.

Challenges to questionnaires

> Indicators need to be reliable and valid and, as both Bowling (2009) and Gray (2009) discuss, to render concepts into measurable and well defined indicators is a challenge.
> They do not allow respondents to represent their own interpretations and experiences.
> They do not allow for explanations or clarification.
> They do not allow for respondents' misunderstanding or confusion.
> People answer as they think you want them to.
> We endeavour to 'represent' ourselves, and identify ourselves in particular ways; thus conforming discourses can influence how we answer questionnaires.
> Postal questionnaires have a low response rate and there is a bias in terms of who responds and who does not – so there are self-selected responses (Calnan 2007).
> When using postal questionnaires you cannot control how people answer the questions; in what order they answer them; if they get someone else to fill it in or they check with other people; and finally if they answer all the questions (Calnan 2007).
> For face-to-face questionnaires and interviews: there is an impact by interviewer characteristics; they can be slow and require the recruitment of other interviewers, which then confounds the control replicable element needed for validity and reliability.

Useful resources: surveys and questionnaires

Calnan, M. (2007) 'Quantitative Survey Methods in Health Research', in M. Saks and
    J. Allsop (eds), *Researching Health: Qualitative, Quantitative and Mixed Methods*.
    London: Sage, pp. 174–96.

Fink, Arlene (2009) How to Conduct Surveys: A Step-by-Step Guide, 4th edn. London: Sage.

Case study 5.8   Using questionnaires

Purpose. The purpose of this piece of research was to develop a psychometric measure of risk factors for obesity that could be used to identify the 'at-risk individual' but also to determine the importance of each risk factor to each individual and the population as a whole. Thus, the research itself was *piloting* a possible tool for measuring these outcomes, with the intention of adapting and amending it depending on the outcomes from this pilot.

Approach. it is very positivist in terms of locating concepts such as risk factors, attitudes, behaviours and other correlated variables as being measurable and definable. It uses *deductive* reasoning as it is looking to measure the impact of various variables on being at 'risk' of developing obesity, i.e. testing a theory and measuring outcomes.

Method. The tool developed was based on a very extensive literature review that looked at risk theory, attitudes and behaviours, social influences and context. The researchers also included some of the elements of a tool known as the Theory of Planned Behaviour (which looks at attitudes, norms and control and their relation to how we behave and act). What this 100 item questionnaire was designed to do was to move beyond simple measurements of behaviours, consumption and outcomes, to include what research has also indicated, which is the importance of informing contexts and social environment on our behaviours.

Findings. There were some useful findings in terms of the association between high BMIs and attitudes, emotions and perceived difficulties in performing behaviours, i.e. adjusting eating consumption and increasing physical activity (hence a need for more categories in the next tool development). This association could explain why exercise and diet programmes that ignore this association don't really work. It had a response rate of 48 per cent, which is not unexpected in terms of questionnaires generally having low response rates. The returns were 67 per cent women with a mean age of 36 overall.

Critique. As a deductive method the anticipated outcomes were generally found though the known relationship between high BMI and what is eaten produced little association. They considered this to be (a) because what we say we eat and what we eat are not always congruent and (b) because of the higher socio-economic population they trialled on. Again as a tool they would consider adjusting this to include measures that would enable this association to be more clearly indicated. While this tool certainly attempts to 'nod its head' to the impact of context and social environment on how individuals may eat, it reduces these, as it does with all the concepts it sets out to measure, to unitary descriptions that can be generalised to all individuals. Meanings and interpretations of individuals are negated, and the ability of individuals to explore ↘

5

and interpret their own experiences is not considered as valid. The article attempts to represent its findings as significant in terms of further development of a risk factor tool and minimises both the low response rate and the fact that the population that was used was self-selected as well as from a very selective population group and location.

Source: Chambers, J. A. and Swanson, V. (2006) 'A Health Assessment Tool for Multiple Risk Factors for Obesity: Results from a Pilot Study with UK Adults', *Patient Education and Counselling*, 62, 79–88.

Systematic review

Systematic reviews are often informed by a positivist framework and associated with EBP, as they are concerned with locating the 'best' studies carried out on, or around, a particular practice. They use existing primary research for secondary data analysis, eliciting common themes and results, and providing a good evidence base to inform policy-making and practice (Smith and Dixon 2009). Bowling's (2009, p. 147) discussion of systematic reviews, like Gomm's (2009), focuses on how they 'aim to be systematic in the identification and evaluation of included literature, objective in their interpretations of this, and have reproducible conclusions. They are prepared with a systematic approach to minimising biases and random errors.'

A systematic review essentially involves a thorough search of research studies that have been done in or around your particular area of research (Bryman 2008; Bowling 2009). its purpose is to describe the most accurate and up-to-date state of knowledge about a specific matter – usually where uncertainty or the need for consistency exists. It is very popular and highly regarded in health care and practice as it seeks out and brings together all the most valid and reliable studies done on particular areas of practice and their effects (Bowling 2009).

Traditionally, and more commonly, it utilises a framework informed by a theory of 'the hierarchy of knowledge'; meaning that more often than not only it will only consider research studies that have used a systemised method of data collection – RCTs are the most popular of these. Have a look at the Cochrane Library on-line, which provides a wide range of up-to-date reviews undertaken within the field of healthcare research (Fox et al. 2007). There has been, you will discover, an emphasis on the utilisation of only quantitative or positivist-based research for systematic reviews, though this bias has not gone unchallenged. A number of disciplines as well as theorists consider it to be limitated in terms of its inability to truly reflect the complexities of phenomena (see also the EBP discussion for further debate on this issue). EBP and the Cochrane Library now include systematic reviews that have drawn on qualitative research and the CEBM has produced guidelines for utilising qualitative research.

Key qualities of (quantitative) systematic reviews

> They have explicit and clearly defined exclusion and inclusion criteria.
> They utilise a large number of resources (databases) as gateways to

searching for relevant literature, e.g. Medline, Cinahl, PsycINFO, Assia, Web of Knowledge; and names them.

> They report their method and strategies of searching for literature (Bowling 2009).
> The research question must be clearly defined (Bowling 2009).
> There is a comprehensive review of literature that is defined as being unbiased, replicable and scientific (Bryman 2008).
> They are sometimes known, when quantitative, as meta-analyses (Bryman 2008), though Gomm (2009) and Bowling (2009) differentiate them, a systematic review being a review of literature utilising a particular criterion, while meta-analysis synthesises and 'pools its results – expressed as effect sizes' (Gomm 2009, p. 201).
> They often use meta-analysis in conjunction as an aspect of the systematic review.
> They present the purpose of the research, particularly when researching the effect of an intervention on a particular phenomenon (EBP).
> They use *all* the possible available research that conforms to the criterion.

Challenges to systematic reviews

> The measures for hierarchy of evidence can be limited and irrelevant to many studies and research areas (Jones 2007) – particularly if you want to explore the why rather than the what of a particular practice, phenomenon or intervention.
> Given the criticism of the narrow confines of RCTs the focus of systematic reviews on RCTs can also be challenged as being confining, exclusive rather than inclusive, and limited in terms of the breadth and depth of the phenomenon under investigation (Jones 2007).
> Publication bias can seriously threaten the validity – if RCTs, for instance, are positioned as the 'gold standard' in research, then potentially publications may only accept material that is located within this method (Smith and Dixon 2009).
> Systematic reviews are only as good as the primary studies available and accessed. Given the challenges of producing a piece of research that is completely replicable, reliable and valid, this throws up a number of potential problems (Smith and Dixon 2009).

5

Useful resources: further exploration of systematic reviews

The NHS National Institute for Health Research provides guidelines for reading and carrying out reviews utilising both quantitative and qualitative research (http://www.york.ac.uk/inst/crd/).

An international source of systematic reviews (http://www.cochrane.co.uk).

The Centre for Evidence Based Medicine (CEBM) guidelines give details in the form of a table of hierarchy of evidence for systematic reviews (http://www.cebm.net/index.aspx?o=5653).

Higgins, J., Green, S. and the Cochrane Collaboration (2008) *Cochrane Handbook for Systematic Reviews of Interventions*. Oxford: Wiley-Blackwell.

Case study 5.9a Systematic reviews

Context. The number of children impacted upon by the death of a parent(s) from AIDS ('over 13 million children under the age of 15 (USAID 2002; UNAIDS 2006)', p. 2) or having a parent with HIV is significant and the researchers contend that, based on previous research, children and young people are vulnerable to a number of psychosocial problems as a result. The potential long-term complex effects of these problems on children are multiple and can reduce their ability to (according to the research accessed by the study) 'play an integral role in society' (p. 3). As a result, various international and government-led organisations have responded in a number of ways – in terms of interventions (e.g. physical, medical, mental, social, therapeutic, care and support) in order to address this issue

Purpose. The researchers had three main purposes in engaging in this piece of research. Primarily they wanted to *assess the efficacy* of interventions that are designed to ameliorate the psychosocial well-being of young people who are affected by HIV/AIDS. Second, they wanted to assess the interventions' effects on various defined psychosocial outcomes: mental health, school attendance, criminal activity and so on. Third, they wanted to see how effective the interventions were on what they term 'adverse outcomes', i.e. criminal activity, suicide and poor mental health. So they were particularly interested in the outcomes of the interventions, which would imply that the studies accessed needed to have in place evaluative and outcome measures of their interventions.

Approach. This is positivist as it positions psychosocial well-being as a known defined concept; it also defines interventions within various meanings and locates the study, and the researchers, as concerned with measurable outcomes in terms of using validated instruments. The inclusion criteria are concerned with locating 'randomised control trials, crossover trials, cluster-randomised trials and factorial trials' (p. 4)

Method. A systematic review was undertaken of available published and unpublished studies in any language and/or country, accessing various databases, websites, research experts, agencies and government organisations, and experts in the fields. They provide a very clear search strategy, utilising multiple search terms, which is useful to look at, as well as an inclusion criteria flow chart – both of these give a very clear insight into what the researchers did, how they did it, what they included and what was excluded (which was eventually everything, as they didn't fulfil their criteria and research aims).

Findings. They found that there were no studies that addressed outcomes in terms of interventions. So while there is a great deal in terms of what is out there and how it works, and what they do and so on, as far as the researchers could ascertain none of these studies had actually assessed the efficacy of their interventions.

Limitations. There were very narrow definitions of what is considered valid and reliable research. By limiting themselves to research that utilised measurement tools they excluded all qualitative and interpretative studies. By defining interventions and psychosocial well-being in such a delineated manner they may have excluded research that engages with well-being and mental health in less defined and measured ways. Given that this is an area that is relatively new in terms of exploration, the potential is that studies that are available will be looking at young people's experiences, understandings, their own stories – or the stories of the people who work with the young people.

Source: King, E., De Silva, M., Stein, A. and Patel, V. (2009) 'Interventions for Improving the Psychosocial Well-Being of Children Affected by HIV and AIDS (Review)', The Cochrane Collaboration Issue 3.

Case study 5.9b Systematic reviews

Context. Obesity is an international concern and the number of older people (over 75) with a BMI of over 30 in the UK has increased significantly in the past ten years. While problems such as an increase in type 2 diabetes and CHD are also evident in the older population, the evidence would indicate that there is a relationship between mortality and obesity in older people. Research has also indicated that intentional weight loss in older people can 'significantly' reduce mortality in males (in particular) (pp. 56–75).

Purpose. To investigate the evidence available on the efficacy of interventions intended to support sustained weight loss in older people. The researchers were particularly interested in finding research that is particularly geared to older people, as they claim that interventions that may work for younger people may not for older people, and need to be designed with the co-morbid diseases that can exist alongside old age.

Approach. This was positivist as they were looking for particular types of study, i.e. RCTs, comparative trials and placebo/non-intervention for control groups trials. They were clear that the intentions of the studies needed to be primarily on weight loss, with a follow-up of a minimum of a year. So their variables and outcomes were well defined and what were considered valid were tools that effectively measure outcomes considered pertinent to the study, e.g. cholesterol, deaths, hospitalisation, fasting glucose and so on, as well as quizzing the trials themselves in terms of capacity, funding, dropouts, capacity and so on.

Method. A large range of electronic databases was examined, with dates ranging from 1966 to 2008. They also 'hand searched four obesity and geriatrics journals' (p. 177) – an interesting touch and indicative of how published studies and information available on the database do not necessarily coincide. Two researchers were utilised and the original 'triallers' contacted. Interestingly, where results from studies could be quantitatively combined then meta-analysis was also undertaken.

Findings. Out of a possible 649 studies that might have been potentially relevant they narrowed it down to nine that fulfilled most or all inclusion criteria. What they found was that interventions did indicate a small but significant weight loss, but that overall there was a lack of studies for people aged over 69 and it is the older range where research is needed.

Limitations. As with the previous study the limits of systematic reviewing using fairly fixed levels of hierarchical evidence are always present. Given that they prioritised weight loss as the main purpose of an intervention this too could have limited their work. Research is clear that 'diets' as a singular intervention can be questionably effective in the long term and instead interventions where weight is one of the purposes, as opposed to the main one, may be more effective. The meta-analysis, producing material that synthesised studies' findings in terms of various outcomes, while certainly insightful, was limited as not all studies carried out their research in similar ways, thus reducing its generalisability.

Source: Witham, M. D. and Avenell, A. (2010) 'Interventions to Achieve Long-Term Weight Loss in Obese Older People. A Systematic Review and Meta-Analysis', *Age and Aging*, 39, 176–84.

5

Randomised control trials (RCTs)

RCTs have been discussed in the EBP epidemiology section (p. 195), so here we only briefly consider some of the qualities of a standardised RCT and then go on to unpack a piece of research that utilised this method. Clearly RCTs are a quantitative method located within the positivist ontological and epistemological frameworks of an independent known that is unaffected by social actors. It is rooted in a deductive reasoning approach and considered, as has already been demonstrated, to be the gold standard of research for much of the healthcare industry (Fox et al. 2007; Bryman 2008; Smith and Ryan 2009).

As a method it is located within an experimental (or quasi-experimental) design where the aim is to test different interventions and/or ways of treating and/or measuring situations (Bryman 2008). Systematic reviews will very often only use RCTs within their inclusion framework, as the ability to stipulate what works and what doesn't is often their main purpose. RCTs compare the impact of an intervention on a group of people (experimental group) with another group of people who do not have the intervention (control group). The crucial randomisation is of the participants to ensure that the research is considered valid, reliable and representative. Allocation to either of the groups is very formalised and systematic; the two groups must be as similar as possible in order for direct comparisons to be made and conclusions to be drawn regarding the efficacy of an intervention (Bryman 2008).

Challenges to RCTs

> Attitudes of the researcher, and therefore the design of the research, cannot impact on the research or the outcomes (Lewith and Little 2007).
> There is a 'cause' of all 'outcomes', i.e. a cause and effect relationship. This is considered reductionist and limited in scope, as well as it being 'impossible' to isolate the independent and dependent variables.
> Enormous skill is needed to set up and define the parameters of the research question.
> Randomisation can be very problematic and difficult to achieve
> The ethics of RCT. In a nutshell you are giving one group a set of interventions and the other group a placebo or no intervention – how do you

ethically justify this if you are applying a 'superior' intervention and the other group doesn't receive it?

> Smith and Ryan (2009) challenge the feasibility of isolating the independent variable as well as the population on which it has an effect, e.g. trying to measure the impact of fast food on children cannot be controlled or randomised practically.

> Bowling (2009) adds that the controlled conditions needed to conduct an RCT may have little similarity with real life and/or common practice.

> There can be too few participants, particularly given the stringent eligibility criteria that are applied; this reduces any chance of the 'extrapolation of results to a broader population group' (Smith and Ryan 2009, p. 157). It can also be too small to measure any infrequent and unexpected adverse outcomes due to the intervention (Bowling 2009).

> They do not account for how the patient and clinician or researcher may actually feel about the intervention itself; for instance, if you have designed a particular diet to reduce obesity (let's say one that is based on the 'combination' diet where carbohydrates and proteins are not mixed) and you are testing its efficacy against a calorie control diet, your investment in the combination diet and belief in its efficacy may impact on how you work with it, and how the patient responds.

> Finally, using the example above, you have randomly sampled a population of obese women and clearly explained to them they will be assigned to either the experimental or the control group: the respondents may respond more positively to being given the combination diet as opposed to the calorie control, even being disappointed or elated at being in one or other of the groups (Bowling 2009)

Case study 5.10 An RCT

Purpose. The purpose of both 'interventions' is to increase adolescents' body satisfaction, with its associated attitudes and behaviours, and to reduce their weight. The primary hypothesis was that those individuals within the experimental group would show improvements in eating disorders (which they associate with body dissatisfaction, which is found to be high in adolescents), attitudes and behaviours as well as their weight compared to the control group; the secondary hypothesis would be that the experimental group's physical activities and dietary behaviours would also improve as compared to the control group.

Approach. The approach used was to look at the outcomes of an Internet designed programme. The Student Bodies 2 (SD2) is a 16-week Internet delivered programme, based on a cognitive behavioural approach to weight loss and developing a more positive body image. There was an experiment and a control group of young people; the outcomes from the control group (who received the baseline information usually available in terms of nutrition and physical activity) and the experimental group (the group who received SD2) were compared. ⌐

Method. The processes and steps involved in working with both groups and within the groups were replicated and controlled. Assessments were made at three points – baseline, post-intervention and four months follow-up – for both groups and the assessors were blinded (i.e. did not know to which group individuals belonged). Measures of satisfaction, an Eating Disorder Examination Questionnaire as well as participants' weight and measurements were all taken at these three points – again assessors were blinded regarding which group individuals belonged to.

How they randomised

- Participants were recruited through various sources, including on-line advertisements, flyers, newspapers and medical centres.
- Inclusion criteria: 12–18 years, overweight or at risk of being overweight, regular and easy access to the Internet.
- Exclusion criteria: medical conditions; past/present clinical eating disorders (anorexia etc.); physical conditions that might limit or prevent physical activity; prescription drugs that might impact on weight.
- From the 155 possible contacts, 83 were deemed eligible (based on previous data it was considered that the number of necessary respondents should be 52, considering drop outs etc., looking for 62).
- The 83 contacts were randomly selected for either the control group (41) or the experimental (42).
- There were four separate cohorts, two in San Diego and two in St Louis.

Limitations. There is a considerable limitation to their sample from a selection point of view, i.e. they were by their nature a self-selected sample that needed to volunteer and then contact the researchers. This small sample were also limited to young people who had regular access to the Internet, who were located within urban settings and who accessed the sites where selection took place. Given that it was looking at changing behaviour it was a very short-term project that was limited in terms of being able to measure any long-term effects. Finally, from an ethical position, they provided one intervention, which the researchers believed to be potentially more effective, to only one of the groups – while intervention studies are very often about measuring efficacy by giving the experimental group the 'improved' intervention to be measured and the 'control' group the usual intervention, this still needs to be supported in ways that justify the inequity.

Source: Doyle, A. C., Goldschmidt, A., Huang, C., Winzelberg, A. J., Taylor, C. B. and Wilfley, D. E. (2008) 'Reduction of Overweight and Eating Disorder Symptoms via the Internet in Adolescents: A Randomized Controlled Trial', *Journal of Adolescent Health,* 43, 172–9.

Documentary and textual research: historical, media and demographic

Documentary research can be quantitative or qualitative (or both) and can include a very wide range of material. Silverman (2006, p. 153) defines all documents, or texts, as data 'consisting of words and/or images which have become recorded without the intervention of a researcher (e.g. through an interview)'. He particularly explores in his work the use of files, statistical records, e-mails, the Internet, records of official meetings or procedures and media headlines. Bowling (2009) suggests that there are three types of documentary research: historical, media and demographic. Gomm (2009) adds life history, and Matthews and Ross (2010) add organisational research.

MacDonald and Tipton (1993) consider there to be four broad categories of documents, and while not dissimilar to Sarantakos's (1998) extensive list, these are worth noting in terms of range and definitions. For them public records, visual records, the media and finally private papers make up the broad spectrum of documents available to us for analysis. Sarantakos (1998, p. 275) provides a very detailed description of the possible documents we may use for documentary research, which include:

> public records, namely census statistics, statistical year-books, court archives, prison records, mass media and literature (novels, poetry, etc.); archival records, such as service records of hospitals, doctors and social workers, and records of organisations; personal documents, such as life histories, diaries, memoranda, confessions, autobiographies, suicide notes and letters; administrative documents, such as proposals, memoranda, progress reports, agendas, minutes of meetings, announcements and other internal documents; formal studies and reports related to the research topic.

Documentary research can be a 'stand alone method' and one that is used in conjunction with other methods (Alaszewski 2007). On the whole the term documentary research is used in relation to 'doing research on' documents that exist already and the bulk of this section is on this form of documentary research. However, it can also be a method where you ask or require people to create a document (MacDonald and Tipton 1993; Silverman 2001; Alaszewski 2007) and below we provide a brief outline of what this might look like, before returning to the former meanings.

The diary or journal as a method of data collection

The intention in using this method of data collection is to involve respondents in a daily recording of their activities and events – a method that can be both structured and semi- or unstructured (Bowling 2009). Examples of this type of documentary research might be to ask respondents to complete a food diary (either one that you have provided or one you ask them to devise themselves), a daily record of a carer's experience of working with someone living with dementia and/or an action research group's reflective account of implementing change within an IVF clinic.

5

Useful resources: using diaries in research

Corti, L. (1993) 'Using Diaries in Social Research' (http://sru.soc.surrey.ac.uk/SRU2.html).

Spowart, L. (2008) '"I Would Have Forgotten about That: Using the Diary-Interview Method in Leisure Research (http://www.arasite.org/diaryresmeths.pdf).

As with all methods of data collection you need to have a reason for using it as your chosen method. Researchers will often access documents because they can give insight into not just what is recorded but how it is recorded, not just what is included but also what is not included (Matthews and Ross 2010). So as documentary researchers we may be interested in finding out how the cause of death has been recorded over the years for people with HIV/AIDS, as our purpose is to consider how meanings of HIV are socially situated and fluid. Or we might consider doing a piece of research that is about 'Doctors' approaches to deciding on surgery for chronically obese people', and part of our research will be concerned with what the case notes say and how doctors have recorded their decisions.

How to work with documents

When accessing any document, critical issues of assessing its authenticity, credibility, reliability and validity must be considered. Some of these qualities may be more appropriate for positivistic frameworks that consider documentary research as a process of coding and synthesising data in particular ways (Silverman 2006). Silverman as a qualitative researcher writes instead of the importance of how theoretical elements of knowledge have informed the writing, creation and representation of the material itself. Alaszewski (2007) differentiates the process and analysis of documents as also being concerned with our theoretical/research paradigm and often being engaged with statistical, content or thematic analysis.

MacDonald and Tipton (1993) discuss the necessity to evaluate the quality of the material you are intending to access. For them this means considering the authenticity, the meaning, the credibility and the representativeness of the document. Representativeness in this instance is an interesting quality as it can refer to the consideration of how 'accurate', true and inclusive is the representation of what has been written – so here discourses of 'truth' can be considered. It may also be considered in terms of how representative this type of document is in comparison to other documents of the same type.

Within documentary research must be embedded a rationale, as well as a clear outline of your sampling technique and exclusion and inclusion criteria. This can be an issue of representativeness but it will also refer to your paradigm and purpose. It is useful at this point to refer back to both the process of systematic review and the literature review, both of which provide you with detailed critical reflection processes that researchers need to engage in when considering your research.

Clearly the range of documents available for documentary analysis is wide, so we have on this occasion provided you with two examples using documentary research. The first uses it as its main method of data collection and analyses meanings and relevance. The second piece of research uses documentary research as a way of providing an even greater insight into a particular way in which a phenomenon is represented and understood.

> ❯ 'The defining characteristic of documentary research is that the researcher draws on documents created by others' (Alaszewski 2007).
> ❯ It is not just a stand-alone method, and is often used in case study research and mixed methods.
> ❯ It can use both document that already exist and those that are created for the research, e.g. diaries, reflective journals.
> ❯ A huge range of documents is available.
> ❯ As the documents have already been produced and are in the 'public realm', issues of ethics may be less problematic.
> ❯ Documents are a rich source of data.
> ❯ Rather than being directly interpretative, as happens in primary data collection, you are in essence interpreting and analysing the interpretation and analysis of the original writer (Robson 2007).
> ❯ It is sometimes possible to access a great deal of material in a relatively short space of time.
> ❯ It is possible to gain insight into a phenomenon historically and how it has developed over a long period of time.
> ❯ Documents whose originals and intentions may be wide ranging can be accessed, thus it is possible to gain insight into a phenomenon from a number of different angles.
> ❯ Robson (2007) considers the need to ascertain how much the original purpose of the document might impact on what is written and published, e.g. media accounts that are designed to shock and/or feed into your prejudices and therefore include that which will appeal to the reader.

Challenges to documentary research

> ❯ Bowling (2009) writes that both positivists and phenomenologist have difficulties with documentary research; positivists because, discounting official documents and measurements, documents are too subjective and potentially impressionistic in terms of how they are produced, written and published.
> ❯ Phenomenologists and critical theorists challenge documents as being too invested in representing society's hegemonic constructs in particular ways, i.e. generalising them and presenting them as taken for granted, 'common sense' truths
> ❯ Concerns are expressed as to how the writers' own prejudices and preconceived priorities and representations of reality will influence how material is recorded and what is identified as being relevant.
> ❯ It can often be seen as being oversimplified, decontextualised and lacking in an in-depth interpretative approach.
> ❯ There are questions of authenticity, credibility, errors within the documents, missed information, limited information and bias (Alaszewski 2007; Bowling 2009).

5

> It might not be possible to access the full range of documents, and there is a potential for material to have been missed out.

> Documentts might be partial – clearly this has particular relevance to media research.

> There might be changes in classifications in terms of statistics (see how Aidsmap has changed recordings of HIV over time).

> There might be changes in terms of classifications and definitions (e.g. changes in how class and occupational category are recorded).

> Bowling (2009, p. 450) states that 'the main sources of bias in document research stem from the selective deposit and selective survival of recorded material, whether the material consists of letters, diaries, official or other documents'.

> Matthews and Ross (2010) add that documents can be lost or changed over time, and finally the context of when and how a document is produced can be lost.

Useful resources: documentary research

Bryman, A. (2008) 'Documents as Sources of Data', in *Social Research Methods*, 3rd edn. Oxford: Oxford University Press, 514–36.

Markham, A. N. (2004) 'The Internet as Research Context', in C. Seale, G. Gobo, J. Gubrium and D. Silverman (eds), *Qualitative Research Practice*. London: Sage, pp. 328–44.

Pink, S. (2004) 'Visual Methods', in C. Seale, G. Gobo, J. Gubrium and D. Silverman (eds), *Qualitative Research Practice*. London: Sage, pp. 361–76.

Prior, L. (2004) 'Documents', in C. Seale, G. Gobo, J. Gubrium and D. Silverman (eds), *Qualitative Research Practice*. London: Sage, pp. 345–60.

Case study 5.11 Documentary research

Purpose. The purpose of this piece of research was to compare the cost of multiple births from IVF and single births from IVF to the NHS using data from published literature and cost data from national sources in the public domain. The ultimate purpose was to look at the overall costs to the NHS and to consider the possible implications of introducing a policy of limiting embryo transfer to a maximum of two (this policy has been advocated by the Human Fertilisation and Embryology Authority since 2004 and is fully supported by NICE 2004).

Approach. This is clearly a positivist piece of work as the researchers absolutely believe that the reality, i.e. costs to the NHS, is measurable and discernable and they engage with methods – using data from published sources – that they situate as being objective, distanced and not impacting upon the setting. They are also starting from a deductive position, i.e. that multiple IVF births are more expensive to the NHS.

Method. Their data was from published sources and national figures from 2000–1 (it is useful as a researcher for you to pay attention to when the research was done as clearly this can and does age the research) and when the up-to-date data wasn't available in terms of UK figures they extrapolated from figures for other countries in situations similar to the UK. They then cross-analysed all sets of data to produce figures that gave the costs to the NHS overall but also considered the possible cost implications of reducing IVF births to singletons.

Findings. They established that the overall cost to the NHS of 'twin' and 'triplet' births is substantially higher than for 'singleton' births; this would and could be used to support the 'two embryos' transfer policy recommended by HFEA as well as potentially indicating the validity of introducing a 'single' embryo transfer policy.

Limitations. There are a number of concerns regarding the range and quality of the clinical trial documentation and representativeness of the documents. First, the research could only be based on the material that was available and recorded, and given that they were accessing material from private clinics, public sources as well as international figures the consistency in recording, obtaining full sets of data and being able to verify its consistency would have been problematic. Clearly, too, there was no standardised way in which data was recorded, particularly as they were accessing material from public and private spheres. An added problem is the international nature of some of their data. Again not only would results potentially be recorded differently but there is the added complication of practices, as well as different political, social and historical meanings, of postnatal care and levels of care varying across nations. Finally, record keeping in terms of post natal care is limited, thus establishing clear consensus of differing practices for 'visits' for twin/triplet births and single births is hard to establish.

Source: Ledger, W. L., Anumba, D., Marlow, N., Thomas, C. M., Wilson, E. C. F. and the Cost of Multiple Births Study Group (COMBS Group) (2006) 'The Costs to the NHS of Multiple Births after IVF Treatment in the UK', *British Journal of Obstetrics and Gynaecology*, 113, 21–5.

Case study 5.12 Documentary research (and interviews – mixed methods)

Context. This piece of research was based in Australia and interested in looking at how women who did not become pregnant and give birth from IVF (2001 figures indicate that only 15.4 per cent of women do 'succeed') made sense of their experience.

Purpose. As a feminist piece of work the researchers were interested in rendering visible the invisible and taken-for-granted discourses of how women were situated in the media. They used mixed methods, accessing a range of documents as well as interviewing women as a way of sharing their findings and exploring how women themselves resisted this positioning.

Approach. This was a feminist piece of research and acknowledged how social discourses constructed IVF in terms of the metaphor of a lottery, with women situated as winners (i.e. mothers) and losers (i.e. infertile), with the latter being invisible and undervalued.

Method. The researchers used two methods: in-depth interviews with women about their own understandings and experiences; and data from multiple document sites. ⇲

They accessed documents that included 'print media articles published throughout an infertility Awareness campaign conducted in Australia three times throughout the 1990s and 26 infertility self-help texts available in public libraries and support group collections across Australia ... supplemented with sex education literature and reproductive biology and human development textbooks' (p. 45). The rational for these varied documents allowed the researchers to look at how women were represented within various medical discourse documents.

Findings. What they found in the documents was that women who became pregnant were seen to have succeeded. Being successful was situated as being focused, strong, persistent and enduring, while those women who didn't 'succeed' but endeavoured to continue to engage and try were seen as addicted, obsessed and compulsive.

Limitations (particularly in reference to the documentary aspect). There was a lack of clarity concerning the sampling framework: while we were told what they chose we were not told how they went about that process or why. They chose to access only documents located within what they identified as 'medical discourses', which would mean that (a) there was only a particular perspective represented in their documents and (b) this was their interpretation of the original writers' stances.

Source: de Lacey, S. (2001) 'IVF as Lottery or Investment: Contesting Metaphors in Discourses of Infertility', *Nursing Inquiry*, 9(1), 43–51.

Focus groups

> A focus group is, quite simply, a small group discussion focused on a particular topic and facilitated by a researcher ... offers a distinctive method for generating qualitative data on the basis of group interaction and discussion. (Tonkiss 2004, p. 194)

Focus groups rely 'on interaction within the group based on topics that are supplied by the researcher' (Morgan 1997, p. 12). The emphasis here is that focus groups are a process by which to gather data from groups of people who are interacting and constructing meanings together. The interest for the researcher is 'how' participants negotiate, discuss and contest each other's attitudes and opinions and also 'how' they socially produce meanings (Foster-Turner 2009). In some ways a focus group reflects the way in which people make sense of ideas in the real world and is often used by social constructivists as a primary method of data collection. As with many interactions within the real world, as we interact and communicate with one another 'participants ask questions of each other, seek clarification, comment on what they have heard and prompt others to reveal more. As the discussion progresses (backwards and forwards, round and round the group), individual response becomes sharpened and refined, and moves to a deeper and more considered level' (Finch and Lewis 2003, p. 171).

A well facilitated and planned focus group, therefore, may reveal not only the individual feelings, values, attitudes and meanings but also how individuals interact and communicate with one another. In other words focus groups are often as interested in the process of knowledge construction as in the actual content of the discussion itself (Morgan 1997). Foster-Turner (2009, p. 211) states that the 'defining quality of the focus group process is that it actively encourages interaction, in the form of dialogue, between the group members themselves'. The skills and planning required to run a focus group are fairly extensive and the ability to work with group dynamics and processes is something that needs to be taken into account when planning to utilise focus groups as a method of data collection.

The size of the group can also vary, and theorists' suggestions range from 6–12 (Green 2007) to no more than 8 or 9 (Morgan 1997). Deciding on how homogeneous or heterogeneous the group members will be, and how you define that, depends on the research question and phenomenon under discussion (Finch and Lewis 2003). Given that focus groups rely on interactive engagement, as well as acknowledging the need to explore shared or conflicting meanings, some thought needs to be given to the 'make-up of the group'.

For instance you may want to carry out a focus group on a care home's approach to working with people living with dementia. Does your focus group involve all the workers, including the managers, families, relatives, friends and 'funders'? If so what is your rationale for this sample and how would you facilitate such a group? Your questions or points of focus may need to be designed to encourage discussion of experiences that are not couched in terms of who does what. Or you may decide that your focus group will only contain the workers from a particular care home; or the relatives of people in a particular care home. Your research question may need to be adjusted to accommodate these different groups, or you may need to consider holding focus groups for all the differing sources of care within a nursing home. As you can see, your knowledge of hierarchies, characteristics and the field itself needs to be well founded in order to make the most of a focus group.

Green (2007) writes about a number of practical considerations to take into account when planning and running a focus group and these include its recruitment, the location, the role of the facilitators, researchers and assistants in the group, ethics of confidentiality, managing anonymity and managing group power and knowledge sharing, costs of transport, location, refreshments, recording and child care. Foster-Turner (2009) also discusses the necessary skills needed to develop and run a group and is a good resource in terms of the practical issues around the planning and running of focus groups.

Useful resource

A podcast with David Morgan about research design using focus groups (http://www.youtube.com/watch?v=CzkmPLMUv9o&feature=related).

> A group of people together in the same place discuss a particular phenomenon.
> The members share experiences and/or knowledge of the 'same' phenomenon.
> It is both how people discuss the issues and the content of the discussion that are of interest to the researcher.
> They rely on rapport and engaged participation.
> They are rich and often in-depth sources of data.
> They can be particularly useful in opening up knowledge in areas that are less well knownor about which little is known.
> The findings are often used to develop other methods of data collection.
> They can be useful with groups of people who are 'hard to reach' or 'hard to access'
> They can be both ongoing and continuous as well as 'one offs'.
> They provide insight into how groups of people make sense of their worlds.
> They are insightful regarding the impact of others on our meanings and responses.
> They can be built on reciprocal notions of shared knowledge; thus people who may think they are 'alone' in thinking or feeling something will find that an experience is shared and understood.
> They can enable individuals to feel less isolated or more isolated (if they don't feel understood).
> they are dynamic.
> They can be made up of people who already know each other or who are strangers (there are strengths and weaknesses of both).

Challenges to focus groups

> They are dependent on rapport within the group, among group members and with the researcher and facilitator and the group dynamic (Foster-Turner 2009).
> Focus groups are created settings and, therefore, artificial constructs – this in itself can be uncomfortable and restrictive for everyone involved (Matthews and Ross 2010).
> It is difficult to manage the group dynamic, with issues of dominance, cliques and scapegoats (very similar to issues addressed by Tuckman's (1965) four (six) stage group structure).
> There is often an assumption that a focus group is cheap, as you have a number of people in one place; however, Green (2007) among others considers the costs in terms of time and money as follows: negotiating, arranging, managing a premise that can suit all and provide appropriate space and safety, transport, child care, potentially food and drink (disputable and can be disruptive), tape recorders and tapes.

5

> It takes a lot of time and skill to set up and work in a focus group.
> Time may be required to establish a relationship with the respondents, and potentially even meet them individually, beforehand.
> Group confidentiality, consent forms and access need to be negotiated.
> The researcher has limited control over what data is generated (Matthews and Ross 2010); thus if you try to control it too much you can limit the discussions, interactions and interpretations of the group members; if you allow it 'free rein' than it can go off tangent
> Matthews and Ross (2010) consider that issues of power, social relations and skills, gender, class, cultural and political positions can impact on how the group functions; while you can endeavour to address this when planning the group you cannot always anticipate the impact of social identities on the group dynamic.
> There is a potential for group think and the influence of wanting other people's good opinions; being ashamed and fear of being shamed.
> There is a conforming effect.
> They can be either difficult or useful with issues that are considered sensitive and laden with contested meanings (Green 2007; Foster-Turner 2009; Matthews and Ross 2010)

Case study 5.13 Using focus groups

Context. Previous research has indicated that mothers, being the main purchasers and providers of food, can have a significant impact on how their daughters in particular make choices of what food to eat, how they feel about their bodies and their dieting behaviours. African-American women in particular are at risk of being obese.

Purpose. The researchers were interested in looking at how information and behaviour regarding food was communicated between mothers and daughters. How this manifests in different cultural groups may differ. The purpose of collecting this data from these women was to 'define [an interesting term given that this is framed as a qualitative and emergent method] criteria that will allow diet and nutrition educators to tailor campaigns' (p. 13).

Approach. This is unclear in some ways. Though the implication seems to be that to truly 'understand' these transgenerational practices the research must be located within the meanings and experiences of the women themselves. The approach identified influence in terms of 'type of information transmitted, the process by which this information is communicated and the influence of this information on diet and behaviour'.

Method. Their sample was recruited from a low-income African-American population from within three African Methodist Episcopal church organisations. Interestingly it was church and/or parish nurses who informed female parishioners about the research. Four focus groups with 21 women were carried out. Two of the groups were with women aged 25–65 and two of the groups with women aged 25–45, and the women were 'not related to one another'; their focus here was on the impact of age differences on women's views. Their rationale for using focus groups, as opposed to other qualitative methods, is not

5

particularly well supported but what they were clear about was that they wanted to offer a space for women to explore and discuss openly their feelings and attitudes to food and diet without the presence of a medical professional.

The design of their focus groups is also somewhat intriguing and again reflects the multiple ways in which we can utilise methods to collect data. They were quite interventionist in terms of their role and commenced the group by asking them all individually to write down three things they learnt from their mothers about healthy eating. The focus was clearly on the relationship between mother and daughter, so meanings were fairly fixed in this way. Their probes and prompts also clearly asked the women to distinguish what they were told from what they saw and were shown. The model they used to 'run' the workshop involved asking the first and last questions individually of each group member and the second and third questions more widely to the group as a whole. Morgan (1997) talks about the possible differences in focus group format; one being focused on group discussion, interaction and meanings and the other focusing on interviewing individually a group of people at the same time. Whichever you decide you need to make sure you are clear in your rationale for this.

Findings. The clear influence of mother–daughter communications can be used by programmes as a way of impacting upon and influencing food choices, and educating families in healthy eating habits.

Limitations. There are a number of limitations to this study and their use of focus groups. The sample was selected from a particular religious affiliation – thereby excluding all other women and, given the religious context, including women who potentially already knew one another or about one another (which can be both a weakness and a strength). Thus there was a potential, particularly given that it was church and parish nurses who told the women about the research, that first this would have potentially immediately located the discussion within medical models of understanding; there is a potential impact of religious affiliation in terms of being a 'good' or 'bad' Christian. Also of concern were the assumptions made about women being the only influencers of their daughter's eating; thus this was a depoliticised piece of work that did not work with the realities of being (low-income) African-American. Given that they focused on the mother's role, they play into notions of inequalities and power dynamics that make up the rest of society, particularly around 'blaming the mother'. No consideration was given to male influences on choices and freedoms around food, and women who accepted their bigger body size were problematised rather than any political contexts being considered. Finally, as a focus group it was fairly interventionist and proscriptive about the content. They were particularly concerned with 'finding out' particular sorts of data and the influence of the facilitator (an 'educator') will have been significant in defining these, but this was not engaged with. Given the differing power dynamics of the facilitator and the women within the group this needed to be considered far more clearly.

Source: Wilson, D. B., Musham, C. and McLellan (2004) 'From Mothers to Daughters: Transgenerational Food and Diet Communication in an Underserved Group', *Journal of Cultural Diversity*, 11(1), 12–17.

Interviews

Interviews are a very popular method of data collection (Silverman 2006; Bryman 2008; Gray 2009; Matthews and Ross 2010) and, as you will see from the research literature, come in all shapes and sizes. They range from very structured to unstructured, and can be focused and in-depth; the terminologies used to describe the range of methods are interchangeable and like much of the language in research you will need to learn to differentiate and work with these terminologies. Essentially an interview is between two people, the researcher and the respondent (sometimes a third in terms of translators), and can be face-to-face, over the phone and/or via a chat room or e-mail facility.

Structured interviews

These can also be described as 'face-to-face questionnaires', and they share most of the same qualities. You may use a structured interview, as opposed to a postal questionnaire, in order to ensure that you get a full complement of responses (Gray 2009). Postal questionnaires have a notoriously low rate of response, which often makes the results derived from them less reliable and generalisable; with structured interviews your response rate and ability to get all the information in the way you want it tends to be more reliable.

With structured interviews the art, so to speak, much as with RCTs, is control. Each interviewer asks the questions in the same order, using exactly the same words and even, if possible, with the same pauses and timings. Should there be a need for possible clarifications, and if this is anticipated, then the responses to this must always use exactly the same words, in the same place in the interview – in other words everything is scripted. The key is not to deviate or in any way corrupt the reliability of the tool you are using. Robson (2007, p. 74) considers that 'in fully structured interviews, most of the thinking work is carried out up front, before the interview itself … They are questions that are going to help you get the answers to the research questions.'

You might use a structured interview if you want to assess the pain levels of an individual with dementia. Structured interviews, because they are predetermined, are usually located within a positivist piece of research; this is because your reasoning is deductive and you believe that there is a truth or a reality that can be empirically measured and ascertained. The position to take on structured questionnaires is distanced and objective, so the actual personal contact is minimal and certainly non-interactive. Gomm (2009) talks about removing the 'confounding' (the potential to attribute the reason for one thing to another – so making sure your sample is as representative as possible) variables. Structured interviews, like questionnaires, usually involve a large sample, with the aim of generating the same amount of data per unit, and therefore allow for comparisons and generalisations (Gomm 2009).

5

> The schedule is followed exactly.
> Anonymity is easily guaranteed.
> They are straightforward to analyse.
> They use random sampling.
> They are quick to capture data.
> They can be used to produce data which is generalisable, replicable, valid and reliable.
> They allow for any measures of body language etc. to be added, if necessary, to the results.
> They can be more flexible than written questionnaires as people who can't read (for whatever reason) can be accessed.

Challenges to structured interviews

> There can be an interviewer effect and impact.
> The voice of the interviewer can carry inflections.
> There are problems with (a) deviating from the order of the schedule because the logic of the response from the respondent demands it; or (b) not deviating and keeping to the schedule when in fact it doesn't make sense in terms of what has come before.
> It is challenging to maintain absolute consistency.
> It is necessary to ensure validity, i.e. your questions actually measure the phenomenon you are seeking to measure.
> Reliability can be impacted upon by interviewer bias.
> Gray (2009) talks about maintaining rapport, and how poor and inconsistent maintenance can weaken reliability and introduce bias.
> How you record the interview must be carefully considered.
> You need to decide who will interview whom, so if your study is on parents and their attitudes to their children's obesity, do you send a man to interview men and a woman to interview women? How then do you control and maintain consistency etc.? Bowling (2009) talks about matching in terms of interviewer/interviewee socio-demographic characteristics.
> They are of limited use in sensitive and complex health and mental health issues, as they only measure particular outcomes and concepts, and people are less likely to explore and discuss these issues in a time limited and predetermined measure (Bowling 2009).
> They measure and validate respondents' answers in specific ways, and therefore can render experiences outside this measure as irrelevant.
> It is not possible for people to explore the unexpected or rare.
> There is an impact by what Bowling calls 'social desirability bias'.
> There can be a response bias, i.e. only people who are willing to have face-to-face and/or telephone interviews are chosen.

5

Case study 5.14　Using structured interviews

Purpose. Their theoretical positioning is clearly positivist and the hypothesis is to test the findings that 'adverse parental attributes' (drug addiction and/or HIV infection) have an adverse effect on child maladjustment and substance abuse and that they also weaken the father–child attachment and a consequence is an increase in adolescent risk taking behaviours.

Approach. This is deductively informed by Family Interaction Theory (FIT), based on previous research and measurements, which is designed to explain the development of sexual risk taking and other maladaptive behaviours as being influenced by various factors within family, peers and personal characteristics – and thus looks at social modelling, the attachment between parent and child, and values and behaviours that are informed by attachment.

Method. The authors used structured interviews with two groups: HIV-negative drug abusing fathers and HIV-positive drug abusing fathers and their children. They interviewed them separately. The interview was structured around FIT measures and psychological scales. The research was designed as longitudinal, in that they interviewed the adolescents twice, once at the same time as their fathers and then a year later. They endeavoured to reduce interviewer effect by using the same interviewer where possible over the time.

Findings. Their findings support their hypothesis and in addition highlight how perceived environmental discrimination is also a contributory factor; though no causal relationship could be confirmed.

Limitations

- A self-selected sample was accessed through treatment programmes and community notices.
- The psychiatric background and mathematical frameworks of the researchers located the research and the respondents in particularly fixed ways.
- Other contextual issues, such as family and friend relationships, class and education level, gender and sexuality, race and class and so on were not accounted for.
- The second interview with adolescents had a 41 per cent attrition rate, which means any claims of longitudinal impacts are rendered unreliable.
- Isolating positive and or negative HIV status as the independent variable (cause) of the dependent variable, i.e. increased adolescent sexual risk taking, is dubious.
- It was a small sample to make any claims about ($n = 296$)
- There are questions of the ethics of paying interviewers in terms of where and how the money was spent.
- Fathers or legal guardians of children under 18 had to give signed permission for the adolescent to contribute; this has a number of implications in terms of choice of adolescent, limiting it to fathers or legal guardians who were 'willing' to allow their child be interviewed.

Source: Brook, D. W., Brook, J. S., Rubenstone, B. A., Zhang, C. and Finch, S. J. (2010) 'A Longitudinal Study of Sexual Risk Behavior among the Adolescent Children of HIV-Positive and HIV-Negative Drug-Abusing Fathers', *Journal of Adolescent Health*, 46, 224–31.

5

Qualitative interviews

Qualitative or interpretative interviews differ considerably from structured interviews, not just in the actually 'doing' of them but in their purpose and design. They range from semi-structured, i.e. containing some predetermined questions (though openly worded and flexibly designed), to unstructured (free flowing and led by the respondent), i.e. simply having a guide or letting the process unfold. Within each of these there is a wide range of approaches; again when reading the literature around this you will find a wide range of understandings and approaches. It is up to you the researcher to choose the method and its design that will best provide you with the data you are looking for. The purpose of qualitative interviews is to gather rich, in-depth data from respondents. You want to explore with them their meanings and understandings, their experiences and beliefs, their attitudes and feelings and so on. Qualitative interviews can be very good at gaining insight into complex issues and offer up opportunities to clarify and check meanings. Often in interviews you will gain access to sensitive and deeply personal views and unexpected emergent data. Clearly the success of an interview and its effectiveness as a method rely a great deal on the interviewer's ability to respond, to listen, to engage, to value and be interested in their respondent; rapport can be an important element in informing how well an interview goes. Clearly the more open and flexible they are the more potential there is for emergent and unexpected information to arise.

Semi-structured interviews

Some semi-structured interviews keep to the questions they have predetermined, in as flexible manner as possible, while others may be far more adaptable and reword questions, put the questions in a different order and/or even discard or add some of the questions. Semi-structured interviews are a very rich and in-depth method of data collection. They are often used when there are particular areas and aspects of a phenomenon that you want to cover – hence the open ended and flexible predetermined questions – but are also intended to be free flowing, guided by the interviewer rather than led as in structured interviews, and completely focused on the respondent's own point of view and perspectives. This means that the questions you may have thought of before the interview may change in how you word them and in which order you engage with them; you will add new ones and potentially omit others because the information has been provided by the respondent in answer to a different question. This is because how the respondent responds and how you listen and engage with the respondent will impact on how it precedes. It is a conversation in which you both engage: you can seek clarification, explanation, extrapolation and expansion – and so can the respondent. The key to the design of the interview schedule is to be open, flexible, responsive and exploratory. You don't want too many specific questions as you may limit your respondents' opportunity to give you their views. The more set questions and structure you work with the more you are restricting exploration and are, instead, indicating your own understandings and views.

Unstructured interviews

Unstructured interviews too can range in their open design, but are largely concerned with responding to the spoken realities of respondents and almost following their lead in terms of what to ask and explore. Generally in unstructured interviews a guide is used, which may simply involve a few key words or terms that you may want to explore – clearly this sort of interview still has a purpose, but the purpose is informed by the exploration of the respondents' meanings, not what you think or anticipate they will discuss. Unstructured interviews are particularly used in phenomenological and feminist research, where the respondent is located as the expert on their own lives and meanings. Thus, the role of the interviewer is to be part of an almost reciprocal conversation, as much as possible focused on the respondent but always informed by responses to their realities and interpretations. Your role is to give them the space to make meaning of the phenomenon, and to be a very engaged, interested and interactive listener.

Key qualities of qualitative interviews

> They are a rich in-depth source of data.
> They are engaged and responsive to respondents.
> 'Control' of interview ranges depending on whether it is semi-structured or open, free-flowing and unstructured.
> They are collaborative (again this can vary) – feminists in particular are concerned with the collaborative nature of interviews (Legard et al. 2003).
> They are like a 'conversation with a purpose' (Robson 2007).
> They are exploratory.
> They open up a field of knowledge.
> They engage with the respondents' world and their understanding of it.
> Semi-structured interviews can be more straightforward to analyse as you have predetermined though very flexible questions, categories or concepts to explore (Robson 2007).
> Semi-structured interviews can have more direction and control than unstructured, but there is a fine balance in allowing the flow of the interview to develop while at same time working within the particular framework of purpose (Matthews and Ross 2010).
> They are often called in-depth interviews (Coombes et al. 2009) with less or more structure; no matter how naturalistic they are there is a purpose.
> They can produce insightful and unexpected data.
> They are flexible and designed to respond to the respondent.
> They can be reciprocal.

5

> Depending on paradigm and purpose, the interviewer may return to the respondent a number of times, sharing the transcripts and analysis as a way of developing theory.

> They are useful for exploring how people talk about their experiences, perceptions, understandings and what they do.

> There is transparent use of transcripts and analysis.

Challenges to qualitative interviews

> They can be very time consuming.

> The skills of the interviewer are paramount, i.e. the ability to respond in the moment, to be a reflective listener, to explain, extrapolate etc. without imposing their own views and beliefs (Matthews and Ross 2010).

> There are large amounts of 'raw' data to analyse

> As with structured interviews, interviewer impact, in terms of mismatching characteristics (this can depend on the subject being explored), but also because, since they are in-depth interviews that are more about a rich engagement with the respondent, rapport is even more important.

> They can often result in respondents talking about things not 'of interest' to researcher (Matthews and Ross 2010). There is a tricky balance here as with semi-structured you may find yourself needing to direct them away from that, while with unstructured you may need to allow it to be followed to see where it takes them and their understandings.

> There can be subjectivities (always a criticism of qualitative methods) and the interviews being subject to bias (something that is a major concern for quantitative researchers but that qualitative researchers acknowledge and then work *with*).

> Analysis is challenging (Coombes et al. 2009) in terms of the amount as well as interpretation and selectivity.

> A great amount of time is committed to an in-depth engagement with respondent; the depth of this will vary according to the amount of 'focus' in the interview as well as the topic.

> The process of transcribing is time consuming.

> Silverman (1998) considers interviews as being problematic as a stand alone method if the intention is to explore what people do or what happened, as what people say they do and what they do does not always match – memory, perspective, partiality and lack of awareness can all affect our ability to recall past events.

> They are retrospective (Silverman 1998), though given that unless we are mapping – as researchers in terms of observations or experiments, action research etc. – the experience or phenomenon as it occurs and in the moment, this is the same with most methods of data collection.

Case study 5.15 Using semi-structured interviews

Context. In 2002, 69 per cent of women diagnosed with HIV in the UK were black Africans. The research available on this particular population and their survival strategies was limited.

Purpose. The purpose of this piece of research was to explore how black African women survived and experienced living with HIV in London.

Approach. They chose focused life history interviews as they acknowledged how past life and experiences and present conditions and life experiences impacted on how people, and on this occasion these women, understood and told their stories. 'Life history researchers recognize the participants as collaborative partners, involved in exploration, discovery, and understanding. The participants actively remember and reconstruct their lives through the telling of their stories. The researcher guides the participant through his or her life history, prompting memories and encouraging the participant's reflections, interpretations, and insights. This approach yields data that help researchers gain insights into how past events and relationships might influence current phenomena and how human beings understand their lives' (Haglund, 2004, p. 1309).

Methods. The researchers used two methods of data collection; the first was a questionnaire that asked for specific information on age, when they were diagnosed with HIV, how long they had been in the country, their children, family, housing, relationships and medical information. Immediately after going through this questionnaire (much of this was done verbally due to potential language difficulties etc.), the researchers did semi-structured, focused life history interviews that utilised some of the data collected in the questionnaire as a way of providing areas that the researchers wanted to explore.

Findings. These were similar to other findings in terms of women negotiating meanings and experiences through socially constructed meanings of gender and biology, but with the added nuance of experiences being shaped by their immigrant status, as well as the countries of origin often being among the poorest and the contrast to being in one of the richest. Spiritual beliefs, who and how they disclosed, and how they managed their health were of concern, as was their location of selves and the possibilities of other relationships. All the women had access to healthcare in the UK, which they probably wouldn't have had back in their countries of origin, and there was a sense of feeling trapped by these services to stay in the country; so their level of choice was impacted upon by this.

Limitations

- The sample was selected from HIV clinics in London: thus the women had already been identified as having HIV and were accessing treatment.
- The research study was introduced by the women's clinician, so how free did the women feel to say no to someone providing care?
- The main research location was in the hospital (not neutral ground), though a choice was given and 20 per cent were interviewed at home.
- One of the researchers worked there in a clinical capacity (though she did not interview anyone in her care, she was nonetheless part of the clinical team).
- The interviewers were white and all the respondents black.
- Westernised ideas were presented, i.e. looking after ourselves, independence and responsibilities, which might differ from other cultural meanings – so introducing a concept that might not be part of their experience.

Source: Doyal, L. and Anderson, J. (2005) '"My Fear Is to Fall in Love Again ..." How HIV-Positive African Women Survive in London', *Social Science and Medicine,* 60, 1729–38.

Case study 5.16 Using unstructured interviews

Context. There has been a lot of research done on early mild dementia in homes, and while others have used interviews, much has been informed by observations and questionnaires. Little has been done on the lived phenomenological experience of people. Research that has been done has revealed that people still have a sense of identity and selfhood (see the dementia case study in Chapter 4 and Kitwood 1997) but this can often be neglected in residential homes.

Purpose. The research in this piece of work is focused on the experiences and meanings of people living with moderate to severe dementia living in residential care.

Approach. Their rationale for using unstructured interviews is very well located within critical discussions of phenomenology in terms of allowing the respondents to fully explore their own meanings and experiences rather than limiting them to particular predetermined or defined concepts and constructs.

Methods. In comparison to Hughes et al. (2008; see also phenomenology, p. 239) there was a far more in-depth engagement with the respondents. Their method involved interviewing 81 people a total of 307 times – ranging from one to eight interviews. This 'matches' far more with phenomenology in terms of the interpreted and ongoing nature of experiences and realities, and how our experiences can be reflected on in a multiple of ways. It also reflects the contexts of communication that take place for people living with dementia. They used unstructured interviews that were, as they say, largely led by the respondents. Moreover, 'alongside the conversation transcripts, field notes made by the researchers and contextual information derived from records kept by the residential homes were also available for consultation. We used these, for example, in those instances in which we needed clarification of events mentioned in the transcripts' (p. 713).

Findings. They used thematic analysis, or as they call it Interpretative Phenomenological Analysis (IPA) (see thematic analysis, p. 326). Their findings were located around four themes, which they represent and discuss in terms of quotes and field notes; they have also endeavoured to represent them in the form of quantitative data in terms of the frequency of being mentioned and by proportion of the respondents – in some ways this is more content analysis, and challenges notions of phenomenology as well as the purpose of unstructured interviews. These four themes – 'Nothing's right now; I'm alright, I'll manage; I still am somebody; It drives me mad' – are used by the researchers to suggest practice improvements to care. The credibility and validity of the method has been strengthened by the use of an outside researcher for analysis and then meeting as a group to discuss and look at emergent themes. They fed the results back, in the form of focus groups, to care workers, family carers and professionals in dementia care; they also held individual discussions with people with early stage dementia – thus addressing some of the criticisms directed at both unstructured interviews and phenomenology.

Source: Clare, L., Rowlands, J., Bruce, E., Surr, C. and Downs, M. (2008) 'The Experience of Living with Dementia in Residential Care: An Interpretative Phenomenological Analysis', *The Gerontologist*, 48(6), 711–20.

Participant and non-participant observation

Observations can be structured, i.e. located within the positivist paradigm, or qualitative or ethnographic in design. There is a wide range of possible ways in which the researcher can use the skills of observation to gather data. What you will find in the literature is that it is likely to be written about in terms of participant and non-participant observation, as well as potentially differentiating between covert and overt observations. Robson (2007) makes a clear distinction between 'structured observation' and 'participant observation', in terms of level of engagement, distance and outcomes. Thus, structured observation is a much more quantitative or 'objective' approach to field or experimental observation (experiences of observing rats, and observing children's play in nursery), where the researcher is separate from the field of research. Participant observation, on the other hand, is more concerned with engaged and open observation, where the observer is part of the field of study.

Observation is used in many different ways within research methods and the form this takes will rely very much on your research paradigm as well as your research aims. Your choices of approach must be, as ever, clearly rationalised and the choices available to you clearly gone through in terms of which will provide you with the most valid and/or credible data.

Bouma and Ling (2004, p. 58) simply describe the method of observation as relying on 'watching' what happens. They go on to emphasise that 'all research observation is guided by a research question. Researchers do not just go and "have a look at their subjects" – they look for something particular that is stated or alluded to in their research hypothesis or objective.' Gray (2004, p. 238) says about observation that it 'is a complex combination of sensation (sight, sound, touch, smell and even taste) and perception; [it] provides an opportunity to get beyond people's opinions and self-interpretations of their attitudes and behaviours towards an evaluation of their actions in practice'.

Being an observer or being a participant observer is one of the key qualitative decisions you need to make when considering your role in the observation. Do you feel that by observing you will obtain the most appropriate data or is it by participating that you will be able to gain insight into the practices, behaviours and relationships that make up what you want to observe?

A participant observer study cannot, by its very intention and design, be structured. The three particular types of observation we explore here are a structured observation, a qualitative observation and finally a participant observation that is covert. In the Ethnography section participant observation has also been considered, but not of a 'covert' nature.

Challenges to observations

> They are time consuming – particularly given how tight time boundaries and expectations in turning round health research are – so this is not a weakness in itself unless you have a tight time frame (Hughes 2007).

> There is sustained contact with participants or the field (this varies depending on type and purpose).
> It is difficult to mediate between being a researcher and a participant – so there is role conflict (relevant for participant observation).
> The ethics of witnessing unethical practice or breaches of codes of practice need to be considered.
> You need to consider your sampling approach in terms of when, where and how often you observe.
> There is a limited scope of observation, i.e. you can't see everything at once.
> The Hawthorne Effect (Mayo 1933; cited in Matthews and Ross 2010) is the effect of the observer on the observed. Mayo's research clearly found that people change their behaviour when being observed. In Mayo's research workers worked harder and in a more productive manner when being observed. The second aspect to this is that this 'changed' behaviour can continue after the research end – one of the theories given for this is that being observed in itself makes us feel validated, or reflect more. Or perhaps if we are observed over a long enough time our behaviour becomes habituated.
> How do you record; where do you record?
> On what are you going to focus?
> A complexity is how to isolate a particular behaviour to denote a particular meaning (see Zwakhalen et al. 2007 and the pain scale).

Structured observation

This is quantitative method, again generally located within positivist frameworks and focusing on measurements, frequency of activity, impact of an intervention and so on (Gray 2009). Bouma and Ling (2004) stipulate that in order to carry out a structured observation you must be, as with all quantitative methods, absolutely clear about what it is you are observing, how you will measure it and the relationship between your hypothesis and the variable to be measured.

Gomm (2009, p. 226) writes that, as with all structured approaches, the researcher needs an instrument, otherwise known as an observation schedule, 'for guiding observation and allowing for its recording'. In effect such instruments ask the researcher questions such as 'What is the time now, and which of the following is true of the subject(s) now?' Bryman (2008, p. 254) too emphasises this characteristic and states that 'Like all structured approaches it requires you to be just that structured' as it is 'a method for systematically observing the behaviour of individuals in terms of a schedule of categories. It is a technique in which the researcher employs explicitly formulated rules for the observation and recording of behaviour.'

Structured observation is non-participant observation: that is, you are observing from a distance and not engaged in or part of the environment you are watching (Gomm 2009). While your physical presence may vary from watching behind one-way glass partitions to sitting with or following the individuals or actions you are observing, the distance and non-involvement remain the same. Although this commitment clearly reflects positivist epistemologies, the challenge here is that the mere presence of someone can impact on what we observe, even if we are doing so covertly (Robson 2007).

A further strength of structured observation is that the observation tool is designed to be replicable, focused, defined, predetermined and reliable. However, Robson (2007) stipulates that very often a predetermined observation schedule will not exactly fit with what you are observing, thus limiting its validity. A further weakness is that it, like other positivist descriptive studies, reduces actions and behaviours to oversimplified concepts, discounting context and complexities of interactions (Matthews and Ross 2010). A final weakness can be how it limits the ability of the researcher to be in the right place at the right time – as it is so planned, controlled and managed that events may well take place outside your arena of observation.

Case study 5.17 Using structured observation

Purpose. Zwakhalen et al.'s (2007) research was designed to measure the efficacy and evaluate the effectiveness of a reduced pain assessment tool used with older people with a limited capacity to speak.

Approach. They chose to specifically measure the efficacy of a Pain Assessment Checklist for Seniors with Limited Ability to Communicate (PACSLAC) tool. Previous research had indicated that the 60-item list within the PACSLAC tool, while valid and reliable, was too cumbersome for clinical practice. Thus, they devised an amended checklist to include fewer items without compromising the psychometric (this refers to a particular branch of psychology that looks at measuring mental traits, abilities and processes) qualities. The PASCLAC is based on four subscales, which include facial expressions, activity and body movement, social and personality mood and physiological aspects.

Method. The research was based on 128 nursing home patients on 12 dementia care wards. The observer did not interact with the patients, nor had they any previous knowledge or relationship with the patients. They observed two different but related interventions and used the PACSLAC and a pain intensity assessment tool, the VAS (Visual Analogue Scale-observer), after each observation. The aim was to collate these observation measurements and to look at the frequency with which each item was used by the observer. The researcher chose two interventions to observe. The first was an influenza jab that was done by the same person, in the same ward, in the same way, within the same time framework. The second incident observed was a particular patient-specific pain moment where again the observer recorded observations after the incident.

Findings. The reduced checklist was effective in measuring pain.

Challenging the research. Once again this is a very small sample on which to make generalised conclusions. They focused on particular occasions of what were identified as 'pain episodes', thereby potentially reducing its applicability to occasions that have not already been so specifically identified or ones that are 'not known' or are part of daily clinical practice. They utilised one researcher and while this will in some ways demonstrate consistency, in other ways it could introduce bias. The PACSLAC tool ❧

5

measures facial expressions, relating particular facial expressions to particular feelings and pain levels. This can be problematised in terms of being able to reduce an array of facial expressions to particular pain levels – cause and effect relationships need to be absolutely clearly indicated in order for meaning to be given to the outcomes. Given that it involved observations with people and their clinicians the Hawthorne Effect must be considered in terms of the intervention itself, and finally validity may be questioned given that the clinicians relied entirely on observations without any 'informant' interviews or checks with either the clinicians or the people living with dementia.

Source: Zwakhalen, S. M. G., Hamers, J. P. H. and Berger, M. P. F. (2007) 'Improving the Clinical Usefulness of a Behavioural Pain Scale for Older People with Dementia', *Journal of Advanced Nursing*, 58(5), 493–502.

Qualitative observations

Given that the main preoccupations and foci of qualitative researchers are often informed by the process, rather than simply outcomes and certainly not measurements, observation is a method that is well tried and popular (Silverman 2001; Gray 2009). Qualitative observation tends to be over a much longer period of time than structured as the practice of becoming engaged within the environment and familiar with the context is an integral aspect of being an observer. Unlike in structured observations, researchers do not always look for specific measurements they intend to 'watch', but instead look at what comes out and happens. The level of open emergent 'watching' can vary depending on the purpose and style of observation, and rather like qualitative interviews they can have more or less of a framework.

The level of immersion within the setting will vary and often relates to whether you are a participant observer or a non-participant observer. It is also worth noting at this point that observation is often used in conjunction with other methods of data collection. You will often find that, within a case study and/or action research design, observations form part of a multiplicity of methods utilised to facilitate as full a picture as possible of the arena and phenomenon.

Robson (1993), Bouma and Ling (2004), Gray (2004) and Bryman (2008) discuss the qualities of both participant and non- participant observations within qualitative and interpretative frameworks. Often observers will 'watch' the whole situation, to get a full flavour of and insight into the setting (Gray 2009). This may mean they would observe a private healthcare setting's work around IVF rather than simply the actual intervention itself as being separate from the context. Observations, due to their contextual nature, will observe all the participants involved whether they have direct interactions or are implicit within the organisation. For instance, within the 'fertility clinic' they may want to observe and/or be part of the work of reception, advertising, care planning, managing treatment and so on.

Qualitative observations acknowledge to a varying degree that what we observe is informed by our perceptions, subjectivities and attitudes (Robson 2007; Matthews and Ross 2010). Thus, being a reflective researcher is vital in this method, as is the ability to read through your field notes and observations and distinguish between your interpretation of events and the event itself.

Key qualities of qualitative observations

> If you are a 'stranger' then observations need to carried out with a sound background knowledge into the setting, phenomenon and environment you are observing. e.g. if you are observing how gay men negotiate safe sex then it is no good being unaware of on-line sites and communities.
> You need to be open to the unexpected and unanticipated.
> They are flexible and responsive to the field; as an participant observer you will become more and more knowledgeable of the setting and the participants within it, often working with what emerges, therefore might need to negotiate access to areas that are connected but that you hadn't planned for and so on.
> They produce rich descriptions and field notes.
> Research observers often rely on and/or need to have access to a gate-keeper, someone who will get them access to the site and environment they want to observe.
> They are long-term and engaged.
> They are often informed by a loose framework of what to observe, as well as having a completely emergent framework.
> They are inductive.
> They are concerned with representing and interpretation.
> They often use informant interviews and other methods to give more insight into what they see.
> They produce a great deal of material to analyse.

Challenges to qualitative observations

> How you record, when and where, which might involve memory bias and false recollection.
> There can be role conflict.
> To get full insight they can take a great deal of time (Taylor 2009).
> The level of involvement will vary depending on whether you are a nonparticipant or participant.
> Relationships can be developed.
> There can be an impact of the observer on what emerges, in terms of being an actor within the setting and a responder.
> What Robson (2007) and Taylor (2009) describe as 'going native', which is relevant particularly for participant observations.
> There are safety issues for both researcher and researched (Robson 2007; Taylor 2009; Matthews and Ross 2010).

> There is an emotional impact and they can be emotionally demanding (Robson 2007).
> There are ethical issues regarding covert observation but also in terms of your relationships, impact and so on (Matthews and Ross 2010).
> There will be partiality as you can't observe and/or be part of everything all the time.
> Sanchez-Jankowski in May (2002) questions the quality of observations in terms of reliability, responsibility and representation: reliability in this context is more concerned with the observer's impact; responsibility is to self, the arena you are researching and the respondents; representation concerns how you represent their realities and activities, i.e. what you include and exclude, what you think is relevant or irrelevant in terms of analysis.

Going undercover

The issue of accessing your field, your participants and so on is, as has already been touched on, an area of research planning that may need considerable thought. This is of particular relevance to observation, where gaining access can be very complicated and long drawn out. Bryman (2008, p. 402) states that 'one way to ease the access problem is to assume a covert role – in other words, not disclose the fact that you are a researcher. This strategy obviates the need to negotiate access to organizations or to explain why you want to introduce into people's lives and make them objects of study'. Fox et al. (2007, p. 103), in their discussion of covert research, locate it within practitioner research and problematise it as transgressing one of the basic duties of care and professionalism, which is gaining 'informed consent'. They go on to say that most organisations and professional bodies would not encourage such an approach due to its deeply problematic compromising of basic ethical principals. However, they also state that 'it is sometimes seen as acceptable if the topic is sufficiently important and there is no other way of collecting the data ... such as health care workers' hygiene practices in the workplace. In this scenario, staff will be likely to change their practice if they know that they are being observed and far more accurate data will be collected by covert research'.

Bouma and Ling (2004, pp. 199–200) echo that most professional bodies will simply not allow covert observation to take place. If they do then the ethical codes of practice and other conditions set out by research divisions require very specific and strict conditions when it is necessary in order to establish scientific validity: 'the researchers are able to accurately define the extent of the covertness; no alternatives exist; participants are not exposed to any increased harm by the covertness of the project; researchers make immediate disclosures to the participants; participants are able to withdraw their data; and the research will not bring notoriety to the research community'. For Gray (2004) it is the validity of the method itself that can be challenged when people know that they are being watched, and therefore adjust their behaviour.

This is when the observer does not become involved in the event, setting or situation they are observing but sits back and observes the whole (Bouma and Ling 2004). As with any observation this requires a great deal of planning, organising and above all negotiation of access. Negotiating access for all methods of data collection is an aspect you will have to factor into your research project and design – the ability to access your intended population and setting is clearly necessary in order for the research to take place.

Non-participant observation can be used for a range of purposes but they all observe people in their natural settings, without any intervention from you. Non-participant observations are often used to gain insight into a particular phenomenon that the researcher cannot be part of (Robson 2007; Matthews and Ross 2010). Whether you want to observe a particular event or a particular setting will inform how you observe. For instance, you may want to observe an A&E department's work with people with dementia and acute health conditions. So you may find yourself moving around, observing different aspects of A&E work, the focus being on people with dementia. Or you may want to want to observe how parents negotiate healthy eating with their obese children; here your observations would be focused on the interactions between parents and children, and this might require you to be with them in their chosen settings.

As previously noted, observation will often involve informant interviews, checking meanings with the participants and following up your observations with interviews (documents) that provide insight into the participants' motivations and understandings of their behaviours. Thus, it is unlikely that non-participant observations will be used as a stand-alone method, though research using this method as its primary source will only use other methods to complement and add depth to the observation itself.

Case study 5.18 Using qualitative non-participant observation

Purpose. This original research was concerned with exploring the social organisation of home care: looking at how care was given; how being cared for was for carried out; experiences and negotiation of space; preferences, routine, privacy etc. The paper itself is more focussed on the process of observing and the issues that emerged and were responded to regarding using this methodology.

Approach. (Non-participant, with flexible responses.) The observers intended to be uninvolved observers in the home setting, but what they often found was that people who were caring, and the 'cared for as well', found it initially challenging to act normally with a silent observer, and what facilitated the normalisation of the observer's presence was being included by being talked to. The observers, while clearly endeavouring not to intervene or engage in the activities of care, found that the process of observation became more interactive and engaged, as they became ⌄

more accepted and trusted within the environment, so their entrance into the environment became richer. The carers in particular saw the observer increasingly as a friend and someone to speak with; the observer was often positioned as a source of support, comfort and a confidant – and interviews with the carers became part of the research process.

(Emergent and responsive) method. Their observations were intended to be over a period of about 12 hours on each site with varying different times of day and lengths of stay. This, however, did not happen for various reasons, not least because either the carer or the 'cared for' communicated in various ways when they wanted the observer to leave. Thus the number of visits required were more than originally planned and the lengths of stay shorter. Interviews were part of the process. Originally they planned to do one in-depth interview with each carer, but due to the interaction in the field and the carers' need to tell their stories they did two interviews. In the first both the carer and the person with dementia could talk about what they wanted in the first instance; in the second interview after the observation clarification could be sought. Another purpose of the intial interview was that it established rapport and facilitated entry into the home.

Challenges and responses. What is interesting about this piece of research is some of the challenges to remaining a non-participant observer and how researchers can and do adjust their research design to accommodate the responses from the field. This latter is a particular strength in qualitative research as its inductive approach allows the researcher to engage with the field in ways that reflect the emerging 'realities' of the setting and respondents within. What is also useful about this piece of research is that carers' need to engage with the researchers fed into the findings in terms of the isolation, loneliness and guilt equated with caring for an individual with dementia.

The researchers note that the ways to address the potential impact and problems associated with non-participant observation are as follows: 'for instance, allowing people to tell their story before the beginning of the observation is helpful, and indeed, encourages cooperation: sustained observation over a period of time does lead people to ignore the researcher after a while; courteous explanation of why we cannot give medical information, for example, is accepted; emotionally drained researchers can be sustained by support from the rest of the research team; final disengagement from the field can be done gradually and time should be allowed for this in research proposals); and researcher values can be recognized and taken into account in analysis' (p. 278).

Source: Briggs et al. (2003) 'Accomplishing Care at Home for People with Dementia: Using Observational Methodology', *Qualitative Health Research*, 13(2), 268–80.

Participant observation

As previously noted participant observation is closely associated with ethnography, and if you go back to the discussion on ethnography (p. 233), you will see that the example of Evans and Lambert (2008) clearly shows that the researchers were deeply embedded and immersed within the setting they were researching. They engaged as part of the setting rather than separate from it and were therefore able to gain insight into the intricacies of the organisation and interlinked context that might have otherwise not been available to them. Gray (2004,

p. 241) considers that the principal intent of participant observation is 'to generate data through observing and listening to people in their natural setting, and to discover their social meanings and interpretations of their own activities. Part of this process is the reporting of the researcher's own experiences, feelings, fears, anxieties and social meanings when engaged with people in the field. With participant observation the researcher becomes a member of the group being researched and so begins to understand their situation by experiencing it.'

Bouma and Ling (2004) also emphasise immersion within the field being researched, becoming part of what is being observed and sharing some of the aspects and experiences of the setting. Bryman (2008) states that participant observation is often used in conjunction with other methods, such as interviews and the use of documents, to gain further insight into the culture of the group or event that is being observed. Evans and Lambert's (2008) use of mixed methods is a good example of this.

The level of involvement within the setting will vary and again will need to be factored in when planning and designing your research. Gray (2004) talks about the challenge of 'insider' and 'outsider' research positions and how to maintain a balance when getting physically and emotionally involved in the setting while at the same time maintaining some sort of professional position and researcher role. The boundaries between these positions can be very difficult to establish and maintain and can be impacted upon by a whole host of variables and conditions.

Other challenges to consider when planning participant observation is the impact you will have within the setting (Bouma and Ling 2004; Bryman 2008). Some individuals may not feel comfortable with you being part of their 'world' and at the same time observing and recording their behaviour; and this can have an effect on how they behave as well as your 'welcome' and access to the environment. Practitioner research, an area that is often concerned with being part of the research setting as a practitioner and a researcher, is a case in point (Gray 2004; Fox et al. 2007; Bryman 2008). While it is a popular way of trying to gain insight into the complex world of healthcare settings, the ethical negotiation for access may have been through a manager rather than all the participants involved. How you negotiate entry to a field can have a great deal of bearing on the quality of the data you gather. Whose choice it is, who knows, how inclusively consensual it is, are all aspects of your ethical framework that will need consideration. The politics of organisations and the motives of your gatekeepers and/or stakeholders must be considered in this issue of access and negotiation.

For instance, you want to observe the culture of care in a dementia care home. In order to gain access the manager (gatekeeper and stakeholder) agrees to you engaging as a healthcare assistant. She does not tell her employees of your role – rationalised on the basis of its impact on care workers' behaviour. Or she does tell the rest of the workers but takes their consent as read; or their consent is not truly consensual due to the assumed interpretations given to not giving consent; she wants it to be semi-covert (i.e. she is in the know but no one else is) because she wants to use your research as a way of assessing quality of care!

5

While it is understood that, given time, many researchers become 'part of the furniture' (Briggs et al. 2003; see Case study 5.18), and indeed this is one of the purposes for prolonged contact within the field, it is also acknowledged that as observers we have an impact on the environment we are watching. While this is a potential problem with observation the impact of the researcher can be greatly reduced by being engaged in the field over a long period of time, developing rapport and trust with the field and participants, being aware of your own role, impact, experience and influence within the field, responding to the field in ways that are sensitive and respectful of the respondents' reality. To simply justify the use of covert observation by saying 'people will change their behaviour' is an insufficient and frankly shoddy and deeply unethical rationale to use – whatever you decide, as in all research, your rationale and justification must be informed by an ethical commitment to your respondents, the data and the field itself.

Case study 5.19 Using covert participant observation

Context. Virtual communities concerned with eating disorders and anorexia have been particular popular since the advent of the world wide web, and hundreds have been formed. The backlash to this from the media, clinicians and families resulted in the closing down of a number of sites that were seen to be 'pro-anorexia', offering advice, suggestions, inspiration and strategies for maintaining anorexic behaviours. As a result these communities are now far more suspicious and defensive and, therefore, hard to enter and research (a key justification for carrying out covert observation).

Purpose. The research intended to look in greater depth at the experiences, behaviours and notions of 'support' provided in what has been dubbed by the media in particular a 'pro-ana website'. The researchers wanted to research, through participation in these communities, notions of support, beliefs and benefits to members of the community.

Method/approach. To be part of what are defined as 'protected synchronous communication environments', where 'live' communication occurs, the researchers needed to enter into the culture of this community. Their justification for covertness was framed in 'hard to enter communities', the hostility and suspicion of these communities to outsiders (including researchers) and 'the charges laid against pro-ana communities (that they are effectively sanctioning self-starvation) and the potential benefit of our findings to the eating disorders clinical field' (p. 96). Their research occurred over two months, based on stages for covert participant observation. The first was to 'create' a plausible anorexic persona, based on a number of sites, descriptors, characteristic membership and identities. The second stage was interaction; the researcher had 38 instant message dialogues, as well as e-mail correspondence, involving an estimate of about 356 individuals. The final stage was withdrawal from the 'ana' communities of which she had become a part. This she accomplished by announcing that her exit was due to her 'entering a recovery programme'.

Challenges to the research. The implication embedded within their research is that they intended to generalise their results to the whole pro-ana community and its pertinence to practice. Given that there were potentially between 200 and 400 sites, and they reduced their sample to 12, this would be very difficult indeed – particularly

5

as the sites themselves varied widely, so representation was difficult to 'prove'. Another challenge to the credibility of this piece of work is the very short period of time given to it; this is particularly problematic given what the researchers already 'know' as being a potentially hostile, suspicious and understandably defensive community. Another drawback to this research in terms of method is around initiating contact in particular ways, thus prompting discussions in particular ways – so how naturally occurring can that be defined as? It seems to be a mix of qualitative and quantitative research and observations that have not been clearly justified or explained.

Further limitations. There are considerable difficulties in terms of validity and reliability with their 'testing' of the consistency of responses and meanings by posting particular statements, e.g. 'I live with ana every day – if she's a disease, disorder, or lifestyle. She is in my life and, for me it is often a love/hate relationship' (p. 99), and then 'seeing' what happened and reducing the responses from this to particular outcomes and meanings: their 'conclusion' is that there is no consistent meaning given to anorexia by the community. They do the same with the exit statement on leaving, testing the response and reducing the data to meaning that people are in the community to support each other once trust has been gained.

They consider their observations a success as the researcher's identity is completely accepted … how can they know that? The reliability of their interpretation is suspect since they cannot clearly ascertain this from the participants themselves. Interestingly, when there is suspicion expressed by community members and doubt about the researcher's authenticity, the researchers problematise this in terms of the respondents being defensive rather than potentially 'seeing through her disguise'. Ethically there are huge problems with this piece of work, and while the researchers acknowledge this they also justify it.

What is intriguing, and somewhat of a concern, is that while the community members' ethical commitment to the researcher is clear in terms of providing on-going support through individuals with whom she can off load and 'come out of the ana community', there is no concern expressed about the participants in terms of how the researcher might have impacted on them. Nor is there any acknowledgement of the development of trust and encouragement of disclosure in others in order to be truly participative and create responses which reflect the archetype anorexic. Finally, and informed by all this, there is concern about exploiting potentially already vulnerable individuals, exploiting their trust, exploiting their need to disclose and belong to a community (which is clearly evidenced in their own findings) by pretending to be a vulnerable, isolated individual themselves.

Throughout, despite this being a 'qualitative' observation, they do not acknowledge their own biases and beliefs. The impact of this is seen in terms of how they dismiss the support and community offered by the 'ana' communities as a 'social mirage' and claim (based on what, we wonder?) that 'they fail to deliver the long-term support that is ultimately required to buffer the physical, psychological, mental, and emotional devastations of anorexia and bulimia. Online cyber-buddies can be dismissed with the click of a mouse; they can never be a substitute for the love and care of friends, partners or family members' (p. 107).

Source: Brotsky, S. R. and Giles, D. (2007) 'Inside the "Pro-ana" Community: A Covert Online Participant Observation', *Eating Disorders*, 15(2), 93–109.

Analysis of your data

As with methods there are a large range of these available to you and the choice of your analytical approach will be guided by your research philosophy, the research question and aims and the methods you chose. They can be roughly divided into qualitative and quantitative methods. As a researcher you have done a piece of research in order to find something out, you have collected or gathered data as a way of getting the information needed in order to 'answer' your question, you now need to do something with that data in order to make sense of it and give it meaning. Once we have analysed the data we can than present and/or discuss our findings.

The research articles that have been discussed throughout this text will have all used various methods to render their data meaningful and relevant. They will tell you what their findings were and what that may mean to practice, or to the population they researched, or their significance in terms of what is already known. This is to a large extent the last stage of your research process and after all the very reason you engaged with the research in the first place – to find something out.

What we present here is only a very brief overview of some of the analytical approaches available to you.

Quantitative analysis

Quantitative analysis is largely concerned (though not exclusively) with managing data in numerical form and explaining the phenomenon under investigation. There are a wide range of computer programs that will do this for you, with varying levels of sophistication. While you can also do this 'manually', the sheer amount of data you may need to manage and the ways in which you want to analyse it may well be best supported through computer programs. Whichever approach you decide upon you will need to consider what it is you want from the data, how you will define the parameters and how you will best establish the validity of your data.

Key qualities of quantitative data analysis

> Systematic.
> Mathematical/statistical.
> Calculated.
> Defines and constructs concepts and theories.
> Reductionist.
> Measured.
> Designed to 'answer' specific questions.
> Tests hypotheses.
> Explains phenomena.
> Makes comparisons.

Descriptive statistics and analysis

These are used with statistical data, which will have been collected from structured methods and recorded measurements and frequencies. Descriptive statistics are used to do just that, describe the basic features of the data in the study. Part of the purpose is to reduce lots of data into simple and more accessible summaries. There are two ways of doing this: one is measures of central tendency and the other is measure of dispersion (Gray 2004; Fox et al. 2007; Bryman 2008). In order to make any significant conclusions from this process you really need to have a very large sample population that is representative of the whole. Briggs et al.'s (2007) research on a pain assessment tool with people with dementia looked at the frequency of the use of items within the tool as indicative of their relevance.

Inferential statistics

This is a more sophisticated way of analysing statistical data as it endeavours to draw conclusions that reach beyond what the data alone actually describe. It makes inferences from the sample data and applies it to what the whole population might be like, i.e. generalisation. Often this is related to an original hypothesis that makes predictions of the relationships between two or more variables. For example, Chambers and Swanson's (2006) research looked at the efficacy of a health assessment tool for measuring risk factors associated with obesity; their preliminary analysis showed a positive relationship between BMI and such factors as attitudes, emotions and perceived difficulties in engaging in physical activities, and they inferred from this that it might explain why exercise and diet programmes that do not take this into account are less successful.

Useful resources

Bowling, A. (2009) 'Preparation of Quantitative Data for Coding and Analysis', in *Research Methods in Health: Investigating Health and Health Services*, 3rd edn. Maidenhead : Open University Press.

Bryman, A. (2008) Chapters 12 to 15, in *Social Research Methods*, 3rd edn. Oxford: Oxford University Press.

Marsh, C. and Elliot, J. (2008) *Exploring Data: An Introduction to Data Analysis for Social Scientists*, 2nd edn. Cambridge: Polity Press.

Qualitative analysis

There are a large number of methods qualitative researchers use to analyse the data they have gathered. Unlike quantitative methods the focus here is on evaluations, interpretations, meanings and insights. Analysis can be in-depth and ongoing and involve an enormous amount of data to work with. Some of the qualities of qualitative data analysis are as follows:

> It involves a large amount of data in the form of recordings, transcripts, field notes, descriptions and visuals.

> The majority of theorists see analysis as 'descriptions of events and of development of concepts, categories' (Sarantakos 1998, p. 314).
> The process is circular and continuous.
> It often involves repetitive reading through of the material, what is known as immersion within the data
> It works with what is emerging as you continue to engage with the data, as well as often being focused on 'a priori' aims.
> It involves being open to what emerges and the subjective nature of analysis.
> It involves making notes and more notes.
> It involves adjusting and readjusting your findings and understandings.

Useful resources

Silverman, D. (2006) *Interpreting Qualitative Data: Methods for Analysing Talk, Text and Interaction*, 3rd edn. London: Sage.

Spencer, L., Ritchie, J. and O'Connor, W. (2003) 'Analysis: Practices, Principles and Processes', in J. Ritchie and J. Lewis (eds), *Qualitative Research Practice: A Guide for Social Science Students and Researchers*. London: Sage, pp. 199–218.

Thematic analysis

This is a very popular approach to take in data analysis, though meanings vary enormously, as do understandings – Bryman (2008, p. 79) acknowledge that the thematic approach 'is a rather diffuse approach with few generally agreed principles for defining core themes in data'. Doyal and Anderson (2005) used thematic analysis in their research, looking at both a priori data and that which emerged in terms of how the women told their stories. They were interested in looking at patterns within the data and interpreting. Aronson (1994, p. 1) says that 'thematic analysis focuses on identifiable themes and patterns of living and/or behaviour'. Braun and Clark (2006, p. 79) describe thematic analysis as 'a method for identifying, analysing and reporting patterns (themes) within data. It minimally organises and describes your data set in (rich) detail. However, while frequency may be significant, it goes further than this, and interprets various aspects of the research topic.' Both Braun and Clark (2006) and Matthews and Ross (2010) provide potential stages and aspects to thematic analysis, which you may find useful to read.

Useful resources

Boeije, H. (2010) *Analysis in Qualitative Research*. London: Sage.

Braun, V. and Clark, V. (2006) 'Using Thematic Analysis in Psychology', *Qualitative Research in Psychology*, 3, 77–101.

Fereday, J. and Muir-Cochrane, E. (2006) 'Demonstrating Rigor Using Thematic Analysis: A Hybrid Approach of Inductive and Deductive Coding and Theme Development', *International Journal of Qualitative Methods*, 5(1), 1–11.

Matthews, B. and Ross, L. (2010) 'Thematic Analysis', in *Research Methods: A Practical Guide for the Social Sciences*. Harlow: Longman.

Case study 5.20 Thematic analysis

This study uses a form of thematic analysis called interpretative phenomenological analysis (IPA), but it bears many of the characteristics of other approaches to thematic analysis. IPA is particularly interested in what they term the internal psychological meanings evident in accounts (p. 713). There can be a challenge to this in terms of phenomenology and their own desire to not impose constructs on the respondents. By using a particular psychological framework they may well have limited alternative interpretations and analyses that could have been more flexible and responsive.

Their approach to analysis was multilayered and included utilising QSR International's NVivo 2.0 software for computer-assisted data analysis (using a computer package to analyse qualitative research is considered contentious by many interpretative researchers). Part of their endeavour is informed by the 'desire' to be as credible as possible, acknowledging the very interpretative nature of thematic analysis. They individually analysed each transcript, coded them, listed key and connecting points, clustered them into groups that reflected emergent themes and then recoded the transcript according to those codes.

Credibility in qualitative research can be a challenge, so the process they went through is clear evidence of the amount of work and rigour required of thematic analysis. They then did a group-level analysis, refined themes and sub-themes in the words of the respondents and cross-referenced with each other, as more than one researcher was doing the analysis. They also brought in an 'independent researcher', i.e. someone who was not involved in the planning and/or doing of the researcher (see the discussion of unstructured interviews, p. 309).

Their analysis resulted in four themes, each with four to six sub-themes. For instance, one theme was 'nothing's right now' and its sub-themes were 'I don't know what's happening; I've lost a lot; It isn't a very happy life; I'm no good now; I'm frightened, please help me' (p. 715). Sub-themes give greater depth and breadth to the main theme, allowing the differing aspects and meanings to emerge and be represented. While they make no claims at all to generalisability, and acknowledge the subjectivity of this thematic analysis, they also see it as a way of potentially informing future practice – largely informed by what Kitwood (1997) would describe as acknowledging the 'person hood of the individual'.

As an interesting final note, they also transfer their research to quantitative data to further demonstrate the rigour and credibility of their data analysis. Essentially what they do is represent the frequency of occurrence of each of the themes and sub-themes and then the mean number of statements made by each individual in relation to the themes. Taking this approach in terms of thematic analysis needs to be robustly defended, as clearly unstructured interviews are not designed (or intended) to quantify participants' responses. As a qualifier for this process, they state that interpretation of the quantitative data needs to be treated with caution – not least because of all the confounding unaccounted for variables.

Source: Clare, L., Rowlands, J., Bruce, E., Surr, C. and Downs, M. (2008) 'The Experience of Living with Dementia in Residential Care: An Interpretative Phenomenological Analysis', *The Gerontologist*, 48(6), 711–20.

5

Narrative analysis is concerned with how people tell stories about their lives and make sense of their experiences. 'Narration or storytelling is one of the fundamental ways that people organise their understanding of the world. In stories they make sense to themselves of their past experience and they share that experience with others. So the careful analysis of topics, content style, context and the telling of narratives will reveal people's understanding of meanings of key events in their lives or their communities and the cultural contexts in which they live' (Gibbs 2007, p. 56). Narrative analysis can emerge both from interview transcripts that did not set out to elicit them and from narrative research itself, the latter being concerned with collecting respondents' stories and narratives (Bryman 2008).

Adamson and Donovan's (2005) research looked at how South Asian and African/African Caribbean women made sense of their caring role with older relatives with dementia. The way in which the researchers analysed the carers drew on the following: 'narratives ... are the stories that relate the unfolding of events, human action, or human suffering from the perspective of the individual's lived experience' (Muller 1999, p. 221). Advocates of this form of analysis claim that 'people perceive their lives in terms of continuity and process and ... attempts to understand social life that are not attuned to this feature neglect the perspective of those being studied' (Bryman 2008, p. 557). So the belief here is that we are telling stories about ourselves and our lives, in terms of life history as well as episodes and particular events in our lives, and then making connections between them in a sense of continuity. Adamson and Donovan's (2005) research therefore elicited material that saw the role of the carer as part of the story; that rather than being an 'extraordinary' event, it was seen and mapped into how the carers understood their lives.

Problems with narrative analysis are the potential to limit people's story telling, whether intentionally or not, to just that – a story – and not pay heed to the social, economic and contextual realities that inform the story (Leonard and Ellen 2008). Robson (2007) challenges this, as for him narrative analysis does locate stories within contexts. Adamson and Donovan's (2005) research also demonstrated this commitment to context. Perhaps the challenge instead is the limited repertoire we might have to tell stories. In other words, if popular representations of 'stories of care' and 'stories of care within marginalised populations' have been already told in various ways, then this can act in some ways as a 'blue print' for how other people may tell their stories. The way we tell stories can also be about how we see ourselves, and how we want to represent ourselves. Leonard and Ellen (2008) discuss the currency in HIV stories to tell a story in a particular way – the 'survivor', the 'victim', the 'learn from my mistakes', the 'playboy' and the 'good boy' story lines.

Narrative analysis uses interviews as its main sources of data, although it can also be used in media research, as well as organisational and case studies. Gray (2009, p. 172) considers that narrative analysis looks at the 'predictive frames that people use to interpret events, and stories that expand on scripts, adding evaluative elements that reveal the narrator's view points'. In this way some of the 'ambiguities', complexities and cultures of organisations etc. can be revealed (Gray 2009). Matthews and Ross (2010, p. 388) look at some of the purposes in telling stories, and the narrative devices that run through people's accounts. These include:

> persuading others;
> justifying past behaviour and decisions;
> rationalising;
> explanations and understanding of events;
> raising pity or concern.

Discourse analysis

This is a mixed and huge field with lots of variations in approaches and, as Matthews and Ross (2010) say, there is no single or simple straightforward definition of discourse analysis. The commonality between the approaches lies in them all being based on 'texts' – what Matthews and Ross (2010) define as being words, either spoken or written, in any medium. One particular approach focuses on the analysis of talk in interaction: that is, what discourses, patterns and forms of talk we draw on and use to accomplish activities in talk. Tonkiss (2004, p. 373) says that 'Discourse analysts are interested in language and texts as sites in which social meanings are formed and reproduced, social identities are shaped, and social facts are secured.'

De Lacey (2002) used discourse analysis to make sense of the data she collected on how women, and a selection of written print material, make sense of IVF 'failure'. She used Foucauldian theory, because she wanted to render visible that which is often familiar and therefore taken for granted in terms of how women are represented in the IVF discourses. She states that discourse analysis 'maps and highlights both the textual dimensions of language that account for the structure of discourses, and the contextual dimensions that account for the social, political or cultural context in which they take place … it … functions to "defamiliarise what is familiar" … and to make explicit the "not-saids".' In this instance the metaphor of lottery emerges as a way to understand the engagement with IVF and the positioning of women who don't become pregnant as losers and those who do become pregnant as winners.

5

Useful resources

DA On-Line is a brand new, international, interactive on-line journal dedicated to the publication of discourse analysis research (http://extra.shu.ac.uk/daol/).

An article on critical discourse analysis (http://www.discourses.org/OldArticles/Critical%20discourse%20analysis.pdf).

Definitions of discourse analysis (http://www.sussex.ac.uk/linguistics/documents/806q1_lecture_01.pdf).

Case study 5.21 Using discourse analysis

The researchers are clearly interested in what they describe as the discourses – i.e. the ways we talk about things and what we draw on to construct our worlds – relationship counsellors draw on when discussing same-sex parenting. Their interest lies in previous research that indicates that how we make sense of same-sex parenting is informed by heterosexual norms and values, both explicitly and implicitly, which can be either affirmative or negative about the issues. They are, in effect, social constructivists – believing that how groups of people makes sense of their world is informed by interaction and sharing and developing meanings (see social constructivism, p. 238). They used three focus groups with 27 counsellors, meeting them twice. They utilised a particular approach to discourse analysis, which asserts that 'we construct our realities . . . through our choice of language and words in our everyday talk, in order to achieve something in our interactions' (p. 3).

Their findings in terms of the main discourses that inform the counsellors are reduced to 'Risking the Kids', an interesting construction that positions any response to same-sex parenting, be it affirmative or negative, in terms of heterosexual parenting as the ideal. Essentialising the roles of 'mother' and 'father' (i.e. female and male role models) is also drawn on and concerns are framed in terms of it being about the children, i.e. peer bullying, lacking role models and/or it not being fair to put children through this (this particularly in reference to same-sex use of IVF). Thus the discourse here positions male and female roles as fairly limited and proscriptive constructions; when same-sex parents somehow 'replicate' or are as 'good as heterosexual parents' they can offer the children double the love. Affirmative discourses also draw on this discourse of 'we are all the same' and that, therefore, makes same-sex parenting and heterosexual parenting equally acceptable – again the implication being here that there is somehow a norm of parenting that we all can access. Difference, and research indicates the diversity of same-sex parenting and relationships, is seen as problematic, i.e. those same-sex couples who are in a committed and stable relationship (which does not necessarily reflect the lives of same-sex relationships) are more acceptable, and therefore more legitimate.

Finally, concern or anxieties about same-sex parenting are often transferred to concern for the children – e.g. 'I am only thinking of the children and what they have to put up with'. Contradictions regarding positing same-sex parenting as potentially 'excellent' yet at the same time exposing the children to risk also ran throughout some of the research.

As a piece of discourse analysis it is fairly clear and gives you examples throughout as to 'how' they analysed the transcripts – this adds to credibility in terms of transparency. However, what is less clear is why only Evans, who also facilitated the groups, did the analysis. While their findings were not unexpected, as their own constructions and understandings were fairly clear in the introduction, what would have been interesting would have been to unpack more of the impact of the facilitator on the discourses and the impact of 'social desirability' on the discussions and outcomes.

Source: Evans, M. and Barker, M. (2006) '"Risking the Kids" versus "Double the Love": Couple-Counsellors in Conversation on LGB Parenting', *Gay and Lesbian Issues and Psychology Review*, 3(1).

Analysing mixed method research

While clearly we have not engaged explicitly with this particular design, the analysis of the results would be just that. It would draw on both quantitative and qualitative methods of data analysis, and then develop the discussion from using both. The purpose of using mixed methods can be for cross-validation and/or increasing credibility, or it can be because different methods are more appropriate for different aspects within your case study. Thus, how you analyse and write up this will again rely on your original intention and design.

Findings, discussion and conclusions

Clearly at this stage of your research journey you are now looking to write up your findings. How you write these up will depend very much on the original purpose of your research. The audience for whom it is intended will also inform how you approach this task. Given this diversity in purpose and audience what we do here is briefly present some of the ways in which you might choose to present your data, findings and discussion. We therefore make references to articles that you will already have accessed throughout this text. What will become apparent is that while style may vary, the content and elements that make up this stage are fairly similar. At the end of this section we suggest some sources that you may find helpful in your writing-up stage.

Presenting and writing up quantitative data

Brook et al. (2010) present their results first in the form of tables, outcomes, measures and data that have been clearly collated and organised into particular categories and variables. They have separated these aspects into 'Data analysis' and then the 'Discussion', where they render meaningful their analysis in particular critical ways. As part of their final discussion they consider the limitations of the research, as well as locating their results within what is already known. Zhakhalen et al. (2007) also analyse their results into tables, indicating particularly the item reduction and factor structure that made up their results and was the main aim of their work. They then discuss these results, relating their findings to significance and the theory that informs the intent. Their limitation section is concerned with acknowledging what has restricted its efficacy, in relation to what they intended it for. In other words their limitation discussion is concerned with issues of validity and reliability, and how these might have impacted on the results as well as how they can address this at a later date. Finally Ledger et al.'s (2006) documentary research, having used a decision tree analytical method, presents their results in the form of two tables. They spend a considerable amount of time discussing the implications, meanings and relevance to what is already 'known' as well as informing the theoretical position they took from the beginning.

The methods that were used to collect this data were structured interviews, structured observations and a quantitative documentary analysis. They also drew on a range of analytical methods and tools, including computer programs designed to analysis statistical data. How you choose to analyse your data and then present your findings needs to be factored into your planning and presentation. You also need to consider issues of validity, reliability and generalisability. So make sure that, if your research was designed to measure the efficacy of a particular intervention using particular scales, how you present your data 'matches' that in the most effective manner possible. This is not just about whether to use tables, graphs, bar charts, pie charts etc., but more about the need to ensure that the data you present accurately represents the data you collected and analysed. Any inferences you make from this need to be clearly demonstrated as well.

Presenting and writing up qualitative data

In contrast qualitative data analysis and the discussion of the findings rests largely on presenting material from the data collected but in the form of words rather than numbers. More often than not findings and discussions are elided (although not always), presenting an ongoing emergent discussion that attempts to render the meaning, interpretations and significance of the data at the same time as presenting the data itself. The purpose of this section is to develop, discuss and represent the realities of the respondents (documents) that have emerged as you, the researcher, have gone along.

Klunklin and Greenwood (2006) utilised interviews as their main method of data collection. Their approach was informed by grounded theory and symbolic interactionism, and the theory that informs symbolic interactionism was clearly used to frame the responses and analysis of the data. They used what they describe as a constant comparative analysis, and individually analysed the transcripts; used a particular Thai Ethnograph software; and carried out group analysis. They present their findings in a number of emergent categories, using direct quotes from the transcripts as well as embedding some literature to further develop the meaning of these categories. They also utilise a discussion section, which brings these categories together in meaningful ways, further supplemented by other literature.

De Lacey (2002) presents her results in two central discourses (she carried out discourse analysis) and interweaves meanings and interpretations with literature to further develop the meanings emerging from her data. As with Klunklin and Greenwood (2006), the writing emphasises the inductive nature of the analysis and the findings, i.e. that it is from the data itself that meanings are highlighted and explored. This clearly contrasts with deductive analysis, which is more concerned with the significance of the results of the predetermined measures in relation to what is already known. De Lacey (2002) also provides a discussion section, which brings together 'the outcomes' of her analysis in ways that are ongoing and certainly exploratory.

Shefer et al. (2002) provide a very in-depth and extensive discussion of their findings, again using sub-headings of the main themes that emerged from the data. Throughout these themes there are direct quotes and within the themes there is evidence of differing elements of each theme; thus they demonstrate how multifaceted meanings are. What Shefer et al. (2002) endeavour to do here is represent, through their analytical discussion, the richness of the data. They have made (as have Klunklin and Greenwood 2006) a great effort to be as 'true' as possible to the stories and wordings of the respondents, clearly allowing the emergent meanings to be inductively told. Their final section is sub-headed 'Conclusion' and this does very much a similar thing to de Lacey's (2002) discussion and elements of Klunklin and Greenwood's (2006) discussion and summary.

General writing up advice

There is no absolute set rule for how we present our findings, our results, our discussion and/or our conclusions. Part of what will inform the style of the articles above will be the requirements of the journal's publisher. Thus, publishers can require particular named elements. Dissertations and published research reports will also usually have a proscribed framework, though interpretation of these elements can vary. However, despite the lack of absolute uniformity of this aspect of the research writing, what are apparent are the elements of rigour, critical analysis and use of the data itself as illustrative of the findings.

All the approaches require you in these sections, in varying degrees, to refer to other sources (i.e. literature) as a way of situating your research. Deductive 'reasoners' *tend* to utilise material as a way of 'reiterating' what was found in the data, i.e. what you set out to measure/ascertain has been tested and found to be 'true' or in need of development, but still within particular parameters of the original theoretical position, unless this has been completely confounded. Inductive researchers *tend* to look to other informing materials to enrich, inform, develop and situate their findings within a bed of ongoing knowledge.

It would be a good idea, as well as looking at research articles, to again look at past dissertations, as well as original research reports, to see how the researchers have written up their findings.

5

Limitations

The limitations of your research need to be considered and, certainly in the writing up stage, you need to demonstrate that you have critically reflected on the quality of your research. Limitations are not just about saying 'I did this wrong' and 'this could have been better'; anything like this needs to be informed by what your intentions were, why these limitations arose, how they have impacted on your results (and indeed your data collection) and in what ways you might address these in future. For instance, if your intention was to provide an in-depth exploration of the experience of professional working women and bulimia, and your sample was eight women, your stated limitation does not have to be the number; having eight as your sample is only a limitation if you were intending to make claims of generalisation or representation. So limitations are related to your research purpose, your paradigm and methods; you may also find yourself questioning the ethics of your research.

The limitation section of your writing may be either clearly sub-headed, as in all three of the quantitative articles mentioned, or embedded in the discussion or conclusion. Very often the concerns of positivistic, interpretative and critical researchers will be different. Thus, researchers coming from a positivistic position will understandably be concerned with validity, replicability, reliability and generalisability. Those with an interpretative background may be more concerned with credibility and their impact on the respondents, how the method might have been too restrictive or even the potential lack of rigour in how they engaged with the population. Feminists will also be concerned with this, as well as the potential for change, empowerment, worries about exploitation and certainly issues of impact and influence.

Meanings for knowledge and/or practice

Finally, and as ever this depends on what your intention was, you may need to write about the implications for practice or knowledge that have arisen from your results. Clearly within EBP this is absolutely essential and you will see in the examples of systematic review that their final recommendations are indeed to do with practice – or more tellingly that nothing is conclusive and more research needs to be done. Zwakhalen et al.'s (2007) results showed that further research was needed to develop a shortened pain scale measure for everyday clinical practice with people living with dementia. For Chambers and Swanson's (2005) research the practice implications are that a straightforward, self-completed assessment tool for risk factors associated with obesity could be useful for health professions. Doyal and Anderson (2005) consider the potential significance of their finding in terms of meanings: that is, African women in the UK receiving a high level of care that was keeping them alive often felt 'trapped' by these services, which were unavailable in their home countries. For Doyal and Anderson (2005) this experience may be rendered even more meaningful, and therefore significant, should female migration to the UK continue, with the added context of inequalities of HIV/AIDS health provision. Jackson et al.'s (2005) research is concerned with highlighting the strategies women adopt as being located within discourses of a family challenge as opposed to individually targeting the obese child. The significance of this is located in the need to do far more research on family life, obese children and mothers' (and fathers') strategies of management within this context.

Thus this section may vary depending on your purpose, paradigm and overall aim for the study. The potential outcomes must only be related to what you have found out. While this may sound very self-evident, the temptation to infer meaning from that which has not been rendered 'visible' through your data collection is mighty. So if you are measuring the efficacy of a 16-week 'health eating programme' and the 'life' of the project is the 16 weeks, then you cannot make any claims to knowing the long-term effects of this programme. As with all stages of your research journey, being a consistent, critical, reflective researcher is an integral aspect of engaging with a rigorous research process.

Useful resources: completing and writing up a research project

Bell, J. (2010) *Doing Your Research Project: A Guide for First-Time Researchers in Education, Health and Social Science*, 5th edn. Maidenhead: McGraw-Hill Open University Press

Matthews, B. and Ross, L. (2010) 'Data Presentation and Reports', in *Research Methods: A Practical Guide for the Social Sciences*. Harlow: Longman

Robson, C. (2007) *How to Do a Research Project: A Guide for Undergraduate Students*. Oxford: Blackwell.

Walliman, N. (2005) *Your Research Project: A Step-by-Step Guide for the First-Time Researcher*, 2nd edn. London: Sage.

Finally

As we said at the beginning of this journey you will often come out with more questions than you went in with. While your study may give insight and enlightenment, or in the case of deductive studies a particular measure or outcome of a 'test', it will also be more than likely to result in a further need to do research. Remember that knowledge is not finite and neither is research. It is a continuous and ongoing journey of exploration and elucidation. It is an exciting world out there, which is constantly changing, and skilled research is always needed to bring 'new' knowledge and insights out into the open.

Good luck and enjoy.

5

6 health and social care careers: from the classroom to the workplace

Tahira Majothi, Careers Consultant, University of Salford, UK

6.1 INTRODUCTION

This chapter explores:

> careers in health and social care;
> working in the third sector;
> skills analysis;
> career planning;
> reflection and continuing professional development (CPD);
> SMART targets;
> interviews;
> employer research and job sources.

In this chapter we take a look at career planning for a successful future within health and social care. This chapter is written in a manner that engages you as an individual, allowing you to reflect on your skills, experiences and practice. In this way we aim to facilitate your career planning on completion of your studies, concluding with the long-term benefits of taking ownership of your professional development, post qualification.

This chapter is in two sections: career planning and career opportunities; and developing your skills: reflective activities. Each section is broken up with a series of questions and reflective activities to prompt personal consideration of the development opportunities open to you.

6.2 CAREER PLANNING AND CAREER OPPORTUNITIES

Overview

Health Studies courses are varied, not only in content, but even in name. They are multidisciplinary and dynamic, covering the following:

> concepts;

> work placements;
> equal opportunity and diversity;
> medical theories, breakthroughs and advances;
> social policy;
> ethical challenges;
> delivery of health and social care initiatives to the individual and community;
> administration and management of projects, services, staff or volunteers;
> analysing and evaluating research;
> commitment to continuous professional development (CPD) during and on completion of your studies.

These courses provide you with a solid grounding in issues pertinent to many careers in health and social care. They can also enable access to a diverse range of further education study, professional development and careers beyond health and social care. Some of these opportunities are spotlighted in this chapter.

Thinking about your career

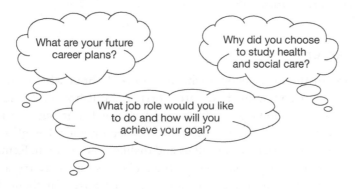

Figure 6.1

Have you asked these questions of yourself before? Can you answer them with confidence? How much have your background, education, work experience and life chances influenced your career choices to date? Have family members, friends, lecturers or careers advisers quizzed you about your career plans?

Do these questions sound all too familiar? If so, it is important to recognise that everyone will have put some thought into their career plans, whether informally, by discussing options with family and friends, or formally, choosing to seek guidance from professionals within the field, careers advisers or lecturers.

On the other hand, you might say 'These are easy questions, I've always

6

known what I would do in the future and how to get there,' in which case you are one of the lucky few people who has it all worked out. Picking the right course at college or university level may have been less stressful for you, but you do still need to consider how you are going to land your dream job and what options are available to you with a health and social care related course. You will also need to consider your continuing professional development (CPD) needs and career opportunities once you are in employment.

Career planning is something that continues, and evolves, throughout your working life. It is important to reflect on your experiences, and connect these experiences to your career ideas. Your dream job may not turn out to be everything you hoped it would be and you may aspire to a new career path or positions of greater responsibility in your current employment. It is therefore useful for you to reflect on your current practice and the opportunities this provides you for the future.

Reflective activity: Post-It exercise

On a Post-It note, in 30 seconds, write down five careers you feel you can progress on to with your qualification.
- How easy did you find this exercise?
- Was it easy to think of five job titles?

Planning your career

If you are one of the many people who is confused about what to do on completion of your course or if you are worried about how and when to start career planning, don't panic. You might not realise it but you have already made some study and career decisions based on your strengths, the opinions of family and friends, your likes and dislikes and so forth. Remember that the majority of people change their choices and may try a few different jobs until they find one that ticks the most boxes for them. This may enrich, not hinder, your life experiences and the subsequent skills you have to offer an employer.

A popular career theory has emerged in recent years, which coined the phrase 'Planned Happenstance' (Mitchell 2003). The planned happenstance approach does not ask you to choose a definitive career and hone in on it. Instead it recognises that many unknowns exist, including things we may have little or no control over (such as government policies, the weather, transport strikes or the economy). Being certain about our career and making fixed choices at an early stage about the rest of our lives may be unrealistic and is likely to be subject to change.

However, planned happenstance is not about taking a back seat in a Zen-like manner and letting careers come to you, but suggests a refocus of our

6

attitude and approaches. It advises you to take the driving seat, taking advantage of *chances* that come your way, however unlikely the source.

Happenstance planning: four key steps

> Think about people or job roles that have intrigued you. Was it the person or the job role that captured your imagination? Follow up on your curiosity, contact the person, call into your careers service and research the idea further.
> How do people (you admire) get to where they want to be? Why shouldn't this be you? What do you need to do? Who is the best person to guide, mentor, advise or help you? Take a different approach: instead of closing off opportunities and putting up barriers or excuses, say yes to new experiences when they come knocking.
> Recognise the opportunities. It may be helping out at work in someone's absence, grabbing the opportunity to work on projects across multidisciplinary teams, writing a paper or a case study, seeing what service is lacking in your community and how to address it, attending conferences. Most importantly, take active steps to meet and speak to new people at conferences or training events, professional social networking groups (as well as family, friends, your manager, human resources department, lecturer, guest speakers etc.) to widen not only your network but also your horizons.
> Once you have generated ideas and made some new contacts, use this information to learn more about yourself, what inspired you, what further skills and ideas need to be developed. Think laterally, as new roles are always emerging, and embrace changes and developments. The more open you are to change, the richer your career trajectory will be and you in turn will inspire future generations.

Personal planning

As a starting point, which of the following statements best describes your career planning to date?

1 I know what I want to do and how I'm going to get there.
2 I have lots of ideas, I need help to decide.
3 I have vague ideas but I'm not sure if it's possible with my qualifications.
4 Clueless. I have no idea, I just picked the subject because I liked it.

SWOT analysis

6

SWOT is an acronym for measuring your *strengths* and *weaknesses*, the *opportunities* open to you (to enable you to succeed) and *threats* to your potential success. Have a look at the example of a SWOT analysis in Table 6.1.

Table 6.1 SWOT analysis

Strengths	Weaknesses
Researching and writing reports Team working Interpersonal skills Commitment Planning and organising Work experience, placements IT Skills Health and social care concepts Empathy Awareness of equal opportunities Being a parent or carer – juggling commitments Budgets Time management Ability to motivate	Problem-solving Public speaking Presentations Lack of work experience within health and social care Psychometric tests and assessment centres
Opportunities	**Threats**
Learner development support Placements/work experience Charity/voluntary work Part-time or supply work Careers service Network contacts Websites/newspapers Careers fairs Employer presentations NHS Private sector Armed forces Educational establishments Work abroad Flexible working: hours and location	Lack of qualifications Shortage of relevant work experience Financial constraints Family commitments Minimal IT skills Seeking opportunities solely in the local area

Reflective activity

The key to effectively marketing your skills to an employer is knowing what you have to offer, and matching your skill set to their requirements.
Use the following SWOT diagram to make a list to suit your present situation.

Strengths	Weaknesses
Opportunities	**Threats**

Other activities to help with your career planning are included later in this chapter.

Now you have identified your strengths and weaknesses, and potential threats, it is important to investigate what opportunities might be available to you in the health and social care sector.

There are three main industries you can progress into:

> the health sector;
> social care;
> the third sector – charities and voluntary work.

The health sector

When you think of jobs within the health and social care industry, it is highly likely that you may have imagined that the majority of opportunities open to you exist solely within the National Health Service (NHS). This is not necessarily the case, but it is useful to look at the emergence of the NHS and how medical advances have developed, as this will help you to research new job opportunities available to you. The health and social care industry is in a constant state of flux, beholden to investment, government initiatives, the diagnosis of new illnesses and diseases and breakthroughs in treatments (DoH 2008a).

The NHS

The NHS is the largest employer in Europe. There are over 300 careers available, and 1.3 million staff work in over 500 different organisations within England alone (NHS Careers 2010a).

The NHS was established in 1948 by the then Health Secretary, Aneurin Bevan, who stated that: 'The collective principle asserts that … no society can legitimately call itself civilized if a sick person is denied medical aid because of lack of means' (Lancet Oncology 2008, p. 809). The Health Secretary opened the first NHS Hospital, Park Hospital in Manchester (now Trafford General Hospital) in July 1948, bringing together key healthcare providers such as doctors, nurses, pharmacists, opticians and dentists under one roof to provide healthcare, funded by the taxpayer, but free of charge at the point of need.

Box 6.1 Key Dates of Medical Breakthroughs and Policy Changes within the NHS

1953   DNA structure discovered
1954   Causal link established between smoking and cancer
1958   Mass vaccinations to tackle polio and diphtheria
1960   First Kidney transplant
1961   Pill made widely available
1967   Abortion Act
1968   First NHS heart transplant

6

1972   CT scans introduced
1978   First test tube baby
1980   Keyhole surgery performed for the first time
1986   AIDS campaign launched
1988   Breast screening introduced
1991   Community health services established
1994   Organ donor registration
1998   NHS Direct launched
2002   Primary care trusts launched
2007   Robotics use to treat patients with irregular heartbeats in a move towards minimally invasive surgery. (NHS Choices 2008)

Today the sector has expanded to incorporate hospitals, surgeries, outreach work, nursing homes, medical and dental work, complementary medicine and government-led initiatives working to tackle issues affecting the community. Services are delivered by organisations working across the public, independent and voluntary sectors (Prospects 2010a).

Future demands on the health service

There is likely to be an increasing focus on joined up working across health and social care careers to offer more comprehensive support to the population, along with an increasing emphasis on prevention (DoH 2008a). Roles may vary but primarily they will be established to educate people on the issues of the day, such as obesity, alcohol abuse, treatable cancers and the effects of smoking.

In addition the number of elderly people is increasing:

Over the last 25 years the percentage of the population aged 65 and over increased from 15 per cent in 1983 to 16 per cent in 2008, an increase of 1.5 million people in this age group. By 2033, 23 per cent of the population will be aged 65 and over compared to 18 per cent aged 16 or younger.

The fastest population increase has been in the number of those aged 85 and over, By 2033 the number of people aged 85 and over is projected to more than double again to reach 3.2 million, and to account for 5 per cent of the total population. (Office for National Statistics 2010)

This raises questions about adequate long-term provision to support the elderly.

6

Reflective activity

Consider the impact of these changing demands on the types of careers and jobs available in the future.

The future workforce entering into the health sector need to offer the following:

A patient-centred approach … reflects changes in approaches to supporting people with chronic illness and major improvements in the quality, cost and accessibility of healthcare.

Improved public health … emphasis in preventing ill health and supporting healthier lifestyles.

Team based approaches to healthcare delivery – through multi-professional and multi-disciplinary working across the sector. (Dresser et al. 2008, p. 4)

All these changes open up opportunities for the future.
The overall job types currently within the NHS fit into three categories:

> Working as part of a team to provide care and treatment in a medical setting.
> Working in the community, either one-to-one or in group sessions.
> Support and infrastructure, e.g. human resources, finance, administration (NHS Careers 2010b).

Advances in technology and medical breakthroughs have helped to modernise the industry and empower patients to make informed decisions on treatments and aftercare. These developments include:

> technological breakthroughs in medicine;
> the Human Genome Project;
> the development of artificial body parts and organs;
> developments in minimally invasive surgery;
> the use of robotics to ensure accuracy and consistency (Healthcare for London n.d.).

As a health studies student, you will have theoretical knowledge or subject-specific information. Experience of work placements may also enable you to apply your knowledge and learn about the different strands of healthcare, such as mental health, paediatrics, midwifery, learning difficulties and adult care. Work experience can provide you with the opportunity of working across multidisciplinary teams, promoting healthcare and offering services to the community.

Health and social care jobs are not only to be found in the NHS, but also with local authorities, social services, educational establishments, charities and voluntary organisations and private healthcare providers. There are more unusual opportunities in areas such as art, play or music therapy, health promotion initiatives within the community and working in sales or in supermarkets and shopping centres offering outreach medical tests to customers.

6

Job roles

Box 6.2 lists some of the job titles that are closely related to your course or degree. This is not an exhaustive list and you must bear in mind that the majority of these roles will require some previous work experience from your studies, paid and unpaid work, voluntary activities and/or further qualifications. In addition, some job roles may require a postgraduate qualification to aid your progression, especially if you are keen to work as an administrator or manager in charge of budgets, projects and staff or volunteers (Prospects 2010b).

Box 6.2 Job Titles

> Nurse: adult, children's or paediatric, mental health, midwifery
> Health promotor
> Health service administrator/manager
> Physiotherapist
> Therapist: art, play, sports
> Further education lecturer
> Dietician or nutritionist
> Personal trainer
> Social worker
> Charity and development worker
> Speech and language therapist
> Biomedical scientist
> Environment health officer
> Working for international aid or non-governmental organisations such as the Red Cross, Médecins sans Frontières

---

Be aware that job titles are likely to change and new ones likely to emerge over time. Always check with your careers service, professional body or occupational job databases for the most recent roles.

In terms of destinations upon graduation, in 2008, 60 per cent of healthcare graduates entered full-time employment six months after graduation, 10 per cent worked part-time, 10 per cent of graduates on a medically related course chose full-time study and 8 per cent of respondents chose a combination of work and further study (Prospects 2010c).

Useful resources

For further information about graduate destinations look on:

http://prospects.ac.uk/links/occupations

http://www.connexions-direct.com/jobs4u/

http://careersadvice.direct.gov.uk/helpwithyourcareer/jobprofiles

Social care and social work

The two key roles within these areas are social workers and care assistants, with different types of work responsibility and requiring different educational and professional qualifications. To become a social worker you will be required to study to degree level as a minimum, with a postgraduate qualification an option if you have a degree in a different discipline.

As a social worker you will need to be familiar with laws and legislation pertaining to protecting the rights of children and vulnerable adults. You are likely to work in multidisciplinary teams made up of colleagues from the local authority, NHS staff, police, courts and probationary services, as well as organisations such as Barnado's or Connexions.

In contrast, a social care (care assistant) role is to provide people with practical support, in their own home, in residential care homes or even in educational establishments. Traditionally, these roles do not require formal qualifications such as a degree but you need to undergo a Criminal Record Bureau (CRB) check and have relevant care work experience, gained through temporary or agency work, and strong interpersonal skills such as empathy, emotional resilience and the ability to motivate are highly valued. In 2010 the Department of Health announced plans to encourage more graduates into social care, particularly graduates who are looking for a rewarding career that will help them progress into management. The National Skills Academy for Social Care (NSA) initiated a management trainee scheme in 2009, developing leadership skills for graduates. The scheme is highly competitive and offers a bursary as part of the 12-month programme, which will see the graduate placed with a local authority, private or independent care service or within the voluntary sector (Qureshi 2010). Job opportunities in both social work and social care are most likely to exist within the statutory, independent or third and voluntary sectors such as local authorities, health centres, education establishments, children's services and residential care, charities such as Barnado's or Age UK and jobs within the Children and Family Court Advisory and Support Service (CAFCASS).

Job roles in social care

There are just under one million people in paid employment in the social care sector. Two-thirds work in services providing support for older people, 19 per cent work with adults with disabilities, 13 per cent are in children's services and the remaining 7 per cent are in mental health (Prospects 2010d). The roles are varied (see Box 6.3) and, again, are likely to require some work experience and/ or further qualifications. Your careers service will be able to advise about this.

6

Box 6.3 Job Roles in Social Care

> Advice worker
> Charity advocate, fundraiser, officer
> Community development worker
> Counsellor
> Homelessness or housing officer
> Mental health nurse
> Occupational therapist
> Probation officer
> Police officer
> Prison officer
> Social worker, social care worker, support worker
> Forensic psychologist
> Health and safety officer
> Youth worker
> Adult guidance adviser, careers personal adviser
> Art therapist
> Administrator

New and emerging careers within health and social change

As mentioned earlier, recent health policy objectives (DoH 2008a) have increasingly emphasised the need to focus on prevention initiatives and this has opened up an extended range of health-related professional roles.

The new roles include:

> health trainer;
> health promotion specialist;
> complementary and alternative medicine (CAM);
> assistant practitioner;
> counselling psychologist;
> primary care graduate mental health worker;
> black and minority ethnic (BME) community development worker;
> psychology associate;
> counsellor in oncology, primary care, genetics;
> emergency care practitioner.

This is by no means an exhaustive list and these job titles are likely to evolve, or even become obsolete and be replaced by new titles and responsibilities as new careers emerge or job roles become amalgamated. Please contact your careers service for help on researching the latest occupations within health and social care.

Third sector: voluntary organisations or charities (social change)

The third sector includes organisations that have emerged to meet the needs of, often, vulnerable individuals and groups and are usually non-profit making organisations. They can range from social enterprises, charities and voluntary organisations to community groups, and offer services to complement both public and private sector organisations.

The Department of Health describes the third sector as sharing 'common characteristics in the social, environmental or cultural objectives they pursue, their independence from government, and the reinvestment of surpluses for those objectives'.

They have a strong track-record of designing services based on insight into a clients' needs, and are often well placed to respond flexibly to those needs. In 2007, it was estimated that around 35 thousand third sector organizations were providing health and/or social care throughout England. (DoH 2010)

There are over 600,000 registered charities in the UK and just under half a million full-time paid staff, which accounts for 2 per cent of the UK's workforce. Jobs are typically not highly paid, but as a number of organisations are likely to be small to medium sized enterprises, there is a real possibility that roles will double up. This way you will be able to gain a multitude of skills because of the different responsibilities you will undertake. In addition, you will find that many organisations will have a comprehensive training programme, a good work–life balance, flexible working hours and the chance to make a difference to people's lives. Job satisfaction in such organisations can be very high.

Often the best way to enter these professions is through voluntary work experience aligned to an issue of importance to you. It may be that you would like to work for an ethical employer who is socially and environmentally friendly, who champions fair trade and the rights of workers and people overseas. If this is the case, you could consider working for a non-governmental organisation (NGO). Working with NGOs provides the opportunity to explore ethical issues first hand, gain a deeper understanding of international issues, such as life expectancy, diseases, promoting safe sex and health clinics, and help to set up infrastructures with other aid agencies and partners overseas.

6

Job roles may include service provision, administrative duties, marketing, fund-raising, managing volunteers, policy and research. They can include working for organisations supporting the third sector such as voluntary placement advisers based in your college or university, government departments, the National Council for Voluntary Organisations and the National Council for Work Experience (Prospects 2010e).

If some of these job roles and opportunities appeal to you, you can research this industry further by visiting your careers service, the not for profit and public sector careers fairs or summer camp organisations who visit your school or university.

Useful resources

For more information, visit http://www.socialchange.org.uk or http://www.ethicalcareers.org or Oxfam, through their website http://www.oxfam.org.uk

Summary

As you can see, there are a huge variety of jobs within the health and social care field. The main challenge for you as an individual is to reflect carefully on your own strengths and weaknesses, and your personal motivations and aspirations. Below, we introduce you to some case studies of people who, like you, chose to study in health and social care. Their stories may provide added inspiration to your career choices.

Case study: Real-life opportunities

Name: Laura
Qualifications: BSc Psychology 2:1
Job title: Trainee Personal Adviser
Location: Manchester

Laura started her education many years ago (with a diploma in social work) but had to leave due to personal circumstances, eventually coming back to university to study psychology. Prior to completing her psychology degree, Laura had worked in adult social care with people with learning difficulties, having started 21 years earlier as a cook/supervisor in a homeless men's project. Laura also worked as a union learning representative.

Laura now works as trainee personal adviser working for Connexions (a non-profit making careers service for young people aged 13–19, up to age 25 for young people with learning difficulties and disabilities). The main focus of her work is to help young people overcome barriers to education and employment, such as drug misuse, mental health problems and low self-esteem. She works with projects for young people who are not in employment, offering them careers appointments in projects such as the Roundhouse and Music Stuff, and circulating relevant information about projects and courses to enable her colleagues to refer other young people too. Previously she worked as an employment support worker with the same organisation, meeting employers, training providers and young people to help the latter to gain qualifications and employment.

To take the job with Connexions, Laura left her permanent employment with the local authority, but feels that the training opportunities offered at Connexions more than make up for the lack of security. For example, she is training for her NVQ level 4 in advice and guidance. Laura also works as a volunteer mediator, a role she started in January 2009. The role at Connexions provides variety, as it is not office based all the time, and she enjoys the challenge of making a positive difference.

She would advise other students to 'get as much experience as possible in a variety of roles – as many paths can lead to the same place. Volunteering shows that you are willing to go the extra mile to meet your goals/aspirations.' In addition her mediation work has provided additional kudos to her skills set as 'mediation gives you skills of impartiality, which are asked for in a variety of roles'.

Her university study provided her with academic and IT skills and a 'high level of interpersonal skills as I need to be sensitive to the needs of others and be aware of issues that may affect individuals'. Laura has not discounted studying further, and has considered cognitive behaviour therapy (CBT) as an option as this will allow her to be a self-employed practitioner.

Names and specific details have been modified to protect identities, although the themes the cases illustrate represent real-life events.

Case study

Name: Julia
Qualifications: Master in Public Health (Ongoing), Master in Public Health Nutrition (PHN)
Job title: Public Health Trainee
Location: Cheshire

Julia initially wanted to become a vet, but later picked a psychology degree and public health master so she could work abroad with NGOs. She has extensive experience working in summer camps in the USA (with people with physical and mental disabilities), as a volunteer at a Romanian orphanage and undertaking voluntary research for Save the Children in Zimbabwe. She also worked at a vet's practice and educational farm.

When she first graduated she worked in a mental health role for a housing association, followed by work in a mental health training and rehabilitation centre. Later she

6

worked as a public health business manager for a regional office in London and as a community nutrition and dietetics manager.

This diversity of experience led to her current role on a five-year training scheme as a public health trainee. For this scheme, she works on placements within the health economy, e.g. the local primary care trusts, acute trusts, local authority schools, community organisations, prisons and the Health Protection Agency. Julia's key responsibilities are researching and auditing health needs assessments and health protection work (e.g. public health responses to disease notifications health promotions). Julia set up a bowel screening programme in her local area, and wrote the emergency plan for a primary care trust, as well as being involved in community health promotion work and conducting a survey of the skills within the sexual health workforce. Julia is currently conducting a survey of immunisation, and writing a review on how effective hand washing is at preventing community outbreaks of disease, among other varied activities.

The least enjoyable part of her job is the revising and report writing, and being office based. Although you are paid, the lengthy training programme requires commitment, and it does involve taking work home. Julia's advice to people interested in public health is that 'You have to be comfortable working outside of your "comfort zone" as the point of the training is to develop skills in areas you are not good at.' Eventually she would like to develop her reputation and career in public health.

In conclusion, Julia's advice to other students and graduates is that public health is 'the type of career that you seem to fall into along the way rather than setting out to be'. If it interests you, 'perhaps start working within the local health community, or with community organisations, and see where it takes you'. It is 'very competitive, if you are not a medic you need at least three years experience of working within public health setting and you may need to repeatedly apply ... try and make opportunities for yourself to get relevant experience, and keep trying, you get there in the end!'

Qualifications for working in healthcare

Skills for Health has produced a breakdown of statistics of the level of educational attainment of the people working within healthcare in England, Northern Ireland, Scotland and Wales. Nearly 70 per cent of staff across all regions had a level 3 (A level equivalent) or higher qualification. The largest proportion of the workforce was described as students in training. The majority of these were classed as being in further education (FE). The courses centred on health, social care and public services. The reminder of the workforce was described as students in higher education (HE) enrolled on courses allied to medicine, biological sciences and medicine and dentistry (Skills for Health 2008).

Entry routes

Job roles are available for direct entry into the NHS or health and social care services. These roles may be entry level routes including cleaners, porters, data entry or administration, care assistants, support workers and so on. These opportunities are likely to be open to people aged 18+ and may require minimal academic qualifications and/or some prior work experience. Check out opportunities in the local and national press or http://www.nhscareers.nhs.uk, http://www.socialworkcareers.co.uk, http://www.socialcarecareers.co.uk.

Access courses

Access courses are usually available to adults aged 19 and over who may have no previous academic qualifications and would like to gain some qualifications and work experience. Courses are available through local colleges and are offered in subjects such as an Introduction to Health and Social Care or Health and Social Care Levels 2 and 3. Alongside the main subject, some providers may also offer the opportunity for you to gain some qualifications in your literacy, numeracy and ICT skills.

The courses can be studied part-time or full-time to cater for those who may have childcare or caring responsibilities as well as those who may be working. You may also be entitled to some help with funding through the Adult Learning Grant or Learner Support funds. For more information contact your local college or access http://www.ucas.ac.uk, http://www.nextstep.direct.org.uk or http://www.direct.gov.uk.

Further study

Some job roles within health and social work in particular will require you to have a degree. It might be worth considering postgraduate study to aid your career progression and enhance your technical skills and specialist knowledge. This may help you to gain the theoretical and practical skills needed for a successful transition to management track careers.

If you are interested in studying a subject closely linked to medicine, such as optometry, physiotherapy, dentistry or prosthetics, then you will need to have a second undergraduate degree if your first degree was not science based. There are accelerated courses for graduates of science-based subjects. Speak with a careers adviser for more information.

If the thought of being an art, drama, music or sports therapist interests you, then it is useful to consider relevant work experience or voluntary work, and then you may need to commit to further specialised postgraduate study.

It might also be possible to convert your degree to subjects such as law or psychology; you will need to check with the university you wish to study at for entry requirements.

For full details of postgraduate courses, how to apply and financial assistance, speak to your careers service or visit http://www.prospects.ac.uk/links/pgstudy.

6

You will be able to research destinations of learners from higher education institutions by accessing the Prospects website (http://www.prospects.ac.uk/links/wdgd, or access http://www.unistats.com and search for destinations by name of subject and college or university).

Destination details are also available from related courses such as social care, social work, psychology, social studies and sociology, social policy and anthropology.

Apprenticeships

Apprenticeships are a combination of work and study. They have been traditionally available to young people aged 16–25. The government, however, is looking to increase the take-up of apprenticeships among young people and adults. Learners are usually required to be working at level 2 which is equivalent to five good GCSEs at grade C or above, including English and maths (or equivalent, e.g. key skills in the application of numbers and communication). It is taught in three parts, the NVQ, a Technical certificate and Key Skills. The training and assessment is led by a training provider working in collaboration with an employer if it is a paid apprenticeship.

Volunteering

There may be opportunities available to help you gain an insight into the healthcare sector and provide you with experience to enhance your studies or help you gain some relevant experience if you have minimal academic qualifications. Access volunteering sites such as http://www.direct.gov.uk, http://www.timebank.org.uk, http://www.do-it.org.uk, http://www.volunteering.org.uk, Volunteer Development Scotland (http://www.vds.org.uk), Wales Council for Voluntary Action (http://www.wcva.org.uk) or the Volunteer Development Agency in Northern Ireland (http://www.northern-ni.org).

Useful resources

For details of opportunities available to you, contact the following:

- In England, the Health Learning and Skills Advice Line (http://www.hlas.careers-advice.org) or (http://www.nhscareers.nhs.uk).
- In Scotland, NHS Scotland Careers and Opportunities (http://www.infoscotland.com/nhs) and NHS Education for Scotland (http://www.nes.scot.nhs.uk/).
- In Wales, the National Leadership and Innovation Agency for Health (NLIAH) (http://www.nliah.wales.nhs.uk) and the NHS Wales Careers Information Service (http://www.wales.nhs.uk).
- In Northern Ireland, the Department of Health, Social Services and Public Safety (DHSSPS) (http://www.dhsspsni.gov.uk), the Careers Service NI (http://www.careersserviceni.com). The Educational Guidance Service for Adults (EGSA) (http://www.egsa.org.uk) provides career pathway information, advice and guidance. Alternatively the Health and Care NI has links to the main education and training organisations in NI which provide health and social care courses.

6.3 DEVELOPING YOUR SKILLS THROUGH REFLECTIVE ACTIVITIES

Skills and competencies: how your course has made you employable

Throughout your studies educational establishments will have worked to encourage you to be a creative and independent thinker, who can self-manage their work and be a reflective learner. In other words, someone who is able to learn from experiences to recall their strengths and identify areas they need to develop.

The skills listed in Box 6.4 are likely to be required by employers regardless of the type of career you choose to enter into. These are called *transferable skills* as they are likely to translate into the main duties of any job role.

Box 6.4 Key Transferable Skills

These include the ability to:

> Work independently and be self-reliant.
> Prioritise and organise.
> Manage your time effectively.
> Be self-motivated, committed and confident.
> Know how to find and use paper and web based resources effectively.
> Reflect on your personal learning and development.
> Understand that you will need to continue to develop your skills beyond university and throughout life.
> Work as part of a team.
> Highlight examples of leadership via group work or projects.
> Understand the demands of the industry you plan to work in.
> Be up to date with new polices, initiatives and medical advances.
> Use strong communication skills.
> Research, analyse and feedback to peers, tutors or professionals.
> Have a good understanding of basic maths, English and ICT skills.
> Be calm, patient, empathetic and have stamina and resilience.
> Work towards a flexible working pattern or adapt to new environments.

The Association of Graduate Recruiters in a survey of employers found that the most important qualities for an employer were for a candidate to show 'commitment, drive, motivation and enthusiasm'. The most sought after skills include 'problem solving, teamwork and oral communication'. Crucially employers felt that the most difficult skills a candidate could demonstrate as attaining included 'commercial awareness, enterprise and leadership' (AGR 2010). The variety of volunteering experiences and so forth, already mentioned, may help you gain experience in these matters.

6

Reflection: a step-by-step approach using the DOTS Model

This section takes you through the use of a reflective tool, a valuable process to help you identify your strengths and weaknesses and guide you towards appropriate career choices.

> ## Reflective activity
>
> - Think about careers that appeal and skills that would complement these careers.
> - Think about how you have developed relevant skills via your studies, placements and work experience.
> - Work on producing examples – you may find the SODT Model and other examples below helpful.

The DOTS Model was originally developed to help effective career planning. The four elements of the DOTS Model represented (Law and Watts 1977):

> D – decision learning;
> O – opportunity awareness;
> T – transition learning;
> S – self-awareness.

However, most people now accept that the four processes do not necessarily flow in this way, and it is now widely referred to as the SODT Model, rearranged in the following order:

> S – self-awareness;
> O – opportunity awareness;
> D – decision learning;
> T – transition learning.

Self-awareness

You will need to reflect on whether your personality and aspirations meet the differing demands that are likely to be placed upon you in your future job role (see Table 6.2). You can also try online careers exercises to filter out unappealing careers, while simultaneously helping you to clarify your ideas. You might try Belbin's team role assessments, using your self-perception to see how you feel you fit in a team with other people (http://www.belbin.com – please note: a charge may be levied in order to receive feedback) or access the buzz online confidence builder for teenagers (http://www.thebuzzbook.co.uk).

Confidence in your skills and abilities is an important part of presenting a positive image. If you value your skills, then employers will too. Knowing your skills and weaknesses is also important. Try the following exercise (McMenamin 2009).

Table 6.2 Skills rating exercise
Read the following statements and rate yourself

	Please circle
1. Working effectively with others Being able to cooperate with others on a shared task, being adaptable to other people's working styles, teamwork.	1 2 3 4
2. Communication Expressing your ideas, explaining something complicated.	1 2 3 4
3. Judgement and decision-making Assessing a problem or situation using appropriate criteria and making a decision.	1 2 3 4
4. Persuading and influencing Using effective communication to convince other people of the value of a particular course of action.	1 2 3 4
5. Ability to solve problems Use of creative or lateral thinking to develop new and different ways of solving a particular problem.	1 2 3 4
6. Time management Use of priority setting skills to manage your time effectively to ensure your most important tasks are completed on time.	1 2 3 4
7. Achieving your goals Setting and achieving your personal goals (SMART).	1 2 3 4
8. Relevant use of IT	1 2 3 4
9. Relevant specialist subject (health and social care) knowledge	1 2 3 4

Note: 1 = *never* good at it; 2 = *sometimes* good at it; 3 = *often* good at it; 4 = *always* good at it.
Amended with kind permission of the University of Westminster Career Development Centre.
J. McMenamin (2009) Job Seeking Strategies for Graduates, Skills Rating Exercise, University of Westminster Career Development Centre. http://www.westminster.ac.uk/business/carer-development-centre.

Online skills questionnaires

It might be worthwhile practising with online questionnaires to help you to identify your strengths, as well as to prepare for assessments by revisiting your maths and English skills as well as logic and aptitude tests. Questionnaires are available on http://www.prospects.ac.uk/links/pplanner, http://www.windmillsonline.co.uk or http://www.connexions-direct.com (careers service website for young people). There is also a national careers advice website for adults: https://nextstep.direct.gov.uk/planningyourcareer/skillshealthcheck/pages/default.aspx.

6

Reflective activity

- What are your strengths – skills that you have rated often or always good at?
- What are your weaknesses – skills you have rated never or sometimes good at?
- These are skills you may need to acquire or develop. Make a note about how will you go about doing this.

Opportunity awareness

Now you have identified your strengths and generated career ideas, consider the following:

> What is out there – what employment opportunities are available?
> Interests – what would you like to be doing in the short term (next 3–6 months)?
> Where you do see yourself in 2–3 years' time?
> How will you go about achieving your short- and long-term objectives?
> Are you able to provide tangible examples of skills and abilities to employers?
> What type of employer and work environment are you looking for?
> What motivates you – work, professional development, financial incentives, geographical location, flexible working, work–life balance?
> What are your current commitments – financial, family, care responsibilities?
> Is further work experience needed to get into your chosen career?
> Is further study necessary too?

If you think it would be helpful, access your college or university careers service. Some university careers services will work with graduates up to 3 years after graduation. Seeing a careers and employability adviser will help you to identify your strengths, clarify your career ideas and better prepare by researching work and study options. Once you are able to establish your career ideas, skills and motivations, you can move on to the following job seeking strategies.

Decision learning

Before you can start working on application forms or CVs (for independent organisations or recruitment agencies) it is worthwhile thinking about the type of employer you would like to work for. Sending out lots of speculative applications may generate some responses, but often employers and human resource officers, in particular, are able to spot a generic CV or application. To make your application form stand out, you will need to research the employer (using the Internet, trade or industry journals or newspapers, and check with your careers service) so that you highlight your skills that are pertinent to the job in question.

Reflective activity

When you do research on a prospective employer look at the following:

- How long have they been established?
- What are their values or strategic objectives for the coming year?
- Who are their main service users or what area do they specialise in?
- Location – are they regional, local, national or international?
- Are they likely to be affected by any social trends, government initiatives or medical breakthroughs?

- Job opportunities – what type of vacancies or voluntary placements do they offer?
- What do they expect from their employees?
- What do they offer their employees in terms of work–life balance, promotions, continued professional development?

Reflect on what this information means to you.

This can help you make an informed decision on the type of work and employer best suited to meet your short-term and longer-term career objectives.

Transition learning

Now you are ready to make your decision, be it work, study or voluntary experience. To help find the appropriate job or career for you the following sources will be of use.

Careers service

Check in with your advisers and/or careers service and sign up for bulletins. You will be able to receive sound advice in relation to your application and it is essential to prepare for potential interviews.

Box 6.5 Your Careers Service

Your careers service may be able to offer some of the following:

> Guidance appointments.
> Targeted support for students with disabilities and additional support needs.
> Telephone or e-mail guidance services.
> Careers-related workshops.
> Details of local and national opportunities.
> Details of recruitment fairs, e.g. COMPASS (http://www.compassjobs-fair.com).
> Help with CVs, application forms, assessment centres.
> Interview preparation.
> Help with your research into current employment trends.
> Help with postgraduate study and funding research.

NHS

There are a broad range of opportunities across the health sector. Check out all vacancies, starting with graduate schemes: www.nhscareers.nhs.uk.

Small and medium-sized enterprises (SMEs) and third sector organisations

Make speculative applications to private hospitals, care homes and surgeries where you feel your skills could be utilised. If they are not currently advertising,

6

they may keep your CV on file. Consider starting up programmes as part of outreach sessions within the local community where there are gaps in provision.

You could approach youth clubs or community centres to run sessions on topics such as diabetes awareness, the dangers of smoking, fitness and healthy eating and looking after your heart, where you could provide culturally appropriate sessions to the community.

Flexible working and short-term contracts: agency work

Very few people are lucky to progress into their dream career straight out of college or university. Be realistic and adaptable in your working patterns, and consider part-time or shift work through agencies to get a footing into your chosen career, where you can establish your credentials and work your way up to a position of responsibility. This is also a good way to ascertain your suitability for certain jobs. Search for recruitment agencies in your chosen sector: www.rec.uk.com.

Networking

Make use of contacts you have built up while at college and university in placements or via lecturers. Ask friends or family if they have any contacts or could put you in touch with any contacts within your chosen industry. Attend recruitment and careers fairs. Reconnect with placement or voluntary work staff to get an update on any opportunities or to look for temporary work to build up your experiences. Do you have social network connections on Facebook, LinkedIn or Twitter?

Web resources

Visit your careers service website or go on local and national newspaper websites. They may have details of vacancies as well as details of training courses relevant to your continued professional development. Researching public, private and voluntary organisations and their websites may also reveal vacancies.

Job websites

Sign up for bulletins from your careers service as well as employment agencies and job search websites where you can upload your CV and save your job choices so you receive e-mail alerts. You can also sign up for alerts from, for example, your local authority, NHS careers and Prospects websites.

Voluntary work

If you do not find a job on completion of your studies or have been unsuccessful in interviews through lack of experience, do not worry. It may be worth dedicating part of your time to voluntary work, in some cases alongside paid work. You could try contacting your former placement or visiting your careers service to discuss opportunities on a local level. Details are likely to be available on your university careers service website or through the national careers website for students (http://www.prospects.ac.uk/links/workexp). If you are aged 16–25, you can search for opportunities via http://www.connexions-direct.com and http://www.vinspired.com. See also http://www.timebank.org.uk and http://www.do-it.org.uk.

Job centres

It is worth contacting your local job centre to search for vacancies; it may also have opportunities or links with local NHS providers. You will also have access to computer portals for job searches and to phones in some cases. You can speak to an adviser and receive information and advice about benefit entitlement. Job centres have access to work schemes for people with disabilities and may have details on funding to support the training of long-term unemployed people.

Professional bodies

It may be worth considering joining a professional body as an affiliated member. You will receive bulletins and updates on the latest training and developments as well as information on career progression and vacancy sources.

Sector skills councils (SSC)

The sector skills councils are useful for researching changes to the industry. Skills for Health is the SSC for the health sector. It has been driven by employers and the government to highlight competencies, qualifications, careers and skills development. It provides advice to employers and training partners as well as news bulletins and labour market information on national and regional trends.

Useful resources

Try http://www.skillsforhealth.org.uk or http://www.skillsforcare.org.uk

For SSCs in Northern Ireland, Wales and Scotland: http://www.skillsforcareanddevelopment.org.uk

---

Going for interviews

We hope all your hard preparation has paid off and you have been invited for an interview. To maximise your success at interview there are certain things that are important to do (see Box 6.6).

Box 6.6 Preparing for an Interview

> Remember to reread your application and be honest about the skills you have. Do not be caught out at the interview!
> Prepare, prepare, prepare! Anticipate likely questions and prepare examples so you are not left floundering in the interview.
> Research the employer again for new developments.
> Read websites and newspapers and watch the news or relevant programmes to keep informed of any changes to the industry.

6

> Find out the format of the interview. Will it be a panel or telephone interview, are there likely to be group or individual assessments, will you be required to deliver a presentation?
> Visit your careers service to help boost your confidence beforehand.
> Try a mock interview with a careers adviser or friends or family first. They may be able to provide feedback on appearance, body language, answers and so forth.

Use of the *STAR* acronym can help you to focus your answers when explaining specific examples or experiences:

> S – situation or background to your example.
> T – task or objective you had to achieve.
> A – action you took, or your contribution if you are discussing multi-agency work.
> R – result. Good or bad, an employer will be keen to hear your reflections. Why did you take the action you took? What was the outcome? What did you learn from it? What would you do differently?

By organising your thoughts you will be able to provide a complete answer with complete confidence.

For instance, tailor the following sentences to your particular recent work placement or in your work history to demonstrate your experience of being part of a team and making a contribution to the team.

S – Whilst on placement with the … *Department of the NHS Trust* … I attended a multi agency meeting with … we discussed a case focusing on …

T – As part of this meeting we discussed high priority cases and in this particular instance we set out to achieve …

A – The team decided to move forward by delegating tasks to the different representatives from the different agencies according to their specialism, with the aim of achieving our objective before the next meeting. I was responsible for …

R – At the next meeting we all came together to discuss the progress/outcome of our actions. The result was … This experience resonated with me because I was able to make a positive contribution to the team. I learnt … If I was able to change anything, I would choose to do things differently by …

Reflective activity

Use the STAR system to provide examples of the following key skills employers look for:

- communication (written and oral);
- problem-solving;

Even though you may not be familiar with the STAR technique, remember that you have lots of experience of reflection. Most courses provide many opportunities to comprehensively detail experiences, provide descriptions of learning and reflect on your skills, strengths and areas of development. These reflections will help you to confidently evidence and articulate your employability skills at interview.

Reflective practice: what's the point?

Keeping a reflective diary or journal or engaging in reflective activities is likely to have been a requirement of your course and you may continue to work on jotting down your thoughts, feelings and descriptions of memorable events once you are in work. A reflective diary is personal; it's about you, your applied learning, your hopes, fears, goals, ambitions and motivating factors. It is a work in progress, to be added to as you journey through life. You may be given guidelines on how to format a reflective journal or diary from your educational establishment, work placement, mentor or supervisor, but how meaningful it will be is down to you and the time you dedicate to filling it in.

At the end of a busy and stressful day, the last thing you may want to do is complete more paperwork; however, writing down your thoughts after an event while it is still fresh in your mind will prove invaluable. You should be honest about situations, the challenges you faced, the decisions you made, your progress, the opinions and actions of the people around you, the impressions of your service users, what you learnt, what you still need to learn, your achievements and frustrations. The full gambit of emotions, actions and reactions will help to inform your future practice. Keeping a diary or journal can also help when preparing for an interview, as a log to remind you of good examples to talk about with the interviewer.

Box 6.7 Completing a Reflective Journal/Activity

1. Reflect on key moments of your studies placements and work. The events, how you felt, the challenges you faced, the decisions you and those around took all add up to valuable learning experiences. Think about how you felt the first time you worked with a patient or you had to report to a doctor: what did you learn, how would you approach things next time?

2. Self-awareness comes with time and experience. You will be familiar with this as reflection and continuing professional development (CPD)

6

are likely to have been mandatory requirements of your course. However, what took you by surprise during a placement? Were your values about people with learning difficulties or mental health issues challenged? How did you find working with someone who didn't speak English? Were you surprised by how well you handled it, your resilience, or did you feel frustrated, scared or impatient?

3. It is important to remember that you will be faced with new challenges, and the demands of your shift, your mood and factors outside of work will all impact on the kind of day you are having. Not all experiences will be rosy and even negative thoughts of others or feelings of inadequacy can help us to learn, to take a different course of action next time. Think about what weaknesses came to light: what do you need to work on?

4. It is important to write down your thoughts or discuss it with someone. Return to your reflections a day later once the emotion of the moment has passed. Read over what you have written: how have things changed in 24 hours? A fresh perspective will help you to tackle things in a different way, it will give you confidence next time you are faced with the scenario and you won't feel as overwhelmed. This shows that you are making the most of reflection and approaching decisions in a measured way, thereby adapting to situations and learning to balance the demands of the role against your personal values and principles. This is what makes you an effective practitioner (Schon 1983).

The process of reflection involves asking yourself some pertinent questions.

Being SMART

To help you in your process of personal and professional development it can be useful to identify and document your goals and attainment in a structured manner. Try using the SMART acronym. By charting your reflections in a journal, action plan or SMART graph, you will be able to personalise and chart your learning.

S – specific objective. The desired outcome/objective.

M – measurable. How can you measure or evidence achievement, e.g. patients' views, your view, the opinion of colleagues.

A – achievable. What help or support will you require? Who can help you attain your goals?

R – realistic Why is the action realistic and relevant to your CPD? How can it help you to achieve your goals?

T – time bound. How long will this take? Set some target dates and times.

You should also consider the outcome of your actions and what you have learnt from this experience. What might you do differently?

Table 6.3 A SMART table

S	M	A	R	T	Outcomes/ reflections
Specific goals	Measurable	Achievable	Realistic	Time-bound	

In your job: continuing professional development (CPD)

It will no doubt be satisfying, and a relief, to have a job, particularly one in which you are working towards a fulfilling career. This does not mean that your career planning is necessarily over though. Once you are in employment, it will be a requirement of most employers and/or professional associations for you to sign up to CPD.

CPD is the way health professionals continue to learn and develop throughout their careers so they can keep their skills and knowledge up to date and are able to work safely, legally and effectively within their evolving scope of practice. (Health Professions Council 2010)

Box 6.8 Managing your career path

Try managing your career path by taking advantage of the following:

> Training and development opportunities.
> Enquire about a mentor at work to guide you in your career.
> Keep up to date with developments that are likely to affect your role or industry.
> Continue to use a diary or reflective journal to keep track of your CPD, such as key tasks, what you enjoyed and the harder aspects of the job role, and what you have learnt so far both professionally and personally about yourself.
> Undertake SWOT analysis of your skills; keep a copy of your old ones as a comparison exercise. What improvements have you made and what you still need to work on?
> Be flexible and adaptable to new technologies, working conditions, locations, careers and duties where appropriate. Network while in the job.

6

> Use your appraisals and personal development reviews to let your manager or supervisor know about your commitment to them and to continue developing and focusing on your longer-term career objectives.
> Be proactive: ask employers about the possibility of work shadowing or secondments once you have been established in your role for a significant amount of time, which may be two to five years down the line.
> Consider postgraduate study to enhance skills gained in the workplace and to aid your career trajectory.
> Consider voluntary work or part-time work if possible to help you gain an insight into third sector opportunities, fill any skills gaps and enhance your CV. Your CV should be regarded as a work in progress, to be updated regularly with your most recent skills and achievements, in preparation for your next job.

Conclusion

In this chapter we have given you examples of job opportunities and the sorts of organisations and agencies that are suitable for, and may be attractive to, students who have studied 'health'. It is certainly the case, and will increasingly be so, that you may have several 'careers' throughout your working life. Gathering information, making the most of opportunities to improve your knowledge and skills and self-awareness, is the key to accessing a successful and fulfilling career and some of the tools in this chapter will guide you in the right direction.

glossary

Abstemious Exercising self-control, and not over-indulging in consumption of, for example alcohol or food.

Audit (in health care) The process by which current care is systematically reviewed against particular criteria with the aim of improving patient care and outcomes. Thus it is situated as a quality improvement process and is regularly undertaken in all practice areas.

Bias In research this refers to having a particular leaning, favouritism or prejudice for or against a particular group, meaning or approach. The impact of bias on research may be, for example, to produce a questionnaire that involves leading and meaning-loaded measures that are presented as neutral. The 'accusation' of research bias is more likely to be levelled at positivist or objective research, which positions itself as neutral, rather than interpretative and qualitative research, which acknowledges and works with their subjectivities.

Categorical need This refers to fundamental factors or assets that are needed by all people to ensure survival and effective human functioning. Nutrition and shelter are often considered categorical needs.

Cause and effect relationship This refers to research that is located within establishing a relationship between the independent and dependent variables. Thus, the source (independent variable) causes the effect (outcome/dependent variable).

Compatabilist/compatibilism This refers to the philosophy that acknowledges that humans have free will and moral responsibilities for their actions (although actions are also 'determined' by causal laws). Free will exists if a person *could* have acted differently if they had chosen differently. Free will cannot exist under conditions of constraint or compulsion.

Contextualised/decontextualised In research this refers to the practice of locating your research within a background informed by historical, political and social discourses. Researchers working within contextual realities claim that nothing exists in a vacuum, and that all knowledge and experience is informed by antecedent and present day circumstances. When knowledge, research or understandings are taken out of this situated arena and considered to exist independently of that arena, it is said to be decontextualised.

Discourse This can refer to verbal or written communication but also a set of values, norms and ideas that shape accepted knowledge and understanding of social matters. They reflect powerful cultural and ideological perspectives.

Empirical (empirical research) Research that uses experimentation and/or observation as its source of data.

Encephalitis lethargica A mysterious worldwide illness that affected mainly young people between 1917 and 1928. It was identified as some sort of brain inflammation, which started with various symptoms including fever, muscle pain and weakness. Increasing sleepiness was a symptom and could ultimately lead to a coma. Nearly a million people died and others who recovered exhibited symptoms of Parkinson's disease. The cause has largely remained unknown but more recent research has linked the condition to a rare form of the streptococcus bacterium.

Epistemology/epistemological This term, when used in reference to (social) research, is about the theory of knowledge: how we 'know' what we know and what we understand to be the nature of knowledge.

Essential meanings/essentialised This refers to the practice of ascribing set qualities and meanings to a particular entity. Thus, the essence of a particular form or substance has particular properties, which are accorded to all cases within each form.

Ethnomethodology This is a methodology concerned with studying the ways (methods) by which people conduct and make sense of their world. One of its main foci is the methods people use to account for the everyday features of life.

Evaluation (in healthcare) (sometimes analogous with **audit**) involves the systematic collection and analysis of data within practice; and the making of judgments and decisions from this process as to the validity and meanings of these findings.

Evidence-based practice This refers to the process of applying evidence to practice to ensure that care and clinical interventions are effective. It involves the integration of clinical expertise with evidence from systematic research.

Existentialist/existentialism Relating to philosophical theory that emphasises the existence of humans as free-thinking, individual agents who are responsible for their own actions and choices.

Fact/factual A fact is an actual state of affairs, a complex of objects, properties or relations. A thing that is known to have occurred or exist, or is verifiable. For example, it is a 'fact' that Suki (my cat) is a cat because she has properties that are recognised constituents of 'cats' (fur, claws, four legs, a tail, the ability to purr etc.) and she is a tangible entity (object). Empirical observation demonstrates this too (I, and others, can see, hear and stroke her).

Free market This refers to an economic system that is free to operate without restriction or governmental legislative control.

Grand narrative This refers to ideologies and theories that provide overarching explanations of how things are, how society is structured and how society works.

Hegemony The domination and/or supremacy of one power, group or meaning over others.

Iatrogenesis This word stems from the Greek for physician, *iatros*, and origin, *genesis*, and thus refers to problems originating from treatment by doctors, other health professionals or within healthcare.

Incidence This refers to the number of new cases of disease or disorders over a given period of time. Incidence will rise during epidemics (e.g. swine flu).

Justice There are several ways of defining justice: justice under the law (fair treatment), justice as rights (e.g. the right to be paid as agreed for one's labour), justice as fairness (equity or equal distribution of resources). John Rawls (1921–2002) presents an interesting discussion of the notion of justice as fairness.

Kyoto Agreement A legally binding agreement (for signatory states) concerning reduction in emissions of greenhouse gases. The first discussions took place in 1997 in Kyoto, Japan. It came into effect in 2005 but not all countries have ratified the agreement, e.g. the USA and most Latin American countries. The UK has set its own legally binding targets on cuts to carbon emissions.

Laissez-faire A French term meaning 'allow to do'. It refers to a political and social organisation in which authority (e.g. the state), has little influence over the actions of individuals. It also refers to free-market economics, in which the government has minimal interference with trade.

L-Dopa (laevo-dihydroxyphenylalanine) A drug used in the treatment of Parkinson's disease.

Local authority This refers to the organisation of local government. Local authorities provide a range of services for the populations of specific areas. These services include social services, educational services and environmental services (such as rubbish collection).

Mandate An official instruction. In the context of government, for example, it refers to the authority to exercise power and decision-making for a population, bestowed onto an elected political party.

Marx, Karl (1818–83) A philosopher, historian and social scientist who produced seminal work on a socialist analysis of industrial, capitalist societies.

Marxism An economic and social system based on the complex and extensive theories of Karl Marx and Friedrich Engels. Very

briefly, emphasis is placed on the struggle between social classes as a dynamic for change and Marxism promotes a socialist state system with public ownership of the means of production (such as industrial production) and distribution of resources and capital.

Mixed method research This generally refers to the practice, in research, of using a number of both quantitative and qualitative methods of data collection to analyse and shed meaning on the phenomenon under investigation.

Morality Often used to refer to a 'code of conduct' within society, and strongly associated with ethical theories. It implies certain virtuous behaviours that are accepted within society, often, but not exclusively, associated with sexual behaviour. Judgements are made about 'right' or 'wrong' behaviour based on these codes of conduct.

Neo-classical economics A theory of economics that emphasises the importance of competition as a means of regulating economic activity and the distribution of resources using market forces of supply and demand.

Neutrality Often associated with objectivity and positivism in that is concerned with maintaining a personally uninvolved stance regarding all aspects of research. Being neutral requires the researcher to be completely impartial and unaligned with any aspect of the research, in particular the respondents and the results. This quality, i.e. not wanting a particular result or seeing the world through a partial lens, is a concern of all researchers.

Objective research/objectivity Concerned with adopting a stance to all aspects of the research that is uninvolved and distant. Thus, research that endeavours to adopt this quality positions the researcher as totally separate from the arena they are researching, the implication being that knowledge, and the pursuit of 'truth', can only truly be established when the researcher is not personally influential (or influenced) or invested in any of the decision-making processes involved. Therefore all aspects of the research are informed by 'scientific' rationales and measures. It is often associated with positivism in terms of epistemological positions, as well as ontological understandings of truth existing independently of human actors and influence.

Ontology/ontological This term, when used in reference to (social) research, is about our beliefs about and understanding of the nature of reality, the known and existence.

Panacea A supposed 'cure-all' for a disease or other problem (from the Greek goddess of healing).

Pandemic A disease that is widespread and prevalent worldwide (or within a continent, land mass, country etc.).

Paradigm In research a set of beliefs that inform understandings of reality(s) and our relationship, as researchers, to that known. Thus, in order to ascertain certain truths certain methodologies are adopted.

Patriarchal/patriarchalism Institutionalised dominance of women by men. Women are regarded as inferior and this might be reinforced by social and cultural systems such as restricting women's access to education.

Practitioner research Refers to research done by practitioners within their practice area and organisations. Often associated with **evidence-based practice** as it is concerned with improving, developing and understanding practice from within the

area. Practitioner research involves ongoing reflective engagement with all elements of practice, including the practitioner's role. Very often the intention of engaging with practitioner research is to implement and manage change with a view to improving practice.

Pre-eclampsia Refers to a medical term or condition that describes a set of symptoms during pregnancy, which give rise to hypertension.

Prevalence Refers to the total number of people with a disease or disorder over a particular period of time. Prevalence itself constitutes both new and existing or old cases of the disease or disorder, and so reflects new diagnoses as well as those living with a particular condition. Prevalence will fluctuate according to the number of new cases *and* the number recovering, or dying, from the condition.

Private sector This refers to services and organisations owned by private individuals and business. The services are provided in order to make money and generate profit.

Proposition This refers to the factual content of a declaration such as 'Sue kissed Barry' or 'Barry was kissed by Sue'. Another example is to state 'I am hungry' or 'Stephen is hungry'. These latter two examples are different propositions as they are referring to two different people, whereas the first two examples contain the same proposition (fact), simply expressed differently.

Public health This is concerned with action to protect the health of populations, rather than individuals. The focus is on action to prevent the occurrence or spread of disease and work to ameliorate factors that negatively impact on the health of populations. This can include actions such as mass immunisation, the provision of clean water and proper sanitation, reducing exposure to environmental pollution and the promotion of health behaviours at a population level, e.g. banning smoking in public places.

Public sector This relates to organisations that provide services by, and for, the state; in other words, services for the citizens of a country. Resources are controlled and owned by the state. People who work for the local authority or NHS, for example, are categorised as public sector workers.

Qualitative This term is used to denote methodological approaches in research that are concerned with an in-depth understanding of phenomena. Thus, engaged and exploratory methods are utilised to gain insight into the complexities of phenomena and their possible meanings.

Quantitative This term is used to denote methodological approaches in research that measure properties and phenomena in mathematical terms. Tools of measurement are used to collect numerical data, while statistical models are usually utilised to explain the outcomes of research.

Randomised control trials, double-blinded Patients or subjects do not know if they are being treated with an active ingredient and neither does the assessor.

Randomised control trials, single-blinded Patients or subjects do not know if they are being treated with an active ingredient but the assessor does.

Randomised control trials, triple-blinded Neither the patient/subject, assessor or statistician/pharmacist knows who is being treated with the active ingredients.

Rationalism The idea that beliefs must be founded on reasoning rather than religious belief or emotion.

Reductionism The process by which we oversimplify complex and sophisticated multilayered concepts to simple individual elements, concepts or meanings: for example, analysing human health on the basis of our genetic profile alone. It is often associated with notions of causality (see **cause and effect relationship**), where these complexities are reduced to singular interactions and/or effects. Simple units, principles and/or components are used as a way of describing and explaining phenomena and behaviour.

Representativeness Used in conjunction with generalisability (see the discussion on this in Chapter 5); it describes a population accessed and researched within a piece of research as representative of the characteristics of the whole population that the research seeks to make theoretical statements about. Thus, to say something is representative of the whole is to believe that there are certain qualities that exist in relation to that population that can be, and have been, embodied.

Romanticism A philosophical and artistic movement originating within Western cultures during the eighteenth and nineteenth centuries that changed the way in which people thought about themselves and the world and had a powerful influence, among other things, on literature, music and painting. The ideas embodied in romanticism recognised the importance of simplicity, subjectivity, emotions, the individual and awe inspired by nature.

Sample population Refers to the units (this term can refer to people, documents, entities, forms etc.) that you do your research on or with. The sample is a selection from, or of, the target population. It may be positioned as being representative of the target population or simply be a number from the possible units available to you.

Sampling framework How you select, and by what criteria, your sample population from the target population. There are different methods of selecting your sample and these roughly fall into random sampling frameworks and non-random sampling frameworks (see the discussion in Chapter 1).

Social capital Initially this term referred to the ability of an individual to acquire the skills necessary for employment. It has more recently been used to refer to the 'resources' within a community, which include people resources (e.g. relationship networks and trust), social participation (sense of belonging) and actual resources (e.g. schools, commercial outlets)

Social construction Essentially this refers to the belief that no value-free sources of knowledge exist. The material world (reality) does not exist as separate from our understanding and interpretations of the world; instead 'facts' and 'knowledge' are 'constructed' through social and cultural discourse.

Subjective research/subjectivity The opposite of **objective research** in that the researcher is invested and personally involved in the research process. Thus, to be subjective is to acknowledge that realities are informed by constructs and experiences, and we are constructors of this reality. Being a subjective researcher acknowledges the contexts, beliefs and values that are brought to bear in all aspects of research. This is not to say that subjective researchers do not strive to limit and reduce their impact on the research, but rather that they openly work with these constructs' potential to influence the research.

Transparency This means that all stages and aspects of the research process are visible and open to the researched, the researchers and 'the audience'.

Triangulation/triangulated In research this is often interchangeable with mixed method research, though in actual fact the purpose of these can differ. Triangulation refers to the practice of using more than one method of data collection to validate and cross-check or verify findings.

User involvement In essence this relates to the principle of working with people who access a service or resource, e.g. as patients they 'use' healthcare resources. It can include involvement in the planning and delivery of services and the importance of rights, partnership, engagement and empowerment of individuals and groups (users).

Well-being In philosophical terms 'well-being' refers to debates around what constitutes a 'good life' and human happiness. This raises the distinction between what is 'morally' good and the sort of life most people want (comfort and enjoyment) and what possible connection there is between 'moral good' and health, wealth, happiness and other components of well-being. Both are important components. What constitutes a *good life* is therefore not confined to 'virtuous' behaviour (currently often construed as being not smoking, drinking alcohol in moderation and so forth).

White paper A white paper is a substantive document that outlines the ideas, philosophy, findings and priorities of a government or organisation about a social, political or organisational matter. It constitutes an official publication of a government (or other organisation) and often indicates specific policy objectives (and actions) for all organisations and individuals involved with the matter in question.

references

Abramson, J. H. (1984) *Survey Methods in Community Medicine: An Introduction to Epidemiological and Evaluative Studies*, 3rd edn. Edinburgh: Churchill Livingstone.

Adams, M. L. (2004) 'The Trouble with Normal: Postwar Youth and the Making of Heterosexuality', in M. Webber and K. Bezanson (eds), *Rethinking Society in the 21st Century: Critical Readings in Sociology*. Toronto: Canadian Scholars' Press Inc.

Adams, S. and de Bont, A. (2007) 'Information Rx: Prescribing Good Consumerism and Responsible Citizenship', *Health Care Analysis*, 15, 273–90.

Adamson, J. and Donovan, J. (2005) '"Normal Disruption": South Asian and African/Caribbean Relatives Caring for an Older Family Member in the UK', *Social Science and Medicine*, 60, 37–48.

Ades, A., Parker, S. and Berry, T. (1991) 'Prevalence of Maternal HIV 1 Infection in Thames Regions Results from Anonymous Unlinked Neonatal Testing', *Lancet* , 337, 1562–5.

Age Concern and The Mental Health Foundation (2006) *Promoting Mental Health and Well-Being in Later Life. A First Report from the UK Inquiry into Mental Health and Well-Being in Later Life*. London: Age Concern and the Mental Health Foundation.

AGR (2010) http://www.agr.org.uk/Content/AGR-Summer-Survey-2006.

Aidsmap.com (accessed throughout 2008, 2009, 2010).

Ainsworth, S. (2006) 'Herceptin and the Case of Ann Marie Rogers: The Price of Victory', *Nurse Prescribing*, 4(4), 138–40.

Ajzen, I. and Fishbein, M. (1980) *Understanding Attitudes and Predicting Social Behavior*. New Jersey: Prentice-Hall Inc.

Alaszewski, A. (2007) 'Using Documents in Health Research', in M. Saks and J. Allsop (eds), *Researching Health: Qualitative, Quantitative and Mixed Methods*. London: Sage.

Alberts, A., Elkind, D. and Ginsberg, S. (2007) 'The Personal Fable and Risk-Taking in Early Adolescence', *Journal of Youth Adolescence*, 36, 71–6.

Alder, B. (1999) *Psychology of Health. Applications of Psychology for Health Professionals*, 2nd edn. Amsterdam: Harwood Academic Publishers.

Allison, D. B., Fountaine, K. R., Manson, J. E., Stevens, J. and VanItallie, T. B. (1999) 'Annual Deaths Attributable to Obesity in the United States', *JAMA*, 282(16), 1530–8.

Allsop, J. (1990) 'Does Socialism Necessarily Mean the Public Provision of Health Care?', in J. Carrier and I. Kendall (eds), *Socialism and the NHS: Fabian Essays in Health Care*. Aldershot: Avebury.

Almond, P. (2001) 'What Is Consumerism and Has It Had an Impact on Health Visiting Provision? A Literature Review', *Journal of Advanced Nursing*, 35(6), 893–901.

Alzheimer's Society (2009) *What is Dementia with Lewy Bodies?* Alzheimers.org.uk (accessed October 2010).

Alzheimer's Society (2010) *The Mini Mental State Examination* (MMSE) www.alzheimers.org.uk/site/scripts/documents_info.php?documentID=121 (accessed 3 December 2010).

Alzheimer's Society and The Mental Health Foundation (2008) *Dementia: Out of the Shadows*. London: Alzheimer's Society.

Andersson, E., Creasy, S. and Tritter, J. (n.d.) 'Does Patient and Public Involvement Matter?', in E. Andersson, J. Tritter and R. Wilson (eds), *Health Democracy: The Future of Involvement in Health and Social Care*. London: Involve and The National Centre for Involvement.

Antonovsky, A. (1987) *Unfavelling the Mystery of Health: How People Manage Others and Stay Well.* New York: Wiley.

Antonovsky, A. (1993) 'The Sense of Coherence as a Determinant of Health', in A. Beattie, M. Gott, L. Jones and M. Siddel (eds), *Health and Wellbeing: A Reader.* Buckingham: Open University Press.

Appel, L. J., Brands, M. W., Daniels, S. R., Karanja, N., Elmer, P. J. and Sacks, F. M. (2006) 'Dietary Approaches to Prevent and Treat Hypertension: A Scientific Statement from the American Heart Association', *Hypertension*, 47(2), 296–308.

Appleton, J. V. (2009) 'Starting a New Research Project', in J. Neale (ed.), *Research Methods for Health and Social Care.* Basingstoke: Palgrave Macmillan.

Armstrong, D. (1994) *Outline of Sociology as Applied to Medicine.* Oxford: Butterworth Heinemann.

Aronson, J. (1994) 'A Pragmatic View of Thematic Analysis', *The Qualitative Report*, 2(1), http://www.nova.edu/ssss/QR/BackIssues/QR2-1/aronson.html).

Atkinson, P. and Coffey, A. (1997) 'Analysing Documentary Realities', in D. Silverman (ed.), *Qualitative Research.* London: Sage.

Ausman, J. I. (2003) 'An Example of Physicians Being Used as Scapegoats for Rising Healthcare Costs: A Socialist Government in Action', *Surgical Neurology*, 60, 88–9.

Avert.org (accessed throughout 2008, 2009, 2010).

Baigis, J. and Hughes, A. (2001) 'Evidence-Based Practice', *Journal of the Association of Nurses in AIDS Care*, 12(suppl.), 9–18.

Baggott, R. (2000) *Public Health: Policy and Politics.* Basingstoke: Macmillan.

Baggott, R. (2005) 'A Funny Thing Happened on the Way to the Forum? Reforming Patient and Public Involvement in the NHS in England', *Public Administration*, 83(3), 533–51.

Bailey, D. (1991) *Research for the Health Professional: A Practical Guide.* Philadelphia: F. A. Davis.

Bailey, L., Vardulaki, K., Langham, J. and Chandramohan, D. (2005) *Introduction to Epidemiology.* Maidenhead: Open University Press.

Baldwin, C. and Capstick, A. (eds) (2007) *Tom Kitwood on Dementia.* Maidenhead: Open University Press.

Baldwin, C. and the Bradford Dementia Group (2008) Narrative(,) Citizenship and Dementia: The Personal and the Political', *Journal of Aging Studies*, 22, 222–8.

Bambra, C., Fox, D. and Scott-Samuel, A. (2007) 'Towards a Politics of Health', in J. Douglas, S. Earle, S. Handsley, C. E. Lloyd and S. Spurr (eds), *A Reader in Promoting Public Health: Challenge and Controversy.* London: Sage Publications in association with the Open University.

Bandura, A. (1998) 'Health Promotion from the Perspective of Social Cognitive Theory', *Psychology and Health*, 13, 623–49.

Bandura, A. (2000) 'Health Promotion from the Perspective of Social Cognition Theory', in P. Norman, C. Abraham and M. Conner (eds), *Understanding and Changing Health Behaviour – from Health Beliefs to Self-Regulation.* Amsterdam: Harwood Academic Publishers.

Bandura, A. (2002) 'Self-Efficacy Assessment', in R. Fernández-Ballesteros (ed.), *Encyclopedia of Psychological Assessment.* London: Sage Publications.

Banister, P. et al. (1994) *Qualitative Methods in Psychology: A Research Guide.* Buckingham: Open University Press.

Baranowski, T., Perry, C. L. and Parcel, G. S. (2002) 'How Individuals, Environments, and Health Behavior Interact: Social Cognitive Theory', in K. Glanz, B. K. Rimer and F. M. Lewis (eds), *Health Behavior and Health Education: Theory, Research and Practice*, 3rd edn. San Francisco: Jossey-Bass.

Baric, L (1995) ' The Singer or the Song – Health Promotion and Health Education vs Healthism', *Journal of the Institute of Health Education*, 33(4), 123–9.

Barnett, T. and Whiteside, A. (2006) *AIDS in the Twenty-First Century*, 2nd edn. Basingstoke: Palgrave Macmillan.

Barratt, H. and Sipos, A. (2005) 'Autonomy – Who Chooses?', *Christian Medical Fellowship*, 25, 1–4, http://www.cmf.org.uk (accessed 2008).

Bartlett, R. and O'Connor, D. (2007) 'From Personhood to Citizenship: Broadening the Lens for Dementia Practice and Research, *Journal of Aging Studies*, 21, 107–18.

Bauman, Z. (1989) *Modernity and the Holocaust*. Cambridge: Polity Press.

BBC News (2002) 'Reading "Can Bring Social Change"', http://news.bbc.co.uk/1/hi/education/2494637.stm (accessed March 2009).

BBC News (2003) 'Infertility "Could Be Wiped Out"', 25 July, http://news.bbc.co.uk/1/hi/health/3094209.stm (accessed April 2010).

BBC News (2008) 'Voters Reject Congestion Charge', 12 December, http://news.bbc.co.uk/1/hi/england/manchester/7778110.stm (accessed April 2010).

BBC News (2009a) 'Recession Moves Migration Patterns', 8 September, http://news.bbc.co.uk/1/hi/8243225.stm (accessed May 2010).

BBC News (2009b) 'Government Targets Obesity Rates', 2 January, http://news.bbc.co.uk/1/hi/health/7791820.stm (accessed May 2010).

Beach, T. (1987) 'The History of Alzheimer's Disease: Three Debates', *Journal of the History of Medicine and Allied Sciences*, 42, 327–49.

Beattie, A. (1993) 'The Changing Boundaries of Health', in A. Beattie, M. Gott, L. Jones and M. Siddel (eds), *Health and Wellbeing: A Reader*. Buckingham: Open University Press.

Beauchamp, T. and Childress, J. (1994) *Principles of Biomedical Ethics*, 4th edn. Oxford: Oxford University Press.

Behuniak, S. M. (2010) 'Toward a Political Model of Dementia: Power as Compassionate Care', *Journal of Aging Studies*, in the press.

Bell, D. (1999) 'Ideology', in A. Bullock and S. Trombley (eds), *The New Fontana Dictionary of Modern Thought*, 3rd edn. London: HarperCollins.

Belsey, C. (2002) *Post-Structuralism: A Very Short Introduction*. Oxford: Oxford University Press.

Bender, M. (2003) *Explorations in Dementia*. London: Jessica Kingsley.

Bennett, P., Murphy, S., Carroll, D. and Ground, I. (1995) 'Psychology, Health Promotion and Aesthemiology', *Health Care Analysis*, 3, 15–26.

Bennett, W. and Gurin, J. (1982) *The Dieter's Dilemma*. New York: Basic Books.

Benton, T. and Craib, I. (2001) *Philosophy of Social Science: The Philosophical Foundations of Social Thought*. Basingstoke: Palgrave.

Benzeval, M., Judge, K. and Whitehead, M. (eds) (1995) *Tackling Inequalities in Health: An Agenda for Action*. London: Kings Fund.

Bergh, C., Sabin, M., Shield, J., Hellers, G., Zandian, M., Palmberg, K., Olofsson, B., Lindeberg, K., Björnström, M. and Södersten, P. (2008) 'A Framework for the Treatment of Obesity: Early Support', in E. M. Blass (ed.), *Obesity, Causes, Mechanisms, Prevention, and Treatment*. Sunderland, MA: Sinauer Associates, Inc.

Bergmann, J. R. (2004) 'Ethnomethodology', in U. Flick, E. Von Kardorff and I. Steinke (eds), *A Companion to Qualitative Research*. London:Sage.

Bernardi, M. (2008) 'Global Climate Change – A Feasibility Perspective of Its Effect on Human Health at a Local Scale', *Geospatial Health*, 2(2), 137–50.

Berofsky, B. (2003) 'Identification, the Self, and Autonomy', *Social Philosophy and Policy Foundation*, 20(2), 199–220.

Bharat, S., Aggleton, P. and Tyrer, P. (2001) *India, HIV and AIDS-Related Discrimination, Stigmatisation and Denial*. Geneva: UNAIDS.

Bilton, T., Bonnett, K., Jones, P., Lawson, T., Skinner, D., Stanworth, M. and Webster, A. (2002) *Introductory Sociology*, 4th edn. Basingstoke: Palgrave Macmillan.

Birenbaum-Carmeli, D. (2004) '"Cheaper than a Newcomer": On the Social Production of IVF Policy in Israel', *Sociology of Health and Illness*, 26(7), 897–924.

Black Report (1980) *Inequalities in Health: Report of a Research Working Group*. London: DHSS, http://www.sochealth.co.uk/Black/black.htm (accessed April 2010).

Blair, S. N. and LaMonte, M. J. (2006) 'Commentary. Current Perspectives on Obesity and Health: Black and White, or Shades of Grey?', *International Journal of Epidemiology*, 35, 69–72.

Blair, S. N. and Nichaman, M. Z. (2002) 'The Public Health Problem of Increasing Prevelence Rates of Obesity and What Should Be Done About It', *Mayo Clinic Proceedings*, 77(2), 109–13.

Bloomberg M. R. and Aggarwala, R. T. (2008) 'Think Locally, Act Globally: How Curbing Global Warming Emissions Can Improve Local Public Health', *American Journal of Preventive Medicine*, 35(5), 414–23.

Boffetta, P., Couto, E., Wichmann, J. and 49 others (2010) 'Fruit and Vegetable Intake and Overall Cancer Risk in the European Prospective Investigation into Cancer and Nutrition (EPIC)', *Journal of the National Cancer Institute*, 120(8), 529–37.

Bogart, L. M., Cowgill, B. O., Kennedy, D., Ryan, G., Murphy, D. A., Elijah, J. and Schuster, M. A. (2008) 'HIV-Related Stigma among People with HIV and Their Families: A Qualitative Analysis', *AIDS and Behavior*, 12, 244–54.

Boncz, I. and Sebestyén, A. (2006) 'Economy and Mortality in Eastern and Western Europe between 1945 and 1990: The Largest Medical Trial of History', *International Journal of Epidemiology*, 35, 796–805.

Bond, J. (1992) 'The Medicalization of Dementia', *Journal of Aging Studies*, 6(4), 397–403.

Bond, V., Chase, E. and Aggleton, P. (2002) 'Stigma, HIV/AIDS and Prevention of Mother-to-Child Transmission in Zambia, *Evaluation and Program Planning*, 25, 347–56.

Booth, W. C., Colomb, G. G. and Williams, J. M. (1995) *The Craft of Research*. Chicago and London: University of Chicago Press.

Bordo, S. (1993) *Unbearable Weight: Feminism, Western Culture and the Body*. Berkeley: University of California Press.

Boulton, M (2009) 'Research Ethics', in J. Neale (ed.), *Research Methods for Health and Social Care*. Basingstoke: Palgrave Macmillan.

Bouma, G. D. and Ling, R. (2004) *The Research Process*, 5th edn. South Melbourne: Oxford University Press.

Bourdieu, P. (1977) *Outline of a Theory of Practice*. Cambridge: Cambridge University Press.

Bovbjerg, V. E. (2008) 'The Epidemiology of Obesity: Causal Roots – Routes of Cause', in E. M. Blass (ed.), *Obesity: Causes, Mechanisms, Prevention, and Treatment*, Sunderland, MA: Sinauer Associates, Inc.

Bowell, T. and Kemp, G. (2010) *Critical Thinking. A Concise Guide*, 3rd edn. London: Routledge.

Bowers, D., House, A. and Owens, D. (2001) *Understanding Clinical Papers*. Chichester: John Wiley.

Bowling, A. (2009) *Research Methods in Health: Investigating Health and Health Services*, 3rd edn. Maidenhead: Open University Press.

Bradshaw, J. (1972) 'The Concept of Social Need,' *New Society*, 30 March, 640–3.

Bradshaw, J. (1994) 'The Conceptualization and Measurement of Need: A Social Policy Perspective', in J. Popay and G. Williams (eds), *Researching the People's Health*. London: Routledge.

Brannelly, T. (2006) 'Negotiating Ethics in Dementia Care', *Dementia*, 5(2), 197–212.

Braun and Clark (2006) 'Using Thematic Analysis in psychology', *Qualitative Research in Psychology*, 3(2), 77–101.

Brewerton, P. and Millward, L. (2001) *Organizational Research Methods*. London: Sage.

Briggs, K., Askham, J., Norman, I. and Redfern, S. (2003) 'Accomplishing Care at Home for People with Dementia: Using Observational Methodology', *Qualitative Health Research*, 13, 268–80.

British HIV Association (2008) http://www.bhiva.org/

Brook, D. W., Brook, J. S., Rubenstone, E., Zhang, C. and Finch, S. J. (2010) 'A Longitudinal Study of Sexual Risk Behavior Among the Adolescent Children of HIV-Positive and HIV-Negative Drug-Abusing Fathers', *Journal of Adolescent Health*, 46, 224–31.

Brotsky, S. R. and Giles, D. (2007) 'Inside the "Pro-ana" Community: A Covert Online Participant Observation', *Eating Disorders*, 15(2), 93–109.

Brown, C. (2005) 'Drugs Firms Turning Britain into "Pill for Every Ill"', *The Independent on Sunday*, 5 April, http://www.independent.co.uk/life-style/health-and-families/health-news/drugs-firms-turning-britain-into-pill-for-every-ill-society-531212.html

Brown, C., Conner, K. O., Copeland, V. C., Grote, N., Beach, S., Battista, D. and Reynold, C. F. (2010) 'Depression Stigma, Race and Treatment Seeking Behaviour and Attitudes', *Journal of Community Psychology*, 38(3), 350–68.

Brown, H. (1994) '"An Ordinary Sexual Life?" A Review of the Normalization Principle as It Applies to the Sexual Options of People with Learning Disabilities', *Disability and Society*, 9(2), 123–44.

Bryman, A. (2008) *Social Research Methods*, 3rd edn. Oxford: Oxford University Press.

Bullock, A. (1999) 'Democracy', in A. Bullock and S. Trombley (eds), *The New Fontana Dictionary of Modern Thought*, 3rd edn. London: HarperCollins.

Butland, B., Jebb, S., Kopelman, P., McPherson, K., Thomas, S., Mardell, J. and Parry, V. (2007) *Foresight Tackling Obesities: Future Choices – Project Report*, 2nd edn. London: Government Office for Science.

Butler, J. (1990) *Gender Trouble: Feminism and the Subversion of Identity*. London: Routledge.

Bynum B., (2008) 'The Art of Medicine. Road Maps to Health', *The Lancet*, 372, 1626–7.

Bywater, J. and Jones, R. (2007) *Sexuality and Social Work*. Exeter: Learning Matters.

Calder, G. (2003) *Communitarianism and New Labour*, http://www.whb.co.uk/socialissues/vol2gc.htm (accessed 27 August 2008).

Calnan, M. (2007) 'Quantitative Survey Methods in Health Research', in M. Saks and J. Allsop (eds), *Researching Health: Qualitative, Quantitative and Mixed Methods*. London: Sage.

Cameron, J. (2004) *The Epistemology of Post Modernism and Post Structuralism*. DSA/ESRC Advanced Training Postgraduate workshop in Development Studies, http://www.devstud.org.uk/studygroups/student/workshop04/Cameron%20paper%20-%20epistemology.doc (accessed 25 July 2007).

Campos, P. (2004) *The Obesity Myth: Why America's Obession with Weight Is Hazardous to Your Health*. New York: Gotham Books.

Campos, P., Saguy, A., Ernsberger, P., Oliver, E. and Gaesser, G. (2006a) 'Response: Lifestyle not Weight Should Be the Primary Target', *International Journal of Epidemiology*, 35, 81–2.

Campos, P., Saguy, A., Ernsberger, P., Oliver, E. and Gaesser, G. (2006b) 'The Epidemiology of Overweight and Obesity: Public Health Crisis or Moral Panic?', *International Journal of Epidemiology*, 35 55–60.

Cannold, L. (2004) 'Who Owns a Dead Man's Sperm?', *Journal of Medical Ethics*, 30, 386.

Cantley, C. (ed.) (2001) *A Handbook of Dementia Care*. Buckingham: Open University Press.

Care, N. S. (1995) 'Individualism, Moral and Political', in T. Honderich (ed.), *The Oxford Companion to Philosophy*. Oxford: Oxford University Press.

Carlisle, S., Hanlon, P. and Hannah, M. (2008) 'Status, Taste Distinction in Consumer Culture: Acknowledging the Symbolic Dimensions of Inequality', *Public Health*, 122, 631–7.

Carr, S., Unwin, N. and Pless-Mulloli, T. (2007) *An Introduction to Public Health and Epidemiology*, 2nd edn. Maidenhead: McGraw Hill and Open University Press.

Carryer, J. (1997) Cited in M. Gard and J. Wright (2005) *The Obesity Epidemic, Science, Morality and Ideology*. London: Routledge.

Cavanagh, S. and Chadwick, K. (2005) *Health Needs Assessment: A Practical Guide*. London: NICE.

Cedar, S. H. (2008) 'Human Biology and Health,' in J. Naidoo and J. Wills (eds), *Health Studies: An Introduction*, 2nd edn. Basingstoke: Palgrave Macmillan.

CGOU (Cross Government Obesity Unit) (2008) The National Child Measurement Programme Guidance of PCTs: 2008109 School Year. London: DoH.

Chambers, J. and Swanson, V. (2006) 'A Health Assessment Tool for Multiple Risk Factors for Obesity: Results from a Pilot Study with UK Adults', *Patient Education and Counseling*, 62, 79–88.

Change4Life (2010) http://www.nhs.uk/Change4Life/Pages/default.aspx?gclid=CNmr-e3L45oCFQ2T3wodB1e-CA (accessed May 2010).

Cheston, R. and Bender, M. (1999) *Understanding Dementia: The Man with the Worried Eyes*. London: Jessica Kingley.

Chisick, H. (2008) 'Looking for Enlightenment', *History of European Ideas*, doi: 10.1061/j.histeuroideas.2008.06.002.

Churchill, L. R. (1999) 'The United States Health Care System under Managed Care: How the Commodification of Health Care Distorts Ethics and Threatens Equity' *Health Care Analysis*, 7, 393–411.

Clare, L., Rowlands, J., Bruce, E., Surr, C. and Downs, M. (2008) 'The Experience of Living with Dementia in Residential Care: An Interpretative Phenomenological Analysis', *The Gerontologist*, 48(6), 711–20.

Clark, Jill Macleod and Hockey, Lisbeth (1979) *Research for Nursing: A Guide for the Enquiring Nurse*. Chichester: HM plus M.

Clark, R. C. and Mytton, J. (2007) 'Estimating Infectious Disease in UK Asylum Seekers and Refugees: A Systematic Review of Prevalence Studies', *Journal of Public Health*, 29(4), 420–8.

Clarke, A. E. (1998) *Disciplining Reproduction: Modernity, American Life, Sciences and the Problems of Sex*. Berkeley and Los Angeles: University of California Press.

Clements, C. D. and Sider, R. C. (1987) 'Medical Caring for the Smoker: Ethical Responsibility Works Both Ways', *Chest*, 91(2), 156–8.

Cochrane Collaboration (2002) 'Publication Bias', http://www.cochrane-net.org/openlearning/html/mod15-2.htm (accessed 3 April 2010).

Cohen, D. (2008) 'Health Economics', in J. Naidoo and J. Wills (eds), *Health Studies: An Introduction*, 2nd edn. Basingstoke: Palgrave Macmillan.

Cohen, M. S. (2004) *HIV Prevention: Rethinking the Risk of Transmission,* http://www.iavireport.org/Issues/1104/HIVPrevention.asp

Cole, T. J. et al. (2000) 'Establishing a Standard Definition for Child Overweight and Obesity Worldwide: International Survey', *British Medical Journal*, 320(7244), 1240.

Coles, T. and Health Evidence Bulletins Wales (1999) *Food and Health (Including Overweight and Obesity)*, http://hebw.cf.ac.uk/healthyliving/chapter3.html (accessed 1 June 2009).

Colquhoun, A., Lyon, P. and Alexander, E. (2001) 'Feeding Minds and Bodies: The Edwardian Context of School Meals', *Nutrition and Food Science*, 31(3), 117–24.

Committee on Environmental Health (2007) 'Global Climate Change and Children's Health', *Pediatrics*, 120(5), 1149–52.

Conner, M. and Norman, P. (eds) (1996) *Predicting Health Behaviour: Researching and Practice with Social Cognition Models*. Buckingham: Open University Press.

Coombes, L., Allen, D., Humphrey, D. and Neale, J. (2009) 'In-depth Interviews', 197–211, in J. Neale (ed.), *Research Methods for Health and Social Care*. Basingstoke: Palgrave Macmillan.

Cooper, C., Balamurali, T. B. S., Selwood, A. and Livingson, G. (2007) 'A Systematic Review of Intervention Studies about Anxiety in Caregivers of People with Dementia', *International Journal of Geriatric Psychiatry*, 22, 181–8.

Corrigan, P. W., Morris, S., Larson, J., Rafacz, J., Wassell, A., Michaels, P., Wilkniss, S., Batia, K. and Rüsch, N. (2010) 'Self-Stigma and Coming out about One's Mental Illness', *Journal of Community Psychology*, 38(3), 259–75.

Couch, D. and Liamputtong, P. (2008) 'Online Dating and Mating: The Use of the Internet to Meet Sexual Partners', *Qualitative Health Research*, 18(2), 268–79.

Coombes, L., Allen, D., Humphrey, D. and Neale, J. (2009) 'In-Depth Interviews', in J. Neale (ed.). *Research Methods for Health and Social Care*. Basingstoke: Palgrave Macmillan.

Cottrell, S. (2005) *Critical Thinking Skills: Developing Effective Analysis and Argument*. Basingstoke: Palgrave Macmillan.

Crawford, D. (2002) 'Population strategies to prevent obesity'. *British Medical Journal*, 325, 5 October, 728–9.

Creighton, S., Sethi, G., Edwards, S. G. and Miller, R. (2004) 'Dispersal of HIV Positive Asylum Seekers: National Survey of UK Healthcare Providers', *British Medical Journal*, 329, 322–3.

Creswell, J. (1998) *Qualitative Inquiry and Research Design: Choosing among Five Traditions*. Thousand Oaks, CA and London: Sage.

Cribb, A. and Duncan, P. (2002) *Health Promotion and Professional Ethics*. Oxford: Blackwell.

Cribb, A. (2002) 'Ethics: From Health Care to Public Policy', in L. Jones, M. Sidell and J. Douglas (eds), *The Challenge of Promoting Health: Exploration and Action*, 2nd edn. Basingstoke: The Open University in association with Palgrave.

Crichton, N. and Mulhall, A. (2008) 'Epidemiology and Health', in J. Naidoo and J. Wills (eds), *Health Studies: An Introduction*, 2nd edn. Basingstoke: Palgrave Macmillan.

Cross, R. (2010) 'Health Promotion Theory, Models and Approaches', in D. Whitehead and F. Irvine (eds), *Health Promotion and Health Education in Nursing*. Basingstoke: Palgrave Macmillan.

Crossley, M. L. (2000) *Rethinking Health Psychology*. Buckingham: Open University Press.

CSIP National Older People's Mental Health Programme (2007) *Strengthening the Involvement of People with Dementia*. London: CSIP.

Cummins, S. and Macintyre, S. (2006) 'Food Environments and Obesity: Neighbourhood or Nation?', *International Journal of Epidemiology*, 35, 100–4.

Cunningham, C. and Archibald, C. (2006) 'Supporting People with Dementia in Acute Hospital Settings', *Nursing Standard*, 20(43), 51–5.

D'Amato, G. and Cecchi, L. (2008) 'Effects of Climate Change on Environmental Factors in Respiratory Allergic Diseases', *Clinical and Experimental Allergy*, 38, 1264–74.

Dahlgren, G. and Whitehead, M. (1991) *Policies and Strategies to Promote Social Equity in Health*. Stockholm: Institute of Future Studies.

Darlington, Y. and Scott, D. (2002) *Qualitative Research in Practice: Stories from the Field*. Buckingham: Open University Press.

Daulaire, N. (1999) 'Globalization and Health', *Development*, 42(4), 22–4.

Davey, B. (1994a) 'Biomedical Research Methods', in K. McConway (ed.), *Studying Health and Disease*. Buckingham: Open University Press.

Davey, B. (1994b) 'The Nature of Scientific Research', in K. McConway (ed.), *Studying Health and Disease*. Buckingham: Open University Press.

Davey, B. and Seale, C. (1994) 'An Historical Approach to Medical Knowledge', in C. Seale and S. Pattison (eds), *Medical Knowledge: Doubt and Certainty*. Milton Keynes: Open University.

Davies, D. (1998) 'Health and the Discourse of Weight Control', in A. Petersen and C. Waddell (eds), *Health Matters: A Sociology of Illness, Prevention and Care*. Buckingham: Open University Press.

Davis, D. (2004) 'Dementia: Sociological and Philosophical Constructions', *Social Science and Medicine*, 58, 369–78.

Davis, M. (2008) 'The "Loss of Community" and Other Problems for Sexual Citizenship in Recent HIV Prevention', *Sociology of Health and Illness*, 30(2), 182–96.

Davis, W. and Porteous, M. (2006) 'Controversial Topics in Surgery: Joint Replacement in the Overweight Patient', *Annals of the Royal College of Surgeons England*, 89, 203–6.

Daykin, N. and Jones, M. (2008) 'Sociology and Health', in J. Naidoo and J. Wills (eds), *Health Studies: An Introduction*, 2nd edn. Basingstoke: Palgrave Macmillan.

de Lacey S. (2002) 'IVF as Lottery or Investment: Contesting Metaphors in Discourses of Infertility', *Nursing Inquiry*, 9(1). 43–51.

de Laine, M. (2000) *Fieldwork, Participation and Practice: Ethics and Dilemmas in Qualitative Research*. London: Sage.

de Zulueta, P. and Boulton, M. (2007) 'Routine Antenatal HIV Testing: The Responses and Perceptions of Pregnant Women and the Viability of Informed Consent. A Qualitative Study', *Journal of Medical Ethics*, 33, 329–36.

Del Ser, T., McKeith, I., Anand, R., Cicin-Sain, A., Ferrara, R. and Spiegel, R. (2000) 'Dementia with Lewy bodies: Findings from an International Multicentre Study', *International Journal of Geriatric Psychiatry*, 15, 1034–45.

Deaton, A. (2006) 'Global Patterns of Income and Health' *Wider Angle*, 1–3.

Deech, R. (2008) 'Gresham Lectures: Everyone Is Interested in Fertility', *Education Guardian*, 15 July.

Deech, R. and Smajdor, A. (2007) *From IVF to Immortality: Controversy in the Era of Reproductive Technology*. Oxford: Oxford University Press.

Dehn, T. (2007) 'Joint Replacement in the Overweight Patient', *Annals of the Royal College of Surgeons of England*, 89(3), 203–6.

Denney, D. (2005) *Risk and Society*. London: Sage Publications.

Dent, M. (2006) 'Patient Choice and Medicine in Health Care: Responsibilization, Governance and Proto-Professionalization', *Public Management Review*, 8(3), 449–62.

Dent, N. (1995a) 'Asceticism', in T. Honderich (ed.), *The Oxford Companion to Philosophy*. Oxford: Oxford University Press.

Dent, N. (1995b) 'Normative', in T. Honderich (ed.), *The Oxford Companion to Philosophy*. Oxford: Oxford University Press.

Denzin, N. K. (2004) 'Symbolic Interactionism', in U. Flick, E. Von Kardorff and I. Steinke (eds), *A Companion to Qualitative Research*. London: Sage.

Denzin, N. K. and Lincoln, Y.S. (eds) (2008) *Collecting and Interpreting Qualitative Materials*, 3rd edn. Thousand Oaks, CA: Sage Publications.

Denzin, N. K. and Lincoln, Y. S. (eds) (2008) *The Landscape of Qualitative Research*, 3rd edn. Thousand Oaks, CA: Sage Publications.

Devine, F. and Health, S. (1999) *Sociological Research Methods in Context*. Basingstoke: Palgrave.

DHSS (1976) *Prevention and Health: Everybody's Business. A Reassessment of Public and Personal Health*. London: DHSS.

DoH (1990) *The NHS and Community Care Act*. London: Department of Health.

DoH (1992) *The Health of the Nation*. London: Department of Health.

DoH (1998) *Independent Inquiry into Inequalities in Health* (The Acheson Report). London: Stationery Office.

DoH (1999a) *Saving Lives: Our Healthier Nation*. London: Department of Health.

DoH (1999b) *National Service Framework for Mental Health*. London: Department of Health.

DoH (2000a) *The NHS Plan. A Plan for Investment, a Plan for Reform*. London: Department of Health.

DoH (2000b) *National Service Framework for Coronary Heart Disease*. London: Department of Health.

DoH (2001) *Better Prevention, Better Services, Better Sexual Health. The National Strategy for Sexual Health and HIV*. London: Department of Health.

DoH (2002) *Health Check: On the State of the Public Health*. Annual Report of the Chief Medical Officer. London: Department of Health.

DoH (2004a) *Choosing Health: Making Healthy Choices Easier*. London: Department of Health.

DoH (2004b) *At Least Five a Week. Evidence on the Impact of Physical Activity and Its Relationship to Health*. London: Department of Health.

DoH (2007) *Who Cares? Information and Support for the Carers of People with Dementia*. London: Department of Health.

DoH (Lord Darzi) (2008a) *High Quality Care for All: The NHS Next Stage Review Final Report*. London: Department of Health, http://www.dh.gov.uk/en/Publicationsandstatistics/Publications/PublicationsPolicyAndGuidance/DH_085825

DoH (2008b) *Health Inequalities: Progress and Next Steps*. London: Department of Health.

DoH (2009) *Health Trainer: Review to Date, June 2009*. London: Department of Health.

DoH (2010) *The Third Sector*. London: Department of Health, http://www.dh.gov.uk/en/Managingyourorganisation/Financeandplanning/Section64grants/StrategicPartnerProgramme/DH_112468

Dooris, M. and Hunter, D. J. (2007) 'Organisations and Settings for Promoting Public Health', in C. E. Lloyd, S. Handsley, J. Douglas, S. Earle and S. Spurr (eds), *Policy and Practice in Promoting Public Health*. London: Sage Publications in association with the Open University.

Dougherty, C. J. (1993) 'Bad Faith and Victim-Blaming: The Limits of Health Promotion', *Health Care Analysis*, 1, 111–19.

Douglas, J., Jones, L. and Lloyd, E. (2007) 'The Development of Healthy Public Policy', in C. E. Lloyd, S. Handsley, J. Douglas, S. Earle and S. Spurr (eds), *Policy and Practice in Promoting Public Health*. London: Sage Publications in association with the Open University.

Dowling, M. (2007) 'Ethnomethodology: Time for a Revisit', *International Journal of Nursing Studies*, 44, 826–33.

Doyal, L. and Anderson, J. (2005) '"My Fear Is to Fall in Love Again £" How HIV-Positive African Women Survive in London', *Social Science and Medicine*, 60, 1729–38.

Doyal, L. and Gough, I. (1991) *A Theory of Human Need*. Basingstoke: Macmillan.

Doyal, L. and Pennell, I. (1979) *The Political Economy of Health*. London: Pluto Press.

Doyle, A. C., Goldschmidt, A., Huang, C., Winzelberg, A. J., Taylor, C. B. and Wilfley, D. E. (2008) 'Reduction of Overweight and Eating Disorder Symptoms via the Internet in Adolescents: A Randomized Controlled Trial', *Journal of Adolescent Health*, 43, 172–9.

Dresser, D., Yeomans, L. and Loughlan, C. (2008) *Skills for Heatlh. A Review of the Independent Health Sector in England. A Labour Market Intelligence Report. Executive Summary*. London: Skills for Health, http://www.skillsforhealth.org.uk/~/media/Resource-Library/PDF/Labour_Market_Intelligence_report_executive_summary.ashx

Dubin, W. R. and Fink, P. J. (1992) 'Effects of Stigma on Psychiatric Treatment', in P. J. Fink and A. Tasman (eds), *Stigma and Mental Illness*. Washington, DC: American Psychiatric Press.

Dubos, R. (1987) 'Mirage of Health', in B. Davey, A. Gray and C. Seale (eds), *Health and Disease: A Reader*, 3rd edn. Buckingham: Open University Press (2001).

Dunning, W. (1993) 'Post-Modernism and the Construct of the Divisible Self', *British Journal of Aesthetics*, 33(2), 132–1.

Durazo-Arvizu, R. A., McGee, D. L., Cooper, R. S., Liao, Y. and Luke, A. (1998) 'Mortality and Optimal Body Mass Index in a Sample of the US Population', *American Journal of Epidemiology*, 147(8), 739–49.

Dyson, A. (1995) *The Ethics of IVF*. New York: Mowbray.

Earle, S. (2007) 'Promoting Public Health: Exploring the Issues', in S. Earle, C. E. Lloyd, M. Sidell and S. Spurr (eds), *Theory and Research in Promoting Public Health*. London: Sage Publications, in association with the Open University.

Earle, S., Lloyd, C. E., Sidell, M. and Spurr, S. (eds) (2007) *Theory and Research in Promoting Health*. London: Sage Publications in association with the Open University.

Earle, S. and O'Donnell, T. (2007) 'The Factors that Influence Health', in S. Earle, C. E. Lloyd, M. Sidell and S. Spurr (eds), *Theory and Research in Promoting Public Health*. London: Sage Publications, in association with the Open University.

Ebbeling, C. B., Pawlak, D. B. and Ludwig, D. S. (2002) 'Childhood Obesity: Public-Health Crisis, Common Sense Cure', *The Lancet*, 360, 473–82.

Editorial (2005) 'Will Consumerism Lead to Better Health?' *The Lancet*, 366, 343.

Elford, J. and Hart, G. (2005) 'HAART, Viral Load and Sexual Risk Behaviour', *AIDS*, 19, 205–7.

Ellaway, E., Macintyre, S. and Bonnefoy, X. (2005) 'Graffiti, Greenery, and Obesity in Adults: Secondary Analysis of European Cross Sectional Survey', *British Medical Journal*, 331, 611–12.

Elliot, L. (2008) 'Environmentalism', *Encyclopaedia Britannica*, http://www.britannica.com/eb/article-9032737/environmentalism (accessed 25 June 2008).

Engeland, A., Bjørge, T., Søgaard, A. J. and Tverdal, A. (2003) 'Body Mass Index in Adolescence in Relation to Total Mortality: 32-Year Follow-up of 227,000 Norwegian Boys and Girls', *American Journal of Epidemiology*, 157(6), 517–23.

Etzioni, E. (1993) *The Spirit of Community: Rights, Responsibilities and the Communitarian Agenda*. London: Fontana Press.

Evans, D. (2003) 'Hierarchy of Evidence: A Framework for Ranking Evidence Evaluating Healthcare Interventions', *Journal of Clinical Nursing*, 12(1), 77–84.

Evans, C. and Lambert, H. (2008) 'Implementing Community Interventions for HIV Prevention: Insights from Project Ethnography', *Social Science and Medicine*, 66, 467–78.

Evans, J. G. (1997) 'The Rationing Debate: Rationing Health Care by Age: The Case Against', *British Medical Journal*, 314, 822.

Evans, M. and Barker, M. (2006) '"Risking the Kids" versus "Double the Love": Couple Counsellors in Conversation on LGB Parenting', *Gay and Lesbian Issues and Psychology Review*, 3(1), 34–43.

Evans Braziel, J. (2001) 'Sex and Fat Chics: Deterritorializing the Fat Female Body', in J. Evans

Braziel and K. LeBesco (eds), *Bodies Out of Bounds: Fatness and Transgression*. Berkeley: University of California Press.

Falconer, M. and O'Neill, D. (2007) 'Profiling Disability within Nursing Homes: A Census-based Approach', *Age and Ageing*, 36, 209–13.

Family Health International (2004) *Behaviour Change: A Summary of Four Major Theories*, http://ww2.fhi.org/en/aids/aidscap/aidspubs/behres/bcr4theo.html (accessed 21 March 2010).

Feldman, S. and Marks, V. (2005) 'Whose Opinion Can We Trust?', in S. Feldman and V. Marks (eds), *Panic Nation: Unpicking The Myths We're Told About Food and Health*. London: John Blake.

Fenton, S. and Sadiq-Sangster, A. (1996) 'Culture, Relativism and the Expression of Mental Distress: South Asian Women in Britain', *Sociology of Health and Illness*, 18(1), 66–85.

Filiault, S. M. (2008) 'Exercise for Obesity Treatment and Prevention: Current Perspectives and Controversies', in E. M. Blass (ed.), *Obesity, Causes, Mechanisms, Prevention, and Treatment*. Sunderland, MA: Sinauer Associates, Inc.

Finch, H. and Lewis, J. (2003) 'Focus Groups', in J. Ritchie and J. Lewis (eds), *Qualitative Research Practice*. London: Sage.

Fink, P. J. and Tasman, A. (eds) (1992) *Stigma and Mental Illness*. Washington, DC: American Psychiatric Press.

Finkel, D. and Garrett, T. (2001) 'Costs of Treating AIDS in Malawi and America', in B. Davey, A. Gray and C. Seale (eds), *Health and Disease: A Reader*. Maidenhead: Open University Press.

Finlayson, A. (2003) *Making Sense of New Labour*. London: Lawrence and Wishart.

Fitzpatrick, M. (2001) *The Tyranny of Health: Doctors and the Regulation of Lifestyle*. London: Routledge.

Fitzpatrick, M. (2008) 'Childhood Obesity Is not a Form of Child Abuse', http://www.spiked-online.com/index.php?/site/article/5797/ (accessed 5 June 2009).

Flegal, K. M., Graubard, B. I., Williamson, D. F. and Gail, M. H. (2005) 'Excess Deaths Associated with Underweight, Overweight and Obesity', *JAMA*, 20 April, 293(15), 1861–7.

Flegal, K. M., Graubard, B. I., Williamson, D. F. and Gail, M. H. (2007) 'Cause-Specific Excess Deaths Associated with Underweight, Overweight and Obesity', *JAMA*, 7 November, 298(17), 2028–37.

Flick, U., Von Kardorff, E. and Steinke, I. (eds) (2004) *A Companion to Qualitative Research*. London: Sage.

Fontaine, K. R., Redden, D. T., Wang, C., Westfall, A. O. and Allison, D. B. (2003) 'Years of Life Lost Due to Obesity', *JAMA*, 289(2), 187–93.

Forder, J. (2008) 'The Costs of Addressing Age Discrimination in Social Care', PSSRU Discussion Paper 2538.

Foster-Turner, J. (2009) 'Focus Groups', in J. Neale (ed.), *Research Methods for Health and Social Care*. Basingstoke: Palgrave Macmillan.

Fotaki, M. (2007) 'Patient Choice in Healthcare in England and Sweden: From Quasi-Market and Back to the Market? A Comparative Analysis of Failure in Unlearning', *Public Administration*, 85(4), 1059–75.

Fox, M., Martin, P. and Green, G. (2007) *Doing Practitioner Research*. London: Sage.

Fox, N. (1998) '"Risks", "Hazards" and Life Choices: Reflections on Health at Work', *Sociology*, 32(4), 665–87.

Francis, B. (2000) 'Poststructuralism and Nursing: Uncomfortable Bedfellows?', *Nursing Inquiry*, 7(1), 20–8.

Franco, A., Álvarez-Dardet, C. and Ruiz, M. T. (2004) 'Effect of Democracy on Health: Ecological Study', *British Medical Journal*, 329, 1421–3.

Frankel, R. M. and Devers, K. J. (2000) 'Study Design in Qualitative Research –1: Developing Questions and Assessing Resource Needs', *Education for Health*, 13(2), 251–61.

Franklin, S. (1997) *Embodied Progress: A Cultural Account of Assisted Conception*. London: Routledge.

Freire, P. (1972) 'Pedagogy of the Oppressed: An Abstract', in M. Sidell, L. Jones, J. Katz and A. Peberdy (eds), *Debates and Dilemmas in Promoting Health: A Reader*. Basingstoke: Macmillan in association with the Open University (1997).

French, J. (2007) 'The Market-Dominated Future of Public Health?', in J. Douglas, S. Earle, S. Handsley, C. E. Lloyd and S. Spurr (eds), *A Reader in Promoting Public Health: Challenge and Controversy*. London: Sage Publications in association with the Open University.

Furedi, F. (2007) 'Environmentalism', http://www.spiked-online.com/index.php/site/article/3817/ (accessed 12 September 2007).

Future Vision Coalition (2008) *A New Vision for Mental Health*. Discussion Paper, The Future Vision Coalition.

Gambrill, E. (1999) 'Evidence-Based Practice: An Alternative to Authority-Based Practice', *Families in Society: The Journal of Contemporary Human Services*, 80(4), 341–50.

Gard, M. and Wright, J. (2005) *The Obesity Epidemic, Science, Morality and Ideology*. London: Routledge.

Garfinkel, H. (1967) *Studies in Ethnomethodology*. Englewood Cliffs, NJ: Prentice-Hall.

Garner, D. and Wooley, S. (1991) 'Confronting the Failure of Behavioural and Dietary Treatments for Obesity', *Clinical Psychological Review*, 11, 729–80.

Gastaldo, D. (1997) 'Is Health Education Good for You: Rethinking Health Education through the Concept of Bio-Power', in A. Petersen and R. Bunton (eds), *Foucault: Health and Medicine*. London: Routledge.

Gergen, Mary McCanney and Gergen, Kenneth J. (2003) *Social Construction: A Reader*. London: Sage.

Gibbs, A. (1997) *Social Research Update*, Issue 19.

Gibbs, G. (2007) *Analysing Qualitative Data*. London: Sage.

Gilbert, N. (ed.) (1993) *Researching Social Life*. London: Sage.

Gill, John, Johnson, Phil (1997) *Research Methods for Managers*. London: Paul Chapman.

Gillam, S., Yates, J. and Badrinath, P. (eds) (2007) *Essential Public Health: Theory and Practice*. Cambridge: Cambridge University Press.

Gilliard, J., Means, R., Beattie, A. and Daker-White, G. (2005) 'Dementia Care in England and the Social Model of Disability', *Dementia*, 4(4), 571–86.

Gilson, L. (2003) 'Trust and the Development of Health Care as a Social Institution', *Social Science and Medicine*, 56, 1453–68.

Gimenez, M. E. (1999) 'For Structure: A Critique of Ontological Individualism', *Alethia*, 2(2), 19–25.

Glanville, J., Glenny, A.-M., Melville, A., O' Meara, S., Sharp, F., Sheldon, T. and Wilson, C. (1997) 'The Prevention and Treatment of Obesity', *Effective Health Care*, 3(2).

Glendon, M. A. (1991) *Rights Talk: The Impoverishment of Political Discourse*. New York: The Free Press.

Gobo, G. (2004) 'Sampling, Representativeness and Generalizability', in C. Seale, G. Gobo, J. Gubrium and D. Silverman (eds), *Qualitative Research Practice*. London: Sage.

Goffman, E. (1963) *Stigma: Notes on the Management of Spoiled Identity*. London: Penguin Books.

Goldsmith, M. (1996) *Hearing the Voice of People with Dementia: Opportunities and Obstacles*. London: Jessica Kingsley.

Goodman, R. (2001) 'A Traveller in Time: Understanding Deterrents to Walking to Work', *World Transport Policy and Practice*, 7(4), 50–4.

Gomm, R. (2009) *Key Concepts in Social Research Methods*. Basingstoke: Palgrave Macmillan.

Gorz, A. (1983) *Ecology as Politics*. London: Pluto Press.

Gould, N. and Kendall, T. (2007) 'Developing the NICE/SCIE Guidelines for Dementia Care: The Challenges of Enhancing the Evidence Base for Social and Health Care', *British Journal of Social Work*, 37, 475–90.

Graham, Nori, Lindesay, James, Katona, Cornelius, Manoel Bertolote, José , Camus, Vincent, Copeland, John R. M., de Mendonça Lima, Carlos A., Gaillard, Michel, Gély Nargeot, Marie Christine, Gray, John, Jacobsson, Lars, Kingma, Mireille, Kühne, Nicolas, O'Loughlin, Anne, Rutz, Wolfgang, Saraceno, Benedetto and Taintor, Zebulon (2003) 'Reducing Stigma and

Discrimination against Older People with Mental Disorders: A Technical Consensus Statement', *International Journal of Geriatric Psychiatry*, 18, 670–8.

Gray, A. (1993) 'Rationing and Choice', in B. Davey and J. Popay (eds), *Dilemmas in Health Care*. Buckingham: Open University Press.

Gray, D. E. (2004) *Doing Research in the Real World*. London: Sage.

Gray, D. E. (2009) *Doing Research in the Real World*, 2nd edn. London: Sage.

Green, J. (2007) 'The Use of Focus Groups in Research into Health', 112–32, in M. Saks and J. Allsop (eds), *Researching Health: Qualitative, Quantitative and Mixed Methods*. London: Sage

Green, J. and South, J. (2006) *Evaluation*. Maidenhead: Open University Press.

Greenfield, S (2002) *In Our Time*, BBC Radio 4, 16 May.

Griffin, A. (2007) 'UK Nears European Average in Proportion of GDP Spent on Health Care', *British Medical Journal*, 334, 442.

Grimmett, C., Croker, H., Carnell, S. and Wardle, J. (2008) 'Telling Parents Their Child's Weight Status: Psychological Impact of a Weight-Screening Program', *Pediatrics*, 122, e688, http://pediatrics.aappublications.org/cgi/content/abstract/122/3/e682 (accessed 5 June 2009).

Grimshaw, A. (1999) 'Feminism', in A. Bullock and S. Trombley (eds), *The New Fontana Dictionary of Modern Thought*, 3rd edn. London: HarperCollins.

Guba, E. G. (1990) *The Paradigm Dialog*. Newbury Park, CA and London: Sage.

Guba, E. G. and Lincoln, Y. S. (1998) 'Competing Paradigms in Qualitative Research', in N. K. Denzin and Y. S. Lincoln (eds), *The Landscape of Qualitative Inquiry*. London: Sage.

Guba, E. G. and Lincoln, Y. S. (2004) 'Competing Paradigms in Qualitative Research: Theories and Issues', 17–38, in S. N. Hesse-Biber and P. Leavy (eds), *Approaches to Qualitative Research: A Reader on Theory and Practice*. New York: Oxford University Press.

Haas, S. (2002) 'Social Support as Relationship Maintenance in Gay Male Couples Coping with HIV or AIDS', *Journal of Social and Personal Relationships*, 19(1), 87–111.

Habermas, J. (2007) 'The Language Game of Responsible Agency and the Problem of Free Will: How Can Epistemic Dualism Be Reconciled with Ontological Monism?', *Philosophy Explorations*, 10(1), 13–50.

Haglund, K. (2004) 'Conducting Life History Research with Adolescents', *Qualitative Health Research*, 14(9), 1309–19.

Hamlin, C. (1995) 'Finding a Function for Public Health: Disease Theory or Political Philosophy?', *Journal of Health Politics, Policy and Law*, 20(4), 1025–31.

Handsley, S. and Sidell, M., incorporating previously published material from Thornley, P. (2007a) 'Working with Communities to Promote Public Health', 287–320, in C. E. Lloyd, S. Handsley, J. Douglas, S. Earle and S. Spurr (eds), Policy and Practice in Promoting Public Health. London: Sage Publications in association with The Open University.

Handsley, S. (2007b) 'Promoting Mental Health and Social Inclusion', in C. E. Lloyd, S. Handsley, J. Douglas, S. Earle and S. Spurr (eds), Policy and Practice in Promoting Public Health. London: Sage Publications in association with the Open University.

Handsley, S., Noguera, A., Beaumont, K. (2007c) 'Gauging the Effectiveness of Community-Based Public Health Projects', 321–51, in C. E. Lloyd, S. Handsley, J. Douglas, S. Earle and S. Spurr (eds), Policy and Practice in Promoting Public Health. London: Sage Publications in association with The Open University.

Handy, C. (1998) *The Hungry Spirit: New Thinking for a New World*. London: Arrow Books.

Hardin, R. (1995) 'Democracy', in T. Honderich (ed.), *The Oxford Companion to Philosophy*. Oxford: Oxford University Press.

Harding, S. (ed.) (1987) *Feminism and Methodology*. Indianapolis: Indiana University Press.

Harper, S. and La Fontaine, J. (2009) 'Ethnography', in J. Neale (ed.) *Research Methods for Health and Social Care*. Basingstoke: Palgrave Macmillan.

Harris, J. (1985) *The Value of Life: An Introduction to Medical Ethics*. London: Routledge.

Harris, M. and Taylor, G. (2004) *Medical Statistics Made Easy*. London: Martin Dunitz.

Harrison, J. and Gill, A. (2010) 'The Experience and Consequence of People with Mental Health

Problems, the Impact of Stigma upon People with Schizophrenia: A Way Forward', *Journal of Psychiatric and Mental Health Nursing*, 17, 242–50.

Hart, C. (1998) *Doing a Literature Review: Releasing the Social Science Research Imagination*. London: Sage.

Hart, N. (1985) *The Sociology of Health and Medicine*. Ormskirk: Causeway Press.

Harvey, J. H. and Wenzel, A. (2002) 'HIV, AIDS, and Close Relationships', *Journal of Social and Personal Relationships*, 19(1), 135–42.

Haslett, D. W. (1995) 'Socialism', in T. Honderich (ed.), *The Oxford Companion to Philosophy*. Oxford: Oxford University Press.

Hattersley, L. (1997) 'Expectations ofLife by Social Class', 73–82, in F. Drever and M. Whitehead (eds), *Health Inequalities: Decennial Supplement*, London: Stationery Office.

Health Improvement Analytical Team – Monitoring Unit (2007) *Health Profile of England 2007*. London: DoH.

Health Professions Council (2010) http://www.hpc-uk.org/registrants/cpd/

Health Protection Agency (2008, 2010) *New HIV Diagnoses Surveillance Tables*. London: HPA.

Healthcare for London (n.d.) *A Framework for Action*, 2nd edn. London: NHS London, http://www.healthcareforlondon.nhs.uk/a-framework-for-action-2/

Hek, G., Judd, M. and Moule, P. (1996) *Making Sense of Research: An Introduction for Nurses*. London: Cassell.

Helman, C. G. (1994) *Culture, Health and Illness*, 3rd edn. Oxford: Butterworth-Heinemann.

Helwig, C. C. (2008) 'Book Review: Don't Blame It on the Enlightenment – Law, S. (2006) The War for Children's Minds', *Journal of Applied Developmental Psychology*, 29, 170–3.

Hesketh, K., Waters, E., Green, J., Salmon, L. and Williams, J. (2005) 'Health Eating, Activity and Obesity Prevention: A Qualitative Study of Parent and Child Perceptions in Australia', *Health Promotion International*, 20(1), 19–26.

Heslop, K. (2010) 'How Does the US Healthcare Compare to the Rest of the World?', http://www.guardian.co.uk/news/datablog/2010/mar/22/us-healthcare-bill-rest-of-world-obama#data (accessed 10 April 2010).

Hills, J., Brewer, M., Jenkins, S., Lister, R., Lupton, R., Machin, S., Mills, C., Modood, T., Rees, T. and Riddell, S. (2010) *An Anatomy of Economic Inequality in the UK: Report of the National Equity Panel*. London: Government Equalities Office and Centre for Analysis of Social Exclusion, LSE.

Hillsdon, M., Foster, C., Cavill, N., Crombie, H. and Naidoo, B. (2005) *The Effectiveness of Public Health Interventions for Increasing Physical Activity Among Adults: A Review of Reviews – Evidence Briefing*, 2 February. London: Health Development Agency.

Hitchcock-Nöel, P. and Pugh, J. A. (2002) 'Management of Overweight and Obese Adults', *British Medical Journal*, 325, 5 October, 757–61.

Hodder, I. (1998) 'The Interpretation of Documents and Material Culture', in N. K. Denzin and Y. S. Lincoln (eds), *Collecting and Interpreting Qualitative Materials*. Thousand Oaks, CA: Sage.

Hoedemaekers, R. and Dekkers, W. (2003) 'Justice and Solidarity in Priority Setting in Health Care', *Health Care Analysis*, 11(4), 325–43.

Holborn, M. (1999) 'Modernity', in A. Bullock and S. Trombley (eds), *The New Fontana Dictionary of Modern Thought*, 3rd edn. London: HarperCollins.

Hong, E. (2000) *Globalisation and the Impact on Health: A Third World View*, prepared for The Peoples' Health Assembly, 4–8 December, Savar, Banglasdesh, http://www.phmovement.org/pubs/issuepapers/hong.html (accessed July 2007).

Hope, V. D., Judd, A., Hickman, M., Sutton, A., Stimson, G. V., Parry, J. V. and Gill, O. N. (2005) 'HIV Prevalence among Injecting Drug Users in England and Wales 1990 to 2003: Evidence for Increased Transmission in Recent Years', *AIDS*, 19(11), 1207–14.

Horan, F. (2006) 'Obesity and Joint Replacement', *Journal of Bone and Joint Surgery*, 88-B(10), 1269–71.

Horne, M. (2003) 'Identifying the Health Needs of Communities and Populations', in J. Costello and M. Haggart (eds), *Public Health and Society*. Basingstoke: Macmillan.

Houston, A. M. and Cowley S. (2002) 'An Empowerment Approach to Needs Assessment in Health Visiting Practice', *Journal of Clinical Nursing Practice*, 11, 640–50.

Huff, J. L. (2001) 'A "Horror of Corpulence": Interrogating Bantingism and Mid-Nineteenth Century Fat-Phobia', 39–59, in J. Evans Braziel and K. LeBesco (eds), *Bodies Out of Bounds: Fatness and Transgression*. Berkeley, University of California Press.

Hughes, A., Davies, B. and Gudmundsdottir, M. (2008) '"Can You Give Me Respect?" Experiences of the Urban Poor on a Dedicated AIDS Nursing Home Unit', *Journal of the Association of Nurses in AIDS Care*, 19(5), 342–56.

Hughes, D. (2007) 'Participant Observation in Health Research', in M. Saks and J. Allsop (eds), *Researching Health: Qualitative, Quantitative and Mixed Methods*. London: Sage.

Hussey, R. (2009) 'Introduction: Health Inequalities and Impact on the Economy', Northwest Regional Development Agency and NHS North West Conference Report compiled by Pathways Consultancy Ltd.

Imperial Cancer Research Fund Oxcheck Study Group (1995) 'Effectiveness of the Health Checks Conducted by Nurses in Primary Care: Final Results of the Oxcheck Study', *British Medical Journal*, 310, 1099–104.

Illich, I. (1976) *Limits to Medicine. Medical Nemesis: The Expropriation of Health*. London: Pelican Books.

Inhorn, M. C. and van Balen, F. (2002) 'Introduction. Interpreting Infertility: A View from the Social Sciences', in M. C. Inhorn and F. van Balen (eds), *Infertility around the Globe: New Thinking on Childlessness, Gender and Reproductive Technologies*. Berkeley and Los Angeles: University of California Press.

Innes, A. D., Campion, P. D. and Griffiths, F. E. (2005) 'Complex Consultations and the "Edge of Chaos"', *British Journal of General Practice*, January, 47–52.

Iphofen, R. (2003) 'Social and Individual Factors Influencing Public Health', in J. Costello and M. Haggart (eds), *Public Health and Society*. Basingstoke: Palgrave Macmillan.

Irvine, F. (2010) 'Contextualising Health Promotion', in D. Whitehead and F. Irvine (eds), *Health Promotion and Health Education in Nursing: A Framework for Practice*. Basingstoke: Palgrave Macmillan.

Jackson, D., Mannix, J., Faga, P. and McDonald, G. (2005) 'Overweight and Obese Children: Mothers' Strategies', *Journal of Advanced Nursing*, 52(1), 6–13.

Janz, N. K., Champion, V. L. and Strecher, V. J. (2002) 'The Health Belief Model', in K. Glanz, B. K. Rimer and F. M. Lewis (eds), *Health Behaviour and Health Education: Theory, Research and Practice*, 3rd edn. San Francisco: Jossey-Bass.

Jarviluoma, H., Moisala, P. and Vilkko, A. (2003) *Gender and Qualitative Methods*. London: Sage.

Jewell, P. (1992) 'Snake Oil, Sophistry and Sterile Syllogisms', in P. Jewell (ed.), *On the Same Premises: Proceedings of the Second National Conference in Reasoning, Flinders University, 1991*. Adelaide: Flinders University Press

Johns, C. (2009) *Becoming a Reflective Practitioner*, 3rd edn. Oxford: Wiley-Blackwell.

Joint United Nations Programme on HIV/AIDS (UNAIDS) and World Health Organization (WHO) (2006) *AIDS Epidemic Update*, December 2006. Geneva Switzerland: UNAIDS.

Jones, E. L. and Pickstone, J. V. (2008) *The Quest for Public Health in Manchester. The Industrial City, the NHS and the Recent History*. Oxford: Manchester NHS Primary Care Trust in association with the Centre for the History of Science, Technology and Medicine, University of Manchester.

Jones, F. R. (2003) 'Can Expert Patients Be Created?', Expert Patient Conference, May, http://www.rpsgb.org/pdfs/exptpatsem6.pdf (accessed 18 May 2007).

Jones, K. (2007) 'Doing a Literature Review in Health', in M. Saks and J. Allsop (eds), *Researching Health: Qualitative, Quantitative and Mixed Methods*. London: Sage.

Jones, L. (2000) 'What Is Health?', in J. Katz, A. Peberdy and A. Douglas (eds), *Promoting Health: Knowledge and Practice*, 2nd edn. Basingstoke: Palgrave in association with the Open University.

Jones, L., Sidell, M. and Douglas, J. (eds) (2002) *The Challenge of Promoting Health: Exploration and Action*, 2nd edn. Basingstoke: Palgrave in association with the Open University.

Jones, R. (2008) http://www.philosopher.org.uk/enl.htm (accessed 2 September 2008).

Kagan, C. (2006) *Making a Difference: Participation and Wellbeing*. RENEW Intelligence Report, January, http://www.RENEW.co.uk

Kalish, R. A. (1966) 'A Continuum of Subjectively Perceived Death', *The Gerontologist*, 6, 73–6.

Katz, J.,(2000) 'Studying Populations', in J. Katz, A. Peberdy and A. Douglas (eds), *Promoting Health: Knowledge and Practice*, 2nd edn. Basingstoke: Palgrave in association with the Open University.

Katz, S. (1994) 'Secular Morality', 297–330, in A. M. Brandt and P. Rozin (eds), *Morality and Health*, New York: Routledge.

Kelman, S. (1988) 'The Social Nature of the Definition Problem in Health', in L. Mackay et al. (eds), *Classic Texts in Health Care*. Oxford: Butterworth Heinemann (1998).

Kernick, D. (2006) 'Wanted: New Methodologies for Health Service Research. Is Complexity Theory the Answer?', *Family Practice*, 23, 385–90.

King, E., De Silva, M., Stein, A. and Patel, V. (2009) 'Interventions for Improving the Psychosocial Well-Being of Children Affected by HIV and AIDS', *Cochrane Database of Systematic Reviews*, Issue 3.

Kitwood, T. (1997) *Dementia Reconsidered*. Maidenhead: Open University Press.

Kitzinger, C. (2004) 'Feminist Approaches', in C. Seale, G. Gobo, J. F. Gubrium and D. Silverman (eds), *Qualitative Research Practice*. London: Sage.

Klein, R. (1978) *The Politics of the NHS*. 2nd edn. London: Longman.

Klein, R. (1984) 'Rationing Health Care', *British Medical Journal*, 289(6438), 143–4.

Klein, R. (1996) *Eat Fat*. London: Picador.

Klein, R. (2001) 'Fat Beauty', in J. Evans Braziel and K. LeBesco (eds), *Bodies Out of Bounds: Fatness and Transgression*. Berkeley, University of California Press.

Klunklin, A. and Greenwood, J. (2006) 'Symbolic Interactionism in Grounded Theory Studies: Women Surviving with HIV/AIDS in Rural Northern Thailand', *Journal of the Association of Nurses in AIDS Care*, 17(5), 32–41.

Kobau, R., Dilorio, C., Chapman, D. and Delvecchio, P. (2010) 'Attitudes about Mental Illness and Its Treatment: Validation of a Generic Scale for Public Health Surveillance of Mental Illness Associated Stigma', *Community Mental Health Journal*, 46, 164–76.

Korkeila, M., Rissanen, A., Kaprio, J., Sørensen, T. I. A. and Koskenvuo, M. (1999) 'Weight Loss Attempts and Risk of Major Weight Gain: A Prospective Study in Finnish Adults, *American Journal of Clinical Nutrition*, 70, 965–75.

Kymlicka, W. (1995) 'Liberalism', in T. Honderich (ed.), *The Oxford Companion to Philosophy*. Oxford: Oxford University Press.

Labonte, R. and Schrecker, T. (2007a) 'Globalisation and Social Determinants of Health: Introduction and Methodological Background (Part 1 of 3)', *Globalisation and Health*, 3(5), http://www.globalizationandhealth.com/content/3/1/5

Labonte, R. and Schrecker, T. (2007b) 'Globalisation and Social Determinants of Health: Promoting Health Equity in Global Governance (Part 3 of 3)', *Globalisation and Health*, 3(7), http://www.globalizationandhealth.com/content/3/1/5

Lacey, A. (1995) 'Positivism', in T. Honderich (ed.), *The Oxford Companion to Philosophy*. Oxford: Oxford University Press.

La Fontaine, J., Ahuja, J., Bradbury, N.M., Phillips, S. and Oyebode, J. R. (2007) 'Understanding Dementia amongst People in Minority Ethnic and Cultural Groups', *Journal of Advanced Nursing*, 60(6), 605–14.

Lai, Y. M., Hong, C. P. H. and Chee, C. Y. I. (2000) 'Stigma of Mental Illness', *Singapore Medical Journal*, 42(3), 111–14.

Lalonde Report (1974) *A New Perspective on the Health of Canadians*. Ottawa: Government of Canada.

Lancet Oncology (2008) 'NHS Infrastructure Is Centre of Attention Again', *The Lancet*, 9, 209, http://www.thelancet.com/oncology (accessed May 2010).

Last, J. M. (ed.) (2007) *A Dictionary of Public Health*. Oxford: Oxford University Press.

Laverack, G. (2005) *Public Health, Power, Empowerment and Professional Practice*. Basingstoke: Palgrave Macmillan.

Laverack, G. (2006) 'Improving Health Outcomes through Community Empowerment: A Review of the Literature', *Journal of Health and Population Nutrition*, 24(1), 113–20.

Laverack, G. (2009) *Public Health, Power, Empowerment and Professional Practice*, 2nd edn. Basingstoke: Palgrave Macmillan.

Law in Action (2009) *The Limits to Rights*, 20 January, http://news.bbc.co.uk/1/hi/programmes/law_in_action/7838424.stm (accessed April 2010).

Law, B. and Watts, A. G. (1977) *Schools, Careers and Community*. London: Church Information Office.

Lawton, L. (1999) 'Approaches to Needs Assessment', in E. R. Perkins, I. Simnett and L. Wright (eds), *Evidence-Based Health Promotion*. Chichester: Wiley.

Leach, M., Neale, J. and Kemp, P. A. (2009) 'Literature Reviews', in J. Neale (ed.), *Research Methods for Health and Social Care*. Basingstoke: Palgrave Macmillan.

Lee, S. H. and Sheon, N. (2008) 'Responsibility and Risk: Accounts of Reasons for Seeking an HIV Test', *Sociology of Health and Illness*, 30(2), 167–81.

Le Fanu, J. (1999) *The Rise and Fall of Modern Medicine*. London: Abacus.

Leatherman, S. and Sutherland, K. (2003) *The Quest for Quality in the NHS: A Mid-Term Evaluation of the Ten-Year Quality Agenda*. London: The Nuffield Trust.

Lechte, J. (1994) *Fifty Key Contemporary Thinkers: From Structuralism to Postmodernity*. London: Routledge.

Ledger, W., Anumba, D., Marlow, N., Thomas, C., Wilson, E. and the Cost of Multiple Birth Study Group (COMBS Group) (2006) 'The Costs to the NHS of Multiple Births after IVF Treatment in the UK', *BJOG: An International Journal of Obstetrics and Gynaecology*, 113, 21–5.

Lee, S. H. and Sheon, N. (2008) 'Responsibility and Risk: Accounts of Reasons for Seeking an HIV Test', *Sociology of Health and Illness*, 30(2), 167–81.

Leedy, P. D., Ertmer, P. A. and Newby, T. J. (1996) *Practical Research: Planning and Design*, 6th edn. Upper Saddle River, NJ: Merrill.

Leeuw, E de (1989) 'Concepts in Health Promotion: The Notion of Relativism', *Social Science and Medicine*, 29(11), 1281–8.

Legard, R., Keegan, J. and Ward, K. (2003) 'In-Depth Interviews', 138–69, in J. Ritchie and J. Lewis (eds), *Qualitative Research Practice: A Guide for Social Research Students and Researchers*. Thousand Oaks, CA: Sage.

Leichter, H. M. (1997) 'Lifestyle Correctness and the New Secular Morality', in A. M. Brandt and P. Rozin (eds), *Morality and Health*. New York: Routledge.

Leonard, L. and Ellen, J. M. (2008) '"The Story of My Life": AIDS and "Autobiographical Occasions"', *Qualitative Sociology*, 31, 37–56.

Letherby, G. (2003) *Feminist Research in Theory and Practice*. Buckingham: Open University Press.

Lewis, J. and Ritchie, J. (2003) 'Generalising from Qualitative Research', 263–86, in J. Ricthie and J. Lewis (eds), *Qualitative Research Practice: A Guide for Social Science Students and Researchers*. London: Sage.

Lewith, G. and Little, P. (2007) 'Randomised Controlled Trials', in M. Saks and J. Allsop (eds), *Researching Health: Qualitative, Quantitative and Mixed Methods*. London: Sage.

Leyshon, S. (2002) 'Empowering Practitioners: An Unrealistic Expectation of Nurse Education?', *Journal of Advanced Nursing*, 40(4), 466–74.

Liddle, R. (2008) 'Laugh at Lard Butts – But Just Remember Fatty Fritz Lives Longer', *Sunday Times*, 27 January, http://www.timesonline.co.uk/tol/comment/columnists/rod_liddle/article3257063.ece (accessed April 2010).

Lilley, R. (1999) 'The Road to Wellville', *British Journal of Health Care Management*, 5(7), 259–60.

Link, B. G. and Phelan, J. C. (2001) 'Conceptualizing Stigma', *Annual Sociology Review*, 27, 363–85.

Liss, P.-E. (1998) 'Assessing Health Care Need: The Conceptual Foundation', in S. Baldwin (ed.), *Needs Assessment and Community Care: Clinical Practice and Policy Making*. Oxford: Butterworth-Heinemann.

Lloyd, C. E., Handsley, S., Douglas, J., Earle, S. and Spurr S. (eds) (2007) *Policy and Practice in Promoting Public Health*. London: The Open University in association with Sage Publications.

Loewy, E. H. (1999) 'Health-Care Systems and Ethics: What Can We Learn?', *Health Care Analysis*, 7, 309–20.

Lomas, J. (1998) 'Social Capital and Health: Implications for Public Health and Epidemiology', *Social Science and Medicine*, 47, 1181–8.

Lomborg, B. (2001) *The Skeptical Environmentalist: Measuring the Real State of the World*. Cambridge: Cambridge University Press.

Lomborg, B. (2007) *Cool It: The Skeptical Environmentalist's Guide to Global Warming*. New York: Random House.

Loughlin, M. (1994) 'Rationalities, Harm and Risk', *Health Care Analysis*, 2, 123–7.

Lowe, J. (1999) 'Relativism', in A. Bullock and S. Trombley (eds), *The New Fontana Dictionary of Modern Thought*, 3rd edn. London: HarperCollins.

Lupton, D. (2000) 'Food, Risk and Subjectivity', in S. J. Williams, J. Gabe and M. Calnan (eds), *Health, Medicine and Society: Key Theories, Future Agendas*. London: Routledge.

Lupton, D. (2003) *Medicine as Culture*, 2nd edn. London: Sage.

Lye, J. (2004) 'Notes on Post-structuralism', http://www.brocku.ca/english/courses/4F70/poststruct.html (accessed May 2007).

Lyotard, J. F. (1984) *The Postmodern Condition: A Report on Knowledge*. Manchester: Manchester University Press.

McConway, K. (ed.) (1994) *Studying Health and Disease*. Buckingham: Open University Press.

Macdonald, K. and Tipton, C. (1993) 'Using Documents', in N. Gilbert (ed.), *Researching Social Life*. London: Sage.

McDonald, R., Mead, N., Cheraghi-Sohi, S., Bower, P., Whalley, D. and Roland, M. (2007) 'Governing the Ethical Consumer: Identity, Choice and the Primary Care Medical Encounter', *Sociology of Health and Illness*, 29(3), 430–56.

MacErlean, N. (2008) 'Bosses Join the IVF Learning Curve', *The Observer*, 20 July.

MacIntyre, A. (1985) *After Virtue: A Study in Moral Theory*, 2nd edn. London: Duckworth.

McKeith, I. and Fairbairn, A. (2001) 'Biomedical and Clinical Perspectives', in C. Cantley (ed.), *A Handbook of Dementia Care*. Buckingham: Open University Press.

McKeown, T. and Lowe, C. R. (1974) *An Introduction to Social Medicine*. Oxford: Blackwell Science.

McKibben, B. (2006) *The End of Nature*. New York: Random House.

McMenamin, J. (2009) Skills Rating Exercise, University of Westminster Careers Service.

MacRae, H. (2008) '"Making the Best You Can of It": Living with Early-Stage Alzheimer's Disease', *Sociology of Health and Illness*, 30(3), 396–412.

Mahoney, Rachel, Regan, C., Katona, C. and Livingston, G. (2005) 'Anxiety and Depression in Family Caregivers of People with Alzheimer Disease: The LASER-AD Study', *American Journal of Geriatric Psychiatry*, 13(9), 795–801.

Mansfield, K. (1977) *Letters and Journals*. London: Pelican Books.

Manson, J. E., Willett, W. C., Stampfer, M. J., Colditz, G. A., Hunter, D. J., Hankinson, S. E., Hennekens, C. H. and Speizer, F. E. (1995) 'Body Weight and Mortality among Women', *New England Journal of Medicine*, 333(11), 677–85.

Marantz, P. (1990) 'Blaming the Victim: The Negative Consequences of Preventive Health Medicine', *American Journal of Public Health*, 80(1), 1187.

Marmot, M., Allen, J., Goldblatt, P., Boyce, T., McNeish, D., Grady, M. and Geddes, I. (2010) *Fair Society, Healthy Lives*. The Marmot Review Executive Summary. Strategic Review of Health Inequalities in England post-2010.

Marmot, M., Friel, S., Bell, R., Houweling, T. A. J. and Taylor, S., on behalf of the Commission on Social Determinants of Health (2008) 'Closing the Gap in a Generation: Health Equity through Action on the Social Determinants of Health', *The Lancet*, 372, 1661–9.

Marshall, L. and Rowland, F. (2006) *A Guide to Learning Independently*, 4th edn. Melbourne: Pearson Longman.

Martin, G. (2005) 'The Global Health Governance of Antimicrobial Effectiveness', *Globalization and Health BioMed Central Globalization and Health*, 2(7), http://www.globalizationandhealth.com/content/2/1/7

Martin, G. P. (2008) '"Ordinary People Only": Knowledge, Representativeness, and the Publics of Public Participation in Healthcare', *Sociology of Health and Illness*, 30(1), 35–54.

Martinez-Lavin, M., Infante, O. and Lerma, C. (2008) 'Hypothesis: The Chaos and Complexity Theory May Help our Understanding of Fibromyalgia and Similar Maladies', *Seminars in Arthritis and Rheumatism*, 37, 260–4.

Martyn, C. (2004) 'Commentary: Politics as a Determinant of Health', *British Medical Journal*, 329, 1423–4.

Mathias, P. (1969) *The First Industrial Nation: An Economic History of Britain 1700–1914*. London: Methuen and Co.

Matthews, B. and Ross, L. (2010) *Research Methods: A Practical Guide for the Social Sciences*. Harlow: Longman.

Maurer, F. A. and Smith, C. M. (2005) *Public Health Nursing Practice: Health for Families and Populations*, 3rd edn. Baltimore: Elsevier Saunders.

May, T. (2002) *Qualitative Research in Action*. London: Sage.

Maynard, M. (1999) 'Gender Relations', in S. Taylor (ed.), *Sociology: Issues and Debates*. Basingstoke: Macmillan.

Maynard, M. (1994) 'Methods, Practice and Epistemology: The Debate about Feminism and Research', in M. Maynard and J. Purvis (eds), *Researching Women's Lives from a Feminist Perspective*. London: Taylor & Francis.

Meerabeau, L. (1998) 'Consumerism and Health Care: The Example of Fertility Treatment', *Journal of Advanced Nursing*, 27, 721–9.

Miller, W. C. (1999) 'Fitness and Fatness in Relation to Health: Implications for a Paradigm Shift', *Journal of Social Issues*, 2, 207–19.

Miller, William L. and Crabtree, Benjamin F. (1999) *Doing Qualitative Research*. Thousand Oaks, CA and London: Sage.

Miller, W. .L, Crabtree, B. F., McDaniel, R. and Stange, K. C. (1998) 'Understanding Change in Primary Care Practice Using Complexity Theory', *Journal of Family Practice*, 46(5), 369.

Mills, M. (ed.) (1993) *Prevention, Health and British Politics*. Aldershot: Avebury.

Mills, M. and Saward, M. (1993) 'Liberalism, Democracy and Prevention', in M. Mills (ed.), *Prevention, Health and British Politics*. Aldershot: Avebury.

Milne, A. (2010) 'The "D" Word: Reflections on the Relationship between Stigma, Discrimination and Dementia', *Journal of Mental Health*, 19(3), 227–33.

Mitchell, K. (2003) *The Unplanned Career: How to Turn Curiosity into Opportunity*. San Francisco: Chronicle Books.

Monaghan, L. F. (2007) 'Body Mass Index, Masculinities and Moral Worth: Men's Critical Understandings of "Appropriate" Weight-for-Height', *Sociology of Health and Illness*, 29(4), 584–609.

Montaño, D. E. and Kasprzyk, D. (2002) 'The Theory of Reasoned Action and the Theory of Planned Behaviour', in K. Glanz, B. K. Rimer and F. M. Lewis (eds), *Health Behaviour and Health Education: Theory, Research and Practice*, 3rd edn. San Francisco: Jossey-Bass.

Mooney, G. (2005) 'Communitarian Claims and Community Capabilities: Furthering Priority Setting?', *Social Science and Medicine*, 60, 247–55.

Mooney, G. and Houston, S. (2008) 'Equity in Health Care and Institutional Trust: A Communitarian View', *Cad. Saúde Pública, Rio de Janerio*, 24(5), 1162–7.

Moore, L. and Davis, B. (2002) 'Quilting Narrative: Using Repetition Techniques to Help Elderly Communicators', *Geriatric Nursing*, 23(5), 262–6.

Morgan, D. (1997) *Focus Groups as Qualitative Research*, 2nd edn. London: Sage.

Morgan, K. and Morley, A. (2002) 'Re-Localising the Food Chain: The Role of Creative Public Procurement', The Regeneration Institute, Cardiff University, cited in K. Morgan and R. Sonnino, *Catering For Sustainability: The Creative Procurement of School Meals in Italy and the UK*, http://www.brass.cf.ac.uk/cateringforsustainability1.pdf

Muennig, P. (2008) 'The Body Politic: The Relationship between Stigma and Obesity-Associated Disease', *BMC Public Health*, 8(128), http://www.biomedcentral.com/content/pdf/1471-2458-8-128.pdf (accessed 5 June 2009).

Myers, D. G. (2007) 'Costs and Benefits of American Corporate Capitalism', *Psychological Inquiry*, 18(1), 43–7.

Naidoo, J. and Wills, J. (1994) *Health Promotion: Foundations for Practice*. Edinburgh: Bailliere Tindall.

Naidoo, J. and Wills, J. (2000) *Health Promotion: Foundations for Practice*, 2nd edn. Edinburgh: Bailliere Tindall in association with the RCN.

Naidoo, J. and Wills, J. (eds) (2008) *Health Studies: An Introduction*, 2nd edn. Basingstoke: Palgrave Macmillan.

NAM (National Aids Manual) (2010) http://www.aidsmap.com

National Audit Office (2001) *Tackling Obesity in England*. London: NAO.

National Centre for Social Research (2003) *Health Survey for England Summary of Key Findings*. London: National Centre for Social Research.

National Crime Prevention Council (1995) *How Communities Can Bring Up Youth Free from Fear and Violence*. Indianapolis: American Legion Child Welfare Foundation; Washinbgton, DC: Department of Justice, Bureau of Justice Assistance, http://www.eric.ed.gov/ERICWebPortal/search/detailmini.jsp?_nfpb=true&_&ERICExtSearch_SearchValue_0=ED389828&ERICExtSearch_SearchType_0=no&accno=ED389828 (accessed 28 August 2008).

National Institute for Health and Clinical Excellence (2007) *Behaviour Change at Population, Community and Individual Levels*. London: NICE.

Navarro, V. (1976) *Medicine under Capitalism*. London: Croom Helm.

Ncayiyana, D. J. (2004) 'Is Democracy Good for People's Health? A South African Perspective', *British Medical Journal*, 329, 1425–6.

Nettleton, S. (1995) *The Sociology of Health and Illness*. Cambridge: Polity Press.

Nettleton, S. (1997) 'Surveillance, Health Promotion and the Formation of a Risk Identity', in M. Sidell, L. Jones, J. Katz and A. Peberdy (eds), *Debates and Dilemmas in Promoting Health: A Reader*. Basingstoke: The Open University in association with Macmillan.

Newman, J. and Kuhlmann, E. (2007) 'Consumers Enter the Political Stage? The Modernization of Health Care in Britain and Germany', *Journal of European Social Policy*, 17(2), 99–111.

Newman, J. and Vidler, E. (2006) 'Discriminating Customers, Responsible Patients, Empowered Users: Consumerism and the Modernisation of Health Care', *Journal of Social Policy*, 35(2), 193–209.

Nguyen, T. A., Oosterhoff, P., Pham, Y. N. and Hardon, A. (2009) 'Health Workers' Views on Quality of Prevention of Mother-to-Child Transmission and Postnatal Care for HIV-Infected Women and Their Children', *Human Resources for Health*, 7(39), 1–11.

NHS Careers (2010a) http://www.nhscareers.nhs.uk

NHS Careers (2010b) http://www.nhscareers.nhs.uk/notSure.shtml

NHS Choices (2008) http://www.nhs.uk/Tools/Documents/HistoryNHS.html

NHS Choices (2010a) *IVF, Your Health, Your Choices* website, http://www.nhs.uk/conditions/IVF/Pages/Introduction.aspx (accessed April 2010).

NHS Choices (2010b) http://www.nhs.uk/conditions/dementia/pages/introduction.aspx (accessed April, 2011).

NICE (2004) *Assessment and Treatment for People with Fertility Problems. Understanding the*

NICE Guideline: Information for People with Fertility Problems, Their Partners and the Public. London: NICE.

Noah, N. (2006) *Controlling Communicable Disease*. Maidenhead: Open University Press.

Noble, T. (2000) *Social Theory and Social Change*. Basingstoke: Macmillan.

Nolan, M., Keady, J. and Aveyard, B. (2001) 'Relationship Centred Care is the Next Logical Step', *British Journal of Nursing*, 10(12), 757.

Nordenfelt, L. (1995) 'On the Nature and Ethics of Health Promotion. An Attempt at a Systematic Analysis', in D. Seedhouse (ed.), *Reforming Health Care. The Philosophy and Practice of International Health Reform*. Chichester: John Wiley and Sons: Chichester.

NPCRDC (2007) Executive Summary 44. *National Evaluation of the Expert Patient Programme: Key findings (Research into Expert Patients – Outcomes in a Randomised Trial)*. London: National Primary Care Research and Development Centre, http://www.npcrdc.ac.uk (accessed 26 April 2007).

Oakley, J. (2004) 'Commentary', *Journal of Medical Ethics*, 30, 385.

O'Brien, M. (1995) 'Health and Lifestyle: A Critical Mess? Notes on the Differentiation of Health', in R. Bunton et al. (eds), *The Sociology of Health Promotion: Critical Analyses of Consumption, Lifestyle and Risk*. London: Routledge.

OECD (2008) *Growing Unequal? Income Distribution and Poverty in OECD Countries*, http://www.oecd.org/els/social/inequality (accessed November 2008).

Office for National Statistics (2010) *Ageing: Fastest Increase in the 'Oldest Old'*, http://www.statistics.gov.uk/cci/nugget.asp?ID=949.

Ogden, J. (1996) *Health Psychology: A Text Book*. Buckingham: Open University Press.

Ogden, J. (2000) *Health Psychology: A Text Book*, 2nd edn. Buckingham: Open University Press.

Ogden, J. (2002) *Health and the Construction of the Individual*. London: Routledge.

Ohlbrecht, H. (2004) 'Resources for Qualitative Researchers', in U. Flick, E. von Kardorff and I. Steinke (eds), *A Companion to Qualitative Research*. London: Sage.

Olapegba, P. O. (2010) 'Empath, Knowledge, and Personal Distress as Correlated of HIV/AIDS-Related Stigmatization and Discrimination', *Journal of Applied Social Psychology*, 40(4), 956–69.

Ollila, E. (2005) 'Global Health Priorities: Priorities of the Wealthy?', *Globalization and Health*, 1(6), doi:10.1186/1744-8603-1-6, http://www.globalizationandhealth.com/content/1/1/6

Olmsted, M. P. and McFarland, T. (2004) 'Body Weight and Body Image', *BMC Womens Health*, 4(suppl. 1), S5, http://www.biomedcentral.com/1472-6874/4/S1/S5

O'Neill, B. (2006) 'Global Warming: The Chilling Effect on Free Speech', http://www.spiked-online.com/index.php?/site/article/1782/

O'Neill, B. (2007) 'Environmentalism: The New Death Cult?', *Guardian Online*, 3 July, http://www.guardian.co.uk/commentisfree/2007/jul/03/environmentalismthenewdeathcult

ONS (2008) *Expenditure on Health Care in the UK*. London: Office for National Statistics.

ONS (2009) Migration: Emigration Reaches Record High in 2008, http://www.statistics.gov.uk/cci/nugget.asp?id=260 (accessed May 2010).

Open University Learning Space (n.d.) *The Enlightenment*, http://openlearn.open.ac.uk/course/view.php?id=2090 (accessed 2 October 2009).

Orbach, S. (2006) 'There Is a Public Health Crisis: It's not Fat on the Body but Fat in the Mind and the Fat of Profits', *International Journal of Epidemiology*, 35, 67–9.

Osborne, D. and Neale, J. (2009) 'Discourse Analysis', in J. Neale (ed), *Research Methods for Health and Social Care*. Basingstoke: Palgrave Macmillan.

Ott, A., van Breteler, M. M. and Harskamp, F. (1995) 'Prevalence of Alzheimer's Disease and Vascular Dementia: Association with Education. The Rotterdam Study', *British Medical Journal*, 15(310), 970–3.

Owen, J. W. and Roberts, O. (2005) 'Globalisation, Health and Foreign Policy: Emerging Linkages and Interests', *Globalization and Health*, 1(12), http://www.globalizationandhealth.com/content/1/1/12 (accessed 13 August 2008).

Palmlund, I. (2006) 'Loyalities in Clinical Research on Drugs: The Case of Hormone Replacement Therapy', *Social Science and Medicine*, 6(2), 540–51.

Pampel, F. C. (2000) *Sociological Lives and Ideas. An Introduction to the Classical Theorists*. New York: Worth Press.

Parker, I. (1992) *Discourse Dynamics: Critical Analysis for Social and Individual Psychology*. London: Routledge.

Parker, J. (2005) 'Constructing Dementia and Dementia Care: Daily Practicies in a Day Care Setting', *Journal of Social Work*, 5, 261–78.

Parker, M. J. (2004) "Til Death Us Do Part: The Ethics of Postmortem Gamete Donation', *Journal of Medical Ethics*, 30, 387–8.

Parsons-Suhl, K., Johnson, M. E., McCann, J. J. and Solberg, S. (2008) 'Losing One's Memory in Early Alzheimer's Disease', *Qualitative Health Research*, 18, 31–42.

Patient UK (n.d.) *Different Level of Evidence (Critical Reading)*, http://www.patient.co.uk/showdoc/40002064/ (accessed 6 July 2009).

Paton, C. (1997) 'Necessary Conditions for a Socialist Health Service', *Healthcare Analysis*, 5(3), 205–16.

Patton, M. Q. (1990) *Qualitative Evaluation and Research Methods*, 2nd edn. London: Sage.

Patz, J. A., Gibbs, H. K., Foley, J. A., Rogers, J. V. and Smith, K. R. (2007) 'Climate Change and Global Health: Quantifying a Growing Ethical Crisis', *EcoHealth*, 4, 397–405.

Patz, J. A., Vavrus, S. J., Uejio, C. K. and McLellan, S. L. (2008) 'Climate Change and Waterborne Disease Risk in the Great Lakes Region of the US', *American Journal of Preventive Medicine*, 35(5), 451–8.

Pawson, R. (1999) 'Methodology', in S. Taylor (ed.), *Sociology: Issues and Debates*. Basingstoke: Macmillan.

Peplau, H. E. (1988) *Interpersonal Relations in Nursing*. Basingstoke: Macmillan.

Perakyla, A. (2004) 'Reliability and Validity in Research Based on Naturally Occurring Social Interaction', 283–304, in D. Silverman (ed.), *Qualitative Research: Theory, Method and Practice,* 2nd edn. London: Sage.

Percy-Smith, J. (ed.) (1996) *Needs Assessment in Public Policy*. Buckingham: Open University Press.

Persson, A. and Newman, C. (2008) 'Making Monsters: Heterosexuality, Crime and Race in Recent Western Media Coverage of HIV', *Sociology of Health and Illness*, 30(4), 632–46.

Philippson, P. (2001) *Self in Relation*. New York: Gestalt Journal Press.

Phillips, C. V. (2004) 'Publication Bias *in situ*', *BMC Medical Research Methodology*, 4(20), http://www.biomedcentral.com/1471-2288/4/20 (accessed 3 March 2009).

Phinney, A. (2002) 'Living with the Symptoms of Alzheimer's Disease', in P. B. Harris (ed.), *The Person with Alzheimer's Disease*. Baltimore: Johns Hopkins University Press.

Pickard, L., Wittenberg, R., Comas-Herrera, A., Davies, B. and Darton, R. (2000) 'Relying on Informal Care in the New Century? Informal Care for Elderly People in England to 2031', *Ageing and Society*, 20, 745–72.

Pilkington, E. (2006) 'The "Untouchables" of US Science', *The Guardian*, 29 December, http://www.guardian.co.uk/science/2006/dec/29/genetics.research (accessed 28 May 2009).

Pink, S. (2004) 'Visual Methods', in C. Seale, G. Gobo, J. Gubrium and D. Silverman (eds), *Qualitative Research Practice*. London: Sage.

Piot, P. (2001) 'Global AIDS Epidemic: Time to Turn the Tide, in B. Davey, A. Gray and C. Seale (eds), *Health and Disease: A Reader*. Maidenhead: Open University Press.

Piterman, H. E. (2006) 'Ethics in Medicine. Consumer Representation: Challenges and Pitfalls', *Internal Medicine Journal*, 36, 378–80.

Pitt, B. and Lloyd, L. (2008) 'Social Policy and Health', in J. Naidoo and J. Wills (eds), *Health Studies: An Introduction*, 2nd edn. Basingstoke: Palgrave Macmillan.

Pitts, M. (1996) *The Psychology of Preventive Health*. London: Routledge.

Plsek, P. E. and Greenhalgh, T. (2001) 'The Challenge of Complexity in Health Care', *British Medical Journal*, 323, 625–8.

Polgar, S. and Thomas, S. (1995) *Introduction to Research in Health Sciences*, 3rd edn. London: Churchill Livingstone.

Politics.co.uk (2005) *NHS Prescription Charges*, http://www.politics.co.uk/briefings-guides/issue-briefs/health/nhs-prescription-charges-$366605.htm (accessed April 2010).

Poole, T. (2006) *Dementia Care: Wanless Social Care Review*. London: Kings Fund.

Porter, R. (1997) *The Greatest Benefit to Mankind: A Medical History of Humanity from Antiquity to the Present*. London: Fontana Press.

Pösö, T., Honkatukia, P. and Nyqvist, L. (2008) 'Focus Groups and the Study of Violence', *Qualitative Research*, 8, 73.

Powell, M. (1997) 'Socialism and the British National Health Service', *Healthcare Analysis*, 5(3), 187–94.

Power, L. (2004) 'HIV and Sexual Health in the UK: Politics and Public Health', *Lancet*, 364, 108–9.

Pratt, R. J. (2003) *HIV and AIDS*, 5th edn. London: Arnold.

Prior, L. (2003) 'Belief, Knowledge and Expertise: The Emergence of the Lay Expert in Medical Sociology', *Sociology of Health and Illness*, 25, 41–57.

Prior, L. (2004) 'Documents', in C. Seale, G. Gobo, J. Gubrium and D. Silverman (eds), *Qualitative Research Practice*. London: Sage.

Prochaska, J. O. and DiClemente, C. C. (1986) 'Towards a Comprehensive Model of Change', in U. Miller and N. Heather (eds), *Treating Addictive Behaviors*. New York: Plenum Press.

Prochaska, J. O., Redding, C. A. and Evers, K. E. (2002) 'The Transtheoretical Model and Stages of Change', in K. Glanz, B. K. Rimer and F. M. Lewis (eds), *Health Behavior and Health Education: Theory, Research and Practice*, 3rd edn. San Francisco: Jossey-Bass.

Prospects (2010a) http://www.prospects.ac.uk/industries_health_overview.htm

Prospects (2010b) http://www.prospects.ac.uk/links/occupations

Prospects (2010c) http://www.prospects.ac.uk/options_health_your_skills.htm

Prospects (2010d) http://www.prospects.ac.uk/industries_social_care_overview.htm

Prospects (2010e) 'Charity and Development Work: Overview', http://www.prospects.ac.uk/plsectors/charities_and_voluntary_work_sector.jsp

Pulsford, D., Rushford, D. and Connor, I. (2000) 'Woodlands Therapy: An Ethnographic Analysis of a Small-Group Therapeutic Activity for People with Moderate or Severe Dementia', *Journal of Advanced Nursing*, 32(3), 650–7.

Quigley, R., Cavanagh, S., Harrison, D., Taylor, L. and Pottle, M. (2005) *Clarifying Approaches to Health Needs Assessment, Health Impact Assessment, Integrated Impact Assessment, Health Equity Audit, and Race Equality Impact Assessment*. London: HDA.

Quinton, A. (1997) 'Positivism', in A. Bullock and S. Trombley (eds), *The New Fontana Dictionary of Modern Thought*, 3rd edn. London: HarperCollins.

Quinton, A. and Porter, R. (1999) 'Mind, Philosophy of', in A. Bullock and S. Trombley (eds), *The New Fontana Dictionary of Modern Thought*, 3rd edn. London: HarperCollins.

Qureshi, H. (2010) 'Social Care for Graduates: Compassionate Embrace', *The Guardian*, 27 February, http://www.guardian.co.uk/money/2010/feb/27/social-care-graduate-careers

Radin, M. (1987) 'Market-Inalienability', *Harvard Law Review*, 100, 1849–937.

Raeburn, J. and Rootman, I. (1998) *People Centred Health Promotion*. Chichester: John Wiley and Sons.

Ramazanoglu, C. with Holland, J. (2003) *Feminist Methodology*. London: Sage.

Rawaf, S. and Bahl, V. (eds) (1998) *Assessing Health Needs for People from Minority Ethnic Groups*. London: Royal College of Physicians of London.

Redwood, H. (2000) *Why Ration Health Care? An International Study of the United Kingdom, France, Germany and Public Sector Health Care in the USA*. London: CIVITAS.

Reich, M. (1994) *Democracy and Health: An Overview of Issues Presented in Four Papers*. Cambridge, MA: Department of Population and International Health, Harvard School of Public Health.

Reinharz, S. (1992) *Feminist Methods in Social Research*. New York: Oxford University Press.

Relman, A. (1980) 'The New Medical-Industrial Complex', *New England Journal of Medicine*, 303, 963–70.

Resnik, D. (1998) 'The Commodification of Human Reproductive Materials', *Journal of Medical Ethics*, 24, 388–93.

Rhodes, T. (1997) 'Risk Theory in Epidemic Times: Sex, Drugs and the Social Organisation of "Risk behaviour"', *Sociology of Health and Illness*, 19(2), 208–27.

Richman, J. (2003) 'Holding Public Health Up for Inspection', in J. Costello and M. Haggart (eds), *Public Health and Society*. Basingstoke: Palgrave Macmillan.

Ridge, D., Williams, I., Anderson, J. and Elford, J. (2008) 'Like a Prayer: The Role of Spirituality and Religion for People Living with HIV in the UK', *Sociology of Health and Illness*, 30(3), 413–28.

Ridge, D., Ziebland, S., Anderson, J., Williams, I. and Elford, J. (2007) 'Positive Prevention: Contemporary Issues Facing HIV Positive People Negotiating Sex in the UK', *Social Science and Medicine*, 65, 755–70.

Rissel, C. (1994) 'Empowerment: The Holy Grail of Health Promotion?', *Health Promotion International*, 9(1), 39–47.

Ritchie, C. and Vitali, S. (2009) 'Why Research?', in J. Neale (eds), *Research Methods for Health and Social Care*. Basingstoke: Palgrave Macmillan.

Ritchie, D., Gnich, W., Parry, O. and Platt, S. (2008) '"People Pull the Rug From under Your Feet": Barriers to Successful Public Health Programmes', *BMC Public Health*, 8(173), http://www.biomedcentral.com/1471-2458/8/173 (accessed April 2010).

Ritchie, J. and Lewis, J. (eds) (2003) *Qualitative Research Practice: A Guide for Social Science Students and Researchers*. London: Sage.

Roberts, E. and Robinson, J. (2000) *Briefing Note: Age Discrimination in Health and Social Care*. London: Kings Fund.

Roberts, M. J. and Reich, M. R. (2002) 'Ethical Analysis in Public Health', *The Lancet*, 359, 1055–9.

Robinson, T. N. (1999) 'Reducing Children's Television Viewing to Prevent Obesity: A Randomized Controlled Trial', *Jama*, 282(16), 1561–7.

Robson, C. (2002) *Real World Research: A Resource for Social Scientists and Practitioner-Researchers*. Oxford: Blackwell.

Robson, C. (2007) *How to Do a Research Project: A Guide for Undergraduate Students*. Oxford:Blackwell.

Rogers, A. (2002) 'Is There a Tension between Doctors' Duty of Care and Evidence-Based Medicine?', *Health Care Analysis*, 10, 277–87.

Rogers, A., Bower, P., Gardner, C., Gately, C., Kennedy, A., Lee, V., Middleton, E., Reeves, D. and Richardson, G. (2006) *The National Evaluation of the Pilot Phase of the Expert Patient Programme: Final Report*. London: NPCRDC.

Rogers, C. R. (1957) 'The Necessary and Sufficient Conditions of Therapeutic Personality Change', *Journal of Consulting Psychology*, 21(2): 95–103.

Rosenhan, D. L. (1973) 'On Being Sane in Insane Places', *Science*, n.s, 179(4070), 250–8.

Rossignol, A. (2007) *Principles and Practice of Epidemiology: An Engaged Approach*. New York: McGraw-Hill.

Rowley, C. (2005) 'Health Needs Assessment', *JCN*, http://www.jcn.co.uk/journal.asp?MonthNum=06&YearNum=2005&Type=backissue&ArticleID=808 (accessed 6 November 2006).

Royce, S., Sharpe, P., Ainsworth, B., Greaney, M., Neff, L. and Henderson, K. (2003) 'Conceptualising Barriers and Supports for Physical Activity: A Qualities Assessment', *International Journal of Health Promotion and Education*, 41(2), 41–8.

Rozin, P. (1997) 'Moralization', 379–401, in A. M. Brandt and P. Rozin (eds), *Morality and Health*. New York: Routledge.

Ruger, J. P. (2005) 'Democracy and Health', *Quarterly Journal of Medicine*, 98, 299–304.

Russo, J., Vitaliano, P. P., Brewer, D. D., Katon, W. and Becker, J. (1995) 'Psychiatric Disorders in Spouse Caregivers of Care Recipients with Alzheimer's Disease and Matched Controls: A Diathesis-Stress Model of Psychopathology', *Journal of Abnormal Psychology*, 104, 197–204.

Sabat, S. R. (2006) 'Implicit Memory and People with Alzheimer's Disease: Implications for Caregiving', *American Journal of Alzheimer's Disease and Other Dementias*, 21(1), 11–14.

Sackett, D. L., Richardson,W. S., Rosenberg,W. and Haynes, R. B. (1998) *Evidence-Based Medicine: How to Practise and Teach EBM*. Edinburgh: Churchill Livingstone.

Sacks, O. (1973) *Awakenings*. London: Duckworth.

Saguy, A. C. and Riley, K. W. (2005) 'Weighing Both Sides: Morality, Mortality, and Framing Contests of Obesity', *Journal of Health Politics, Policy and Law*, 30(5), 869–921.

Sandel, M. J. (1982) *Liberalism and the Limits of Justice*. Cambridge: Cambridge University Press.

Sandelowski, M. and de Lacey, S. (2002) 'The Uses of a "Disease": Infertility as a Rhetorical Vehicle', in M. C. Inhorn and F. van Balen (eds), *Infertility around the Globe: New Thinking on Childlessness, Gender and Reproductive Technologies*. Berkeley and Los Angeles: University of California Press.

Sander, R., (2002) 'Continuing Professional Development: Standing and Moving: Helping People with Vascular Dementia', *Nursing Older People*, 14(1), 20–6.

Sarafino, E. P. (1990) *Health Psychology: Biopsychosocial Interactions*. New York: John Wiley.

Sarantakos, S. (1998) *Social Research*, 2nd edn. Basingstoke: Macmillan.

Sarantakos, S. (2005) *Social Research*, 3rd edn. Basingstoke: Macmillan.

Sartorius, N. (2002) 'Iatrogenic Stigma of Mental Illness', *British Medical Journal*, 324, 1470–1.

Saunders, Mark N. K., Lewis, Philip and Thornhill, Adrian (2000) *Research Methods for Business Students*. Harlow: Financial Times/Prentice Hall.

Scambler, G. and Paoli, F. (2008) 'Health Work, Female Sex Workers and HIV/AIDS: Global and Local Dimensions of Stigma and Deviance as Barriers to Effective Interventions', *Social Science and Medicine*, 66, 1848–62.

Scheff, T. J. (1990) *Microsociology: Discourse, Emotion and Social Structure*. Chicago: University of Chicago Press.

Scholes, S. (2008) 'Children's BMI, Overweight and Obesity', in R. Craig and N. Shelton (eds), *Health Survey for England 2007. Volume 1, Healthy Lifestyles: Knowledge, Attitudes and Behaviour*, http://www.ic.nhs.uk/webfiles/publications/HSE07/HSE%2007-Volume%201. pdf (accessed 5 June 2009).

Schon, D. A. (1983) *The Reflective Practitioner*. London: Basic Books.

Schoub, B. D. (1999) *AIDS and HIV in Perspective*, 2nd edn. Cambridge: Cambridge University Press.

Schrecker, T., Labonté, R. and De Vagli, R. (2008) 'Globalisation and Health: The Need for a Global Vision', *The Lancet*, 372(8), 1670–6.

Schrimshaw, E. W. and Siegel, K. (2002) 'HIV-Infected Mothers' Disclosure to Their Infected Children: Rates, Reasons, Reactions', *Journal of Social and Personal Relationships*, 19(1), 19–43.

Schwartz, H. (1986) *Never Satisfied: A Cultural History of Diets, Fantasies and Fat*. New York: Free Press.

Schwarzer, R. (1992) 'Self-Efficacy in the Adoption and Maintenance of Health Behaviours: Theoretical Approaches and a New Model', in R. Schwarzer (ed.), *Self Efficacy: Thought Control of Action*. Washington, DC: Hemisphere.

Scottish Intercollegiate Guidelines Network (2003) *Management of Obesity in Children and Young People: A National Clinical Guideline*. Edinburgh: Scottish Intercollegiate Guidelines Network, http://www.sign.ac.uk (accessed 4 June 2009).

Scott-Jones, R. (2002) 'Medicine, Government and Capitalism', *Journal of the American College of Surgeons*, 2, 111–20.

Scrimshaw, E. W. and Siegel, K. (2002) 'HIV-Infected Mothers' Disclosure to Their Uninfected

Children: Rates, Reasons, and Reactions', *Journal of Social and Personal Relationships*, 19, 19–43.

Scruton, R. (2001) *The Meaning of Conservatism*, 3rd edn. Basingstoke: Palgrave.

Seedhouse, D. (1986) *Health: The Foundations for Achievement*. Chichester: John Wiley and Sons.

Seedhouse, D. (1988) *Ethics: The Heart of Health Care*. Chichester: John Wiley and Sons.

Seedhouse, D. (1994) *Fortress NHS: A Philosophical Review of the National Health Service*. Chichester: John Wiley and Sons.

Seedhouse, D. (1997a) *Health Promotion. Philosophy, Prejudice and Practice*. Chichester: John Wiley and Sons.

Seedhouse, D. (1997b) 'Is a Socialist Health Service Possible?', *Healthcare Analysis*, 5(3), 183–5.

Seedhouse, D. (1998a) *Ethics: The Heart of Health Care*, 2nd edn. Chichester: John Wiley and Sons.

Seedhouse, D. (1998b) 'Death's Moral Sting', *Health Care Analysis*, 6, 273–6.

Seedhouse, D. (2000) *Practical Nursing Philosophy. The Universal Ethical Code*. Chichester: John Wiley and Sons.

Seedhouse, D. (2001) *Health: The Foundations for Achievement*, 2nd edn. Chichester: John Wiley and Sons.

Seedhouse, D. (2002) *Total Health Promotion: Mental Health, Rational Fields and the Quest for Autonomy*. Chichester: John Wiley and Sons.

Seedhouse, D. (2004) *Health Promotion: Philosophy, Prejudice and Practice*, 2nd edn. Chichester: John Wiley and Sons.

Seedhouse, D. (2009) *Ethics: The Heart of Health Care*, 3rd edn. Chichester: John Wiley and Sons.

Sharpe, V. A. (2008) *Policy and Politics 'Clean' Nuclear Energy? Global Warming, Public Health and Justice*. Hastings Center Report, July–August.

Shaw, R. L. and Giles, D. C. (2009) 'Motherhood on Ice? A Media Framing Analysis of Older Mothers in the UK News', *Psychology and Health*, 24(2), 221–36.

Shea, K. M., Truckner, R. T., Weber, R. W. and Pedem, D. B. (2008) 'Climate Change and Allergic Disease', *Journal of Allergy and Clinical Immunology*, 122(3), 443–53.

Sheaff, R. (1996) *The Need for Health Care*. London: Routledge.

Shefer, T., Strebel, A., Wilson, T., Shabalala, N., Simbayi, L., Ratele, K., Potgieter, C. and Andipatin, M. (2002) 'The Social Construction of Sexually Transmitted Infections (STIs) in South Africa Communities', *Qualitative Health Research*, 12(10), 1373–90.

Sherr, Lorraine , Fox, Zoe, Lipton, Michelle , Whyte, Patricia , Jones, Patricia , Harrison, Ursula and Camden Islington Steering Group (2006) 'Sustaining HIV Testing in Pregnancy – Evaluation of Routine Offer of HIV Testing in Three London Hospitals over 2 Years', *AIDS Care*, 18(3), 183–8.

Shiell, A. and Hawe, P. (1996) 'Health Promotion Community Development and the Tyranny of Individualism', *Health Economics*, 5, 242–7.

Shircore, R. (2009) *Guide for World Class Commissioners. Promoting Health and Well-Being: Reducing Inequalities*. London: Royal Society for Public Health in Partnership with the National Social Marketing Centre.

Shiu, M. (2001) 'Refusing to Treat Smokers Is Unethical and a Dangerous Precedent', in B. Davey, A. Gray and C. Seale (eds), *Health and Disease: A Reader*, 3rd edn. Buckingham: Open University Press.

Shoff, S. M. and Newcomb, P. A. (1998) 'Diabetes, Body Size and Risk of Endometrial Cancer', *American Journal of Epidemiology*, 148(3), 234–40.

Silverman, D. (2000) *Doing Qualitative Research*. London: Sage.

Silverman, D. (2004) *Qualitative Research: Theory, Method and Practice*, 2nd edn. London: Sage.

Silverman, D. (2006) *Interpreting Qualitative Data*, 3rd edn. London: Sage.

Singh G.K., Kogan M.D., Van Dyck P.C., and Siahpush M., (2008) Race/Ethnic, Socioeconomic, and Behavioural Determinants of Childhood and Adolescent Obesity in the United States: Analyzing Independent and Joint Associations *Annals of Epidemiology* 18(9), 682–95.

SIRC (Social Issues Research Centre) (2005) *Obesity and the Facts. An Analysis of Data from the Health Survey for England 2003*. Oxford: Social Issues Research Centre February.

Skills for Health (2008) *LMI Resource June 2008*, http://www.skillsforhealth.org.uk

Sloman, A. (1999) 'Normative', in A. Bullock and S. Trombley (eds), *The New Fontana Dictionary of Modern Thought*, 3rd edn. London: HarperCollins.

Smith, Dorothy E. (2002) 'Institutional Ethnography', 150–61 in Tim May (ed.), *Qualitative Research in Action: An International Guide to Issues in Practice*. London: Sage.

Smith, L. and Dixon, L. (2009) 'Systematic Reviews', in J. Neale (ed.), *Research Methods for Health and Social Care*. Basingstoke: Palgrave Macmillan.

Smith, L. and Ryan, T. J. (2009) 'Randomised Controlled Trials', in J. Neale (ed.), *Research Methods for Health and Social Care*. Basingstoke: Palgrave Macmillan.

Snape, D. and Spencer, L. (2003) 'The Foundations of Qualitative Research', in J. Ritchie and J Lewis (eds), *Qualitative Research Practice: A Guide for Social Science Students and Researchers*. London: Sage.

Speedy, J. (2008) *Narrative Inquiry and Psychotherapy*. Basingstoke: Palgrave Macmillan.

Spicker, S. F. (1993) 'Going off the Dole: A Prudential and Ethical Critique of the "Healthfare" State', in D. Seedhouse (ed.), *Reforming Health Care: The Philosophy and Practice of International Health Reform*. Chichester: John Wiley and Sons.

Spriggs, M. (2004) 'Woman Wants Dead Fiancé's Baby: Who Owns a Dead Man's Sperm', *Journal of Medical Ethics*, 30, 384–5.

Stampar, A. (2008) 'Voices from the Past: On Health Politics', *American Journal of Public Health*, 96(8), 1382–5 (originally written in 1966).

Stansfield, S. K., Harper, M., Lamb, G. and Lob-Levyt, J. (2002) *Innovative Financing of International Public Goods for Health*. CMH working paper series WG2:22. Commission on Macroeconomics and Health, http://www.cmhealth.org/docs/wg2_paper22.pdf

Stationery Office Ltd, The (2008) *Human Fertilisation and Embryology Act (2008)* Crown Copyright http://www.opsi.gov.uk/acts/acts2008/ukpga 20080022 en 1 (accessed 28.5.09).

Steele, T. (1999) 'Consumerism', in A. Bullock and S. Trombley (eds), *The New Fontana Dictionary of Modern Thought*, 3rd edn. London: HarperCollins.

Steinberg, D. (1990) 'The Depersonalisation of Women through the Administration of "in Vitro Fertilisation', in M. McNeil, I. Varcoe and S. Yearly (eds), *The New Reproductive Technologies*. Basingstoke: Macmillan.

Strabanek, P. (1994) 'The Emptiness of the Black Box', *Epidemiology*, 5, 553–5.

Strathern, P. (1996a) *Hume in 90 Minutes*. London: Constable.

Strathern, P. (1996b) *Locke in 90 Minutes*. London: Constable.

Street, C. and Powell, C. (2008) 'Empowering Patients: The Role of the Expert Patient Programme in Promoting Health amongst Those with Long Term Conditions', in M. Presho (ed.), *Managing Long Term Conditions: A Social Model for Community Practice*. Chichester: Wiley-Blackwell.

Stroebe, W. and Stroebe, M. S. (1995) *Social Psychology and Health*. Buckingham: Open University Press.

Sudnow, D. (1967) *Passing On: The Social Organisation of Dying*. Englewood Cliffs, NJ: Prentice Hall.

Summerbell, S., Kelly, S. and Campbell, K. (2002) 'The Prevention and Treatment of Childhood Obesity', *Effective Health Care*, 7(6).

Sutcliffe, A. (2008) 'Spinoza, Bayle, and the Enlightenment Politics of Philosophical Certainty', *History of European Ideas*, 34, 66–76.

Swanton, K. and Frost, M. (2007) *Lightening the Load: Tackling Overweight and Obesity. A Tool Kit for Developing Local Strategies to Tackle Overweight and Obesity in Children and Adults*. London: National Heart Forum in association with the Faculty of Public Health and Department of Health.

Sweeting, H. and Gilhooly, M. (1997) 'Dementia and the Phenomenon of Social Death', *Sociology of Health and Illness*, 19(1), 93–117.

references

Swingewood, A. (1999) 'Sociological Theory', in S. Taylor (ed.), *Sociology: Issues and Debates*. Basingstoke: Macmillan.

Syrett, K. (2007) *Law, Legitimacy and the Rationing of Health Care: A Contextual and Comparative Perspective*. Cambridge: Cambridge University Press.

Szwarc, S. (2003) 'Where's the Epidemic?', http://www.techcentralstation.com/073003Chtml

Taylor, B. (2009) 'Participant Observation', in J. Neale (ed.), *Research Methods for Health and Social Care*. Basingstoke: Palgrave Macmillan.

Taylor, S. (1999a) 'Introduction', in S. Taylor (ed.), *Sociology: Issues and Debates*. Basingstoke: Macmillan.

Taylor, S. (1999b) 'Health, Illness and Medicine', in S. Taylor (ed.), *Sociology: Issues and Debates*. Basingstoke: Macmillan.

Tee, S. (2008) 'Partnership for Public Health: User Involvement to Improve Health and Wellbeing', in L. Coles and E. Porter (eds), *Public Health Skills: A Practical Guide for Nurses and Public Health Practitioners*. Oxford: Blackwell.

ten Have, H. (1994) ' Responsibilities and Rationalities: Should the Patient Be Blamed?', *Health Care Analysis*, 2, 119–73.

Ter Meulen, R. and Dickenson, D. (2002) 'Into the Hidden World Behind Evidence-Based Medicine', *Health Care Analysis*, 10, 231–41.

Terrence Higgins Trust (2010) *Information resources – Criminal Prosecutions for Transmitting HIV*, http://www.tht.org.uk/informationresources/prosecutions (accessed 13 December 2010).

Thirlaway, K. and Upton, D. (2009) *The Psychology of Lifestyle: Promoting Healthy Behaviour*. London: Routledge.

Thomas, D. and Woods, H. (2003) *Working with People with Learning Disabilities: Theory and Practice*. London: Jessica Kingsley Publishers.

Thomas, N. E., Baker, J. S. and Davies, B. (2003) 'Established and Recently Identified Coronary Heart Disease Risk Factors in Young People: The Influence of Physical Activity and Physical Fitness', *Sports Medicine*, 33(9), 633–50.

Thomas Pocklington Trust (2009) *Obstacles to Improving Visual Health in Older People*. Occasional Paper no. 18. London: Thomas Pocklington Trust.

Thompson, E. P. (1968) *The Making of the English Working Class*. Middlesex: Pelican Books.

Thompson, N. and Thompson, S. (2008) *The Social Work Companion*. Basingstoke: Palgrave Macmillan.

Throsby, K. (2001) '"No-One Will Ever Call Me Mummy": Making Sense of the End of IVF Treatment', London School of Economics, Gender Institute: New Working Paper Series, issue 5, November.

Titterton, M. (2005) *Risk and Risk Taking in Health and Social Welfare*. London: Jessica Kingsley.

Tod, A. M. and Lacey, A. (2004) 'Overweight and Obesity: Helping Clients to Take Action', *British Journal of Community Nursing*, 9(2), 59–66.

Tolson, D., Smith, M. and Knight, P. (1999) An Investigation of the Components of Best Nursing Practice in the Care of Acutely Ill Hospitalized Older Patients with Coincidental Dementia: a Multi-Method Design', *Journal of Advanced Nursing*, 30(5), 1127–36.

Tones, K. and Green, J. (2004) *Health Promotion: Planning and Strategies*. London: Sage.

Tonkiss, F. (2004) 'Using Focus Groups', in C. Seale (ed.), *Researching Society and Culture*. London: Sage.

Torûn, B. (2005) 'Protein-Energy Malnutrition', in M. E. Shils, M. E. Shike, A. C. Ross, B. Caballero and R. J. Cousins (eds), *Modern Nutrition in Health and Disease*, 10th edn. Philadelphia: Lippincott Williams and Wilkins.

Travassos, C. (2008) 'Forum: Equity in Access to Health Care. Introduction', *Cad. Saúde Pública, Rio de Janeiro*, 24(5), 1159–61.

Travers, M. (2001) *Qualitative Research through Case Studies*. London: Sage.

Tritter, J. (2007) 'Mixed Methods and Multidisciplinary Research in Health Care', in M. Saks and J. Allsop (eds), *Researching Health: Qualitative, Quantitative and Mixed Methods*. London: Sage.

Trochim, W. M., Cabrera, D. A., Milstein, B., Gallagher, R. S. and Leishchow, S. J. (2006) 'Practical Challenges of System Thinking and Modeling in Public Health', *American Journal of Public Health*, 96(3), 538–46.

Tuchman, G., Daniel, A. K. and Benet, J. (eds) (1978) *Hearth and Home: Images of Women in the Mass Media*. New York: Oxford University Press.

Tudor, K. (1996) *Mental Health Promotion: Paradigms and Practice*. London: Routledge.

Ulrich, M. and Weatherall, A. (2000) 'Motherhood and Infertility: Viewing Motherhood through the Lens of Infertility', *Feminism and Psychology*, 10(3), 323–36.

Unicef (n.d.) *Kenya: Statistics*, http://www.unicef.org/infobycountry/kenya_statistics.html (accessed April 2010).

Unwin, N., Carr, S. and Leeson, J., with Pless-Mulloli, T. (1997) *An Introductory Study Guide to Public Health and Epidemiology*. Buckingham: Open University Press.

Van Balen, F. (2008) 'Involuntary Childlessness: A Neglected Problem in Poor-Resource Areas', *Human Reproduction*, 25–8, doi:10.1093/humrep/den141.

Verkerk, M. A. (1999) 'Care Perspective on Coercion and Autonomy', *Bioethics*, 13(3/4), 358–68.

Victor, C. (2005) *The Social Context of Ageing: A Textbook of Gerontology*. London: Routledge.

Viney, D. (1999) 'Normalisation', in A. Bullock and S. Trombley (eds), *The New Fontana Dictionary of Modern Thought*, 3rd edn. London: HarperCollins.

Visscher, T. L. S., Seidell, J. C., Menotti, A., Blackburn, H., Nissinen, E. J. M. and Kromhout, D., for the Seven Countries Study Research Group (2000) 'Underweight and Overweight in Relation to Mortality among Men Aged 40–59 and 50–69: The Seven Countries Study', *American Journal of Epidemiology*, 151(7), 660–6.

Von Schirnding, Y. (2005) 'The World Summit on Sustainable Development: Reaffirming the Centrality of Health', *Globalization and Health*, 1(8), doi:10.1186/1744-8603-1-8, http://www.globalizationandhealth.com/content/1/1/8

Voydanoff, P. (2001) 'Conceptualising Community in the Context of Work and Family', *Community, Work and Family*, 4(2), 133–56.

Walker, R. (2009) 'Mixed Methods Research: Quantity Plus Quality', in J. Neale (ed.), *Research Methods for Health and Social Care*. Basingstoke: Palgrave Macmillan.

Waller, B. N. (2005) 'Responsibility and Health', *Cambridge Quarterly of Healthcare Ethics*, 14, 177–88.

Walliman, N. (2001) *Your Research Project*. London: Sage.

Walsh, F. (2008) '30th Birthday for First IVF Baby', BBC News, http://news.bbc.co.uk/1/hi/health/7505635.stm (accessed 5 September 2008).

Walsh, P. (1995) 'Well-Being', in T. Honderich (ed.), *The Oxford Companion to Philosophy*. Oxford: Oxford University Press.

Walton, D. (2006) *Fundamentals of Critical Argumentation*. Cambridge: Cambridge University Press.

Walzer, M. (1983) *Spheres of Justice*. Oxford: Blackwell.

Wanless, D. (2004) *Securing Good Health for the Whole Population: Final Report 2004*. London: HM Treasury and Department of Health, http://www.dh.gov.uk/en/Publicationsandstatistics/Publications/PublicationsPolicyAndGuidance/DH_4074426

Warin, M., Turner, K., Moore, V. and Davies, M. (2008) 'Bodies, Mothers and Identities: Rethinking Obesity and the BMI', *Sociology of Health and Illness*, 30(1), 97–111.

Warnock, M. (1998) *An Intelligent Person's Guide to Ethics*. London: Duckworth.

Waterman, H. (2007) 'Action Research and Health', in M. Saks and J. Allsop (eds), *Researching Health: Qualitative, Quantitative and Mixed Methods*. London: Sage.

Watson, M. and Coombes, L. (2009) 'Surveys', in J. Neale (ed.), *Research Methods for Health and Social Care*. Basingstoke: Palgrave Macmillan.

Watt, R. G. (2007) 'Emerging Theories into the Social Determinants of Health: Implications for Oral Health Promotion', in J. Douglas, S. Earle, S. Handsley, C. E. Lloyd and S. Spurr (eds), *A Reader in Promoting Public Health – Challenge and Controversy*. London: Sage.

Weale, A. (1998) 'Rationing Health Care: A Logical Solution to an Inconsistent Triad', *British Medical Journal*, 316, 410.

Webster, C. (1994) 'Tuberculosis', in C. Seale and S. Pattison (eds), *Medical Knowledge: Doubt and Certainty*. Buckingham: Open University Press.

Wenzel, L., Glanz, K. and Lerman, C. (2002) 'Stress, Coping and Health Behaviour', 210–39, in K. Glanz, B. K. Rimer and F. M. Lewis (eds), *Health Behavior and Health Education. Theory, Research and Practice*, 3rd edn. San Francisco: Jossey-Bass.

White, K. (2002) *An Introduction to the Sociology of Health and Illness*. London: Sage.

White K. (2009) *An Introduction to the Sociology of Health and Illness*, 2nd edn. London: Sage.

WHO (2003) *Community-Based Initiatives Series: Community Empowerment for Health and Development*. Cairo: WHO Regional Office for the Mediterranean.

WHO (2009a) 'Obesity', http://www.who.int/topics/obesity/en/ (accessed 4 June 2009).

WHO (2009b) 'BMI/Overweight/Obesity United Kingdom WHO Global InfoBase', http://apps.who.int/infobase/reportviewer.aspx?rptcode=ALL&uncode=826&dm=5&surveycode=101069a11&print=1 (accessed 4 June 2009).

WHO (2009c) 'Obesity and Overweight', http://www.who.int/mediacentre/factsheets/fs311/en/index.html (accessed 4 June 2009).

Wilkinson, D. (2005) 'Is There a Double Standard When It Comes to Dementia Care?', *Journal of Clinical Practice*, 59(suppl. 146), 3–7.

Wilkinson, R. G. (1996) *Unhealthy Societies: The Affliction of Inequality*. London: Routledge.

Wilkinson, S. (2000) 'Commodification Arguments for the Legal Prohibition of Organ Sale', *Health Care Analysis*, 8(2), 189–201.

Williams, R. (1983) 'Concepts of Health: An Analysis of Lay Logic', *Sociology*, 17(2), 185–205.

Williams, S. J. (2003) *Medicine and the Body*. London: Sage.

Wills, J. (2005) 'Community Development in Public Health and Primary Care', in D. Sines, F. Appleby and M. Frost (eds), *Community Health Care Nursing*, 3rd edn. Oxford: Blackwell.

Wilson, D. B., Musham, C. and McLellan (2004) 'From Mothers to Daughters: Transgenerational Food and Diet Communication in an Underserved Group', *Journal of Cultural Diversity*, 11(1), 12–17.

Wilson, P. N. (2002) 'The Expert Patient: Issues and Implications for Community Nurses', *British Journal of Community Nursing*, 7(10), 514–19.

Wilson, T. and Holt, T. (2001) 'Complexity and Clinical Care', *British Medical Journal*, 323, 685–8.

Wilton, T. (2000) *Sexualities in Health and Social Care*. Buckingham: Open University Press.

Wolitski, R. J., Pals, S. L., Kidder, D. P., Courtenay-Quirk, C. and Holtgrave, D. R. (2009) 'The Effects of HIV Stigma on Health, Disclosure of HIV Status, and Risk Behavior of Homeless and Unstably Housed Persons Living with HIV', *AIDS Behavior*, 13, 1222–32.

Wood, A. (1995) 'Capitalism', in T. Honderich (ed.), *The Oxford Companion to Philosophy*. Oxford: Oxford University Press.

Wood, M. J., Brink, P. J. and Kerr, J. C. (2006) *Basic Steps in Planning Nursing Research: From Question to Proposal*. Sudbury, MA and London: Jones and Bartlett.

Woodward, D., Drager, N., Beaglehole, R. and Lipson, D. (2001) 'Globalisation and Health: A Framework for Analysis and Action', *Bulletin of the World Health Organisation*, 79(9), 875–81.

Wooffit, R. (1993) 'Analysing Accounts', in N. Gilbert (ed.), *Researching Social Life*. London: Sage.

Woolf, S. (2004) 'Analysis of Documents and Records', in U. Flick, E. von Kardoff and I. Steinke (eds), *A Companion to Qualitative Research*. London: Sage.

Woolhouse, R. (1995) 'Locke, John (1632–1704)', in T. Honderich (ed.), *The Oxford Companion to Philosophy*. Oxford: Oxford University Press.

Wright, C. (2001) 'Community Nursing: Crossing Boundaries to Promote Health', in A. Scriven and J. Orme (eds), *Health Promotion: Professional Perspectives*, 2nd edn. Basingstoke: Palgrave in association with the Open University.

Wright, C. M., Parker, L., Lamont, D., Craft, A. W. (2001) Implications of Childhood Obesity for Adult Health: Findings from Thousand Families Cohort Study', *British Medical Journal*, 323, I December, 1280–4.

Wyatt, J. (1998) *Matters of Life and Death*. Leicester: IVP.

Yach, D. (2005) 'Globalization and Health: Exploring the Opportunities and Constraints for Health Arising from Globalization', *Globalization and Health*, 1(2), doi:10.1186/1744-8603-1-2, http://www.globalizationandhealth.com/content/1/1/2

Yin, R. (2001) *Case Study Research: Design and Methods*. London: Sage.

Young, R. F. (2002) 'Medical Experiences and Concerns of People with Alzheimer's Disease', in Harris, P. (ed.), *The Person with Alzheimer's Disease*. Baltimore, Maryland: Johns Hopkins University Press.

Zaccagnini, M. (2010) *HIV and AIDS Stigma and Discrimination*. AVERT, http://www.avert.org/hiv-aids-stigma.htm (accessed April 2010).

Zaninotto, P., Wardle, H., Stamatakis, E., Mindell, J. and Head, J. (2006) *Forecasting Obesity to 2010*. London: National Centre for Social Research.

Zarrilli, S. (ed.) (1998) *International Trade in Health Services: A Development Perspective*. Geneva: United Nations and WHO.

Zwakhalen, S. M. G., Hamers, J. P. H. and Berger, M. P. F. (2007) 'Improving the Clinical Usefulness of a Behavioural Pain Scale for Older People with Dementia', *Journal of Advanced Nursing*, 58(5), 493–502.

index

Note: Page numbers in *italics* denotes a
figure/table.

A

abstemious lifestyle 12, 365
access courses 351
Acheson Report (1998) 52, 129
action research 261–2
activities of daily living (ADL) 103
Adams, S. 75
Adamson, J. 180, 328
Adult Learning Grant 351
Age Concern 172
ageism
    and dementia 172–3, 174
agency work 358
Aggarwala, R. T. 42
AIDS *see* HIV/AIDS
Ainsworth, S. 88, 90
Ajzen, I. and Fishbein, M. 111
Alaszewski, A. 296
Alberts, A. 156
alcohol
    and heavy drinking 11–12
Almond, P. 76
Alzheimer's disease (AD) 165, 167, 217–17
    see also dementia
Alzheimer's Society 166, 171
Anderson, J. 162, 274, 277, 326, 334
anthropology 234
anti-retroviral therapy 149, 158
Antonovsky, A. 15
application forms 356
apprenticeships 352

Archibald, C. 167, 169, 181
Aristotle 12, 35
Aronson, J. 326
ARTs (artificial reproductive technologies)
    124–5, 140–7
    biology of process 141–2
    consumer exploitation issue 145–6
    cost of 143
    documentary research case studies
        298–300
    effectiveness of 142–3
    emergence of 141–3
    ethics of 142, 144–7
    funding of 143, 146
    historical overview 140–1
    posthumous use of sperm 144–5
    restriction on access to and rights 146–7
    risks of 142
    and social construction of motherhood
        and fertility 143–4
asceticism 12–13
Association of Graduate Recruiters 353
Augustine, St 12
Ausman, J. I. 53
authenticity
    and research 259
autonomy 55–8, 59, 153, 163
    as a basic need 102–3
    creating 56–7
    and health 17–18, 56–8
    respecting 56, 57, 58
    and rights 117
autonomy flip 57
Avert 149, 164

B

Bacon, Francis 38, 39
bad faith 59
Baggott, R. 77
Bailey, L. 188
Baldwin, C. 178
Bandura, A. 63, 64
Barnett, T. 152
Barratt, H. 56, 57
Bartlett, R. 178
Beauchamp, T. 57
behaviour change 58–67, 68, 111, 123
    and health 59–60
    importance of 59–60
    limitations of as a means of promoting
        health 65–7
    models of 60–4
    value of theory of 64–5
Behuniak, S. M. 179–80
Belsey, C. 50–1
Bentham, Jeremy 93, 116
Berofsky, B. 58
Bevan, Aneurin 341
beyond-the-facts judgements 11–12, 13
Bharat, S. 159
bias 191, 251, 252, 298, 306, 365
Bilton, T. 231
biomedical model 13–15, 17, 18, 20, 22, 40,
        94, 99, 136–7
    critique of 14–15
Birenbaum-Carmeli, D. 143, 144
Black Report (1980) 21, 22, 52
Bloomberg, M. R. 42
body mass index (BMI) 126, 134–5, 136,
        232–3
Boffetta, P. 66–7
Bogart, L. M. 159, 160, 161
Bond, V. 159
Bouma, G. D. 204, 213–14, 270, 314, 318, 321
Bourdieu, Pierre 139
Bovbjerg, V. E. 131, 132, 135, 140
Bowell, T. 26, 27, 28
Bowling, A. 189, 234, 242, 248, 250, 254, 258,
        261, 268, 286, 288, 293, 294–5, 297, 298

bracketing 239
Bradford Dementia Group 178
Bradshaw, J. 101–2, 111
Brannelly, T. 178
Braun, V. and Clark, V. 326
Briggs, K. 180, 273
Brook, D. W. 331
Brotsky, S. R. 273
Brown, C. 119
Brown, H. 112
Brown, Louise 140
Bryman, A. 191, 221, 248, 249, 250, 252–3,
        255, 258, 261, 268, 270–1, 274, 314,
        318, 321, 326
budgetary control
    handing over of to GPs 193
Bullock, A. 36
butterfly effect 68
Bynum, B. 98

C

Campos, P. 136, 138, 139
cancer 25, 87, 96, 196
Cantley, C. 168
capabilities approach 174
capitalism 32–3, 42, 44, 52, 174
    benefits 32–3
    and individualism 33
    nature and features of 32
    negative impact of on health 33
carbon emissions 42
care assistants 345
Care Services Improvement Partnership –
        Older People's Mental Health
        Programme 175
careers/career planning 336–64
    application forms 356
    case studies 348–50
    continuing professional development
        363–4
    emergence of new health-related roles
        346–7
    graduate destinations 344
    and interviews 359–61

job roles 344
pathways 341–2
personal planning 339
planned happenstance approach 338–9
qualifications 350–2
reflective activities 340, 342, 348, 354, 355, 356–7, 360–1
researching prospective employers 356–7
skills rating exercise 355
social care and social work 345–6
sources for finding a job 357–9
SWOT analysis 339–40, *340*, 363
voluntary organisations/charities 347–8
careers advisers 337, 351
careers service 339, 345, 346, 348, 351, 357, 358
college and university 356
Connexions 345, 349
carers
and dementia 165, 180–1
Carryer, J. 134
Carson, Rachel
Silent Spring 40
case-control studies 197–8, *198*
case study research 262–3
Chadwick, Edwin
Report on the Sanitary Conditions of the Labouring Classes 95, 96
Chambers, J. 325, 334
Changing Minds campaign 121
chaos/complexity theory 67–71
and health 70
and healthcare 68, 69–70
and organisational change 69
and unpredictable outcomes 68–9
charities, working for 347–8
Child B 88, 89
children
decline in exercise 129–30
impact of global warming on 42
monitoring weight of 137
and obesity 126, 135–6

Children and Family Court Advisory and Support Service (CAFCASS) 345
Childress, J. 57
China 37, 84–5
choice 59, 66
and fertility treatment 145–6
freedom of 34, 45
see also communitarianism; free will
cholera 10, 194
Choosing Health – Making Healthier Choices Easier (2004) 24, 25, 94, 95
Churchill, L. R. 72
Churchill, Winston 37
Citizen's Juries 106
Clare, L. 182, 275
Clark, J. M. and Hockey, L. 188
Clarke, A. E. 47
Clean Air Act (1956) 53
climate change 41–2
Cochrane Library 288
Cohen, D. 104
cohort studies 197, 198
Coles, T. 134
commodification 71–3, 75
of health 71–2, 139
quest for bodily enhancement 72–3
communitarianism 33–5
criticisms of 35
establishing 34
and health 35–6
nature and features of 33–4
compassion
role of in dementia 179–83
compatibilist/compatibilism 80, 365
complexity theory *see* chaos/complexity theory
Comte, Auguste 227–8
condoms 155
confidence interval (CI) 202–3
confirmability
and research 258
Connexions 345, 349
consultations, medical 69–70
consumer-friendly 76

consumerism 47, 73–7, 139
  benefits 77
  complexities of 75–6
  criticisms of 74–5, 76
  establishing 76
  and healthcare 73–4
content validity 253–4
continuing professional development
  (CPD) 363–4
Cooper, C. 180
coronary artery bypass graft (CABG) 90
Corrigan, P. W. 121
Cottrell, S. 189–90
covert observation 318
Cowley, S. 108
Crabtree, B. F. 263
credibility
  in qualitative research 257–9
Cresswell, J. 221
Creutzfeldt-Jakob disease (CJD) 168
Cribb, A. 56, 67
Crichton, N. 110, 111`
Criminal Record Bureau (CRB) check
  345
critical analysis 26–8, 29, 204
critical realism 224
critical reasoning
  and research 189–90
critical theoretical research 224, 225–6,
  227, 251, 262, 297
cues to action 60–1, 132
Cunningham, C. 167, 169, 181
CV 356, 364

D

Dahlgren, G. 95–6
Darzi Report (2008) 24, 25, 58
data analysis 324–31
  qualitative 325–9
  quantitative 324–5
  using mixed methods 331
Daulaire, N. 83
Davey, B. 232
Davis, W. 91, 137

DDT (dichlorodiphenyltrichloroethane)
  40, 41
de Bont, A. 75
De Lacey, S. 142–3, 145–6, 329, 332,
  333
de Tracy, Destutt 31
death rates *see* mortality rates
Deaton, A. 85
decision learning 356–7
deductive reasoning 248–9, 284, 292
Deech, R. 142, 145
dementia 125, 157, 165–83
  and ageism 172–3, 174
  biomedical definitions 165–6
  carers and caring 165, 180–1
  challenging meanings and responses
    170–1
  costs of care 175–6
  directing and measuring 166
  and ethnographic research 233–4
  forms of 167–8
  funding for research 183
  and healthcare equality and rationing
    174–5, 176
  interview research case study 312
  living with and difficulties faced 176–8
  models of practice 173–4
  and personhood 170, 177–8, 182, 183
  prevalence and demographics 169
  quality and range of care 178, 181–2
  role of compassion 179–83
  and stigma 171–2, 180
  symptoms of 168–9, 176
democracy 35–7
  and ancient Greeks 35
  criticisms of 35
  and health 37
  principles and characteristics 36
dependability
  and research 258
dependent variable 250–1
depression 14, 115
Derrida, Jacques 50
Descartes, René 37, 70, 93, 99, 179

descriptive statistics 325
descriptive study 260
designer babies 141, 145
diaries
    reflective 361–2, 363
    using in research 295
diet
    focus group research on impact of
        mothers on daughters choice of
        303–4
dieting
    and obesity 130–1
discourse analysis 329–30
discrimination 119, 120
    age 172–3
    tackling 121–2
    see also stigma
disease
    and Enlightenment 39, 40
    health as absence of 12, 13, 14, 15, 17,
        22, 25, 71, 94
    impact of social class on 96
diversity 48, 49
documentary research 294–300
    case studies 298–300
    challenges to using and limitations
        297–8, 299, 300
    diary/journal 295
    key qualities of 297
    reasons for using 296
    types of 294–5
    useful resources 298
    working with documents 296
Donovan, J. 180, 328
Dooris, M. 108
DOTS Model 254–9
Doyal, L. 33, 102–3, 105, 162, 274, 277,
    326, 334
drug promotion 74–5
drugs
    controls on spending on 88
Dubin, W. R. 119
Dubos, R. 17, 18
Duncan, P. 56, 57

Dunning, W. 48
Durazo-Arvizu, R. A. 136
Durkheim, Émile 111
Dyson, A. 144

E
Earle, S. 74, 75
Earth Summit (1992) 41
eating disorders
    and virtual communities case study 322–3
EBP see evidence-based practice
Edwards, Robert 140
elderly 86, 222, 342 see also ageism
Ellen, J. M. 328
Employment Equality (Age) Regulations
    (2006) 173
empowerment 77–80, 99
    and communities 78, 79
    and health 78, 80
    implications for work for health 78–9
    limitations and difficulties 79–80
    meaning 77–8
    and needs assessment 108
    and people with mental illness 122
    personal 77
    social/political 77
encephalitis lethargica 16, 365–6
Engeland, A. 136
Enlightenment 37–40, 43, 46, 54, 55, 93,
    99, 115, 228
    criticisms of 39
    guiding principles behind 38
    and health 39
    key attributes of 38
environmentalism 40–3
    anthropocentric 40
    biocentric 40
    criticisms of 41–2
    and health 42–3
    impact of 41
    nature and features 40–1
epidemiology/epidemiological studies 22,
    194–204, 229, 366
    basic statistics 199–203

definition 194
drawing conclusions and making
    recommendations 203–4
and evidence-based practice 194–5,
    231
and heavy drinking 11–12
and HIV/AIDS 148–50
rates 195–7
types of studies 197–9
epistemology 7, 9, 10, 174, 223–4, 366
ethics
    and covert observation 318
    and fertility treatment 142, 144–7
    getting research approval 274–7
    issues to be considered 272–3
    and participant observation 321
    political nature of 274–5
    and RCTs 292–3
    in research 272–7
    'ten commandments' on 276
    useful resources 276–7
    and vulnerability issues 275
ethnography 233–7
    challenging aspects and limitations
        235–6, 237
    HIV case study 236–7
    key qualities of 235
    methods 234
    and participant observation 234, 236–7,
        320
    purpose 234
ethnomethodology 191
Etzioni, E. 34, 35, 93
evaluative study 260–1
Evans, M. 154, 197, 320, 321
evidence-based practice (EBP) 11, 91, 159,
    173, 192–5, 366
    and action research 262
    and beyond-the-facts 11–12, 13
    drivers informing 192
    and epidemiology 194–5, 231
    and health 192
    and healthcare rationing 88–9, 91, 193
    and systematic review 288

exercise 58
    obesity and decline in 129–30
existentialism/existentialist 4, 366
experimental research 261
Expert Patient Programme (EPP) 60, 65
explanatory study 260
exploratory study 259–60

F
face validity 253–4
facts 11, 140, 188, 366
    beyond-the-facts 11–12, 13
Fairbairn, A. 167, 168, 169, 177
Family Interaction Theory (FIT) 307
Feldman, S. 26, 27
female circumcision 48
female sex workers (FSWs) 154–5,
    236–7
feminism/feminist methodology 39, 43–4,
    153, 225–6, 244–7, 273, 309, 334
    case study 247
    and fertility treatment 141, 143–4
    and health 44
    key components 43–4
    purpose and features of 245–6
    useful resources 245
Fenton, S. 114
fertility treatment see ARTs (artificial
    reproductive technologies)
Filiault, S. M. 132, 135
Fink, P. J. 119
flexible working 358
Floyer, Sir John 39
focus groups 262, 300–4
    case study 303–4
    key qualities 302
    limitations 302–3, 304
    practical considerations to take into
        account 301
    useful resources 301
Fontaine, K. R. 136
Forder, J. 174, 175, 285
Foster-Turner, J. 301
Foucault, Michel 48, 49, 111, 139

foundations concept of health 18–21, 58, 153, 170–1

Fox, M. 190, 191, 192, 222, 223, 234, 238, 252–3, 255, 269, 270

Frankel, R. M. 263, 264

free market 31, 44, 366

free will 56, 59, 66, 80–3
  and health 81–3

freedom 31, 35, 36, 44–5, 54, 57, 58, 92, 114 *see also* Enlightenment

Freire, Paulo 78

Furedi, F. 42

G

Gaia theory 40

Gard, M. 138

Garfinkel, H. 191

gastric bypass 133

gatekeepers 280–1

gender 44, 156
  and HIV/AIDS 162
  see also feminism/feminist
    methodology

General Medical Council (GMC) 76

generalisability
  and research 255–7

Gergen, M. and Gergen, K. 238

GHR (waist circumference divided by height) 135

Giles, D. 273

Gilhooly, M. 170, 180

Gill, A. 122

Gill, J. and Johnson, P. 205

Gillam, S. 101, 103, 104, 106, 108

Gimenez, M. E. 95

Glanville, J. 135

global warming 41, 42

globalisation 83–5
  definition 83
  and health 84–5
  and inequalities 84

Goffman, E. 171
  Stigma 118

Goldsmith, Edward 40–1

Gomm, R. 190, 191, 249, 251, 253, 255, 257, 288, 295, 305, 314

'good life' 12–13, 137, 139

Goodman, R. 129

Gough, I. 102–3, 105

Gould, N. 174

government
  priorities 4
  responses to HIV/AIDS 160–1

graduate destinations 344

grand narratives 32, 47, 49, 366

Gray, David 205, 206, 221, 223, 242, 249, 252, 255, 259, 260, 261, 263, 265, 266, 269, 272–3, 286, 306, 313, 318, 320–1, 328–9

Greece, ancient 35

Green, J. 301, 302

Greenhalgh, T. 68, 69

Greenwood, J. 332, 333

grey literature 210–11

Grimmett, C. 137

Grimshaw, A. 111

Guba, E. G. 222, 223

H

Haas, S. 277–8

Hamlin, C. 29

Handsley, S. 79

happenstance approach 338–9

Hardin, R. 36

Harper, S. 234

Harris, J. 56

Harris, M. 201

Harrison, J. 122

Hart, C. 212, 266

Hawthorne Effect 314

health
  as ability to adapt 17–18
  as absence of disease 12, 13, 14, 15, 17, 22, 25, 71, 94
  as an ideal state 15–18
  biomedical model 13–15, 17, 18, 20, 22, 40, 94, 99, 136–7
  commodification of 71–2, 139

concepts of 10–13
as a contested concept 9–30
definition 15–16, 106
foundations concept of 18–21, 58, 153,
   170–1
as the 'good life' 12–13
importance of defining 20–1
key factors influencing 95–6
miasma theory of 10
salutogenic 15
studying 26–9
theories of 13–20
Health Belief Model (HBM) 60–1, 63
health education 22
health equity audit (HEA) 107
health impact assessment (HIA) 106, 107,
   109
health needs assessment (HNA) 106, 107,
   108
health policy documents
  reference to health promotion and public
     health 22, 23–4
Health Professions Council (HPC) 363
health promotion 20, 21–4
  and HIV/AIDS 157, 162–3
  origins 21–2
  reference to in policy documents 22,
    23–4
  work to promote health 25
Health Protection Agency (HPA) 149, 164
health sector, careers in 341, 343, 357
health service, future demands on 342–3
Health Studies courses 336–7
health trainers 65
healthcare rationing 82, 85–92, 123, 137,
   165
  control of expenditure on drugs/
    treatments 88
  and cost of healthcare 86–7
  criticisms of 91–2
  and dementia 175, 176
  by evidence-based practice 88–9, 91, 193
  and five Ds 86
  and IVF 143

by lifestyle 89, 91
and obesity 137–8
by postcode 89–90, 91–2
purpose of and mechanisms for 86–7
by quality adjusted life years (QALYs) 90–1
healthism 45
heart disease 25, 96
Heidegger, Martin 239
Helsinki Declaration 274
Hemingway, Ernest 12
Herceptin 90
HFEA (Human Fertilisation and
   Embryology Authority) 141–2, 147
Hill, Sir Bradford 203, 229, 230
Hills, J. 97
HIV/AIDS 25, 125, 148–64
  anti-retroviral therapy 149, 158
  biomedical discourses 150–2
  conditions and variables for transmission
    153–5
  and disclosing 161–2
  epidemiological perspectives 148–50
  ethnographic research case study 236–7
  government responses 160–1
  groups most affected by 151
  ignorance and misinformation relating to
    121
  interventions and treatments 157–63
  interview research case study on black
    Africans and 311
  main methods of transmission 152–3
  media representation 157, 163
  mother to child transmissions (vertical)
    157–8, 159
  National Guidelines for HIV Testing
    (2008) 160–1
  phenomenology research case study on
    people living with 241–2
  prevalence 149–50, 151–2
  prevention of transmission 155–7, 159
  researching 206–8
  responsibilities and rights 162–3
  social constructivism research case study
    238–9

stigma and tackling of issue 119, 120, 121, 122, 150, 154, 159–60, 161, 162
symbolic interactionism case study on women and 243–4
systematic review on impact of on young people 290
useful resources 164
holistic approach 17, 51, 231
home care
and non-participant observation case study 319–20
Horan, F. 137
Horne, M. 101
Houston, A. M. 108
Huff, J. L. 139
Hughes, A. 154
Human Fertilisation and Embryology Authority *see* HFEA
Human Organ Transplants Act (1989) 72
Human Rights Act 147
Human Tissue Act (2004) 72
humanism 17
Hume, David 93, 114
Hunter, D. J. 108
Hunter, John 39–40
Huntingdon's disease 168
Husserl, Edmund 239
Hussey, R. 97
hypothesis 229–31
testing of 268–9

I

iatrogenesis 14–15, 73, 366
ideology/ideologies 3–4
key 31–54
term of 31
Illich, Ivan 14, 17, 18
incidence data 196–7, 366
independent variable 250–1
individualism 38–9, 46, 52, 92–5, 162, 163
and capitalism 33
and health 94–5
see also liberal individualism
inductive reasoning 248–9

Industrial Revolution 32, 52
inequalities (in health) 84, 95–9, 153
causes of 97
implications for policy and action 97–9
infant mortality rate (IMR) 195–6
inferential statistics 325
informed consent 134, 273–4, 318
Inhorn, M. C. 144
Innes, A. D. 69
Internet, research sources on 210
Interpretative Phenomenological Analysis (IPA) 312, 327
interpretative research 224, 225, 226–7, 260, 334
interpretivism 222–3
interviews 299, 305–12
going for 359–61
qualitative 308–12
case studies 311–12
key qualities of 309–10
limitations 310, 311
purpose of 308
semi-structured 308–9, 311
unstructured 309, 312
structured 305–7
case study 307
key qualities 306
limitations 306, 307
intra-cytoplasmic sperm injection (ICSI) 141
IVF (in vitro fertilisation) *see* ARTs (artificial reproductive technologies)

J

Jackson, D. 274, 277, 334
Jarviluoma, H. 245
jejunoileal bypass 133
Jewell, Paul 3
job centres 359
job websites 358
Johns, C. 190
Jones, E. L. 22
judgements, beyond-the-facts 11–12, 13
justice 35, 117, 366–7

K

Kalish, R. A. 182

Kant, Immanuel 29, 44, 93

Kasprzyk, D. 65

Katz, J. 138

Kemp, G. 26, 27, 28

Kendall, T. 174

Kernick, D. 69

Kitwood, Thomas 170, 174, 175–6, 177, 183

Klein, R. 87, 91, 98, 139

Klunklin, A. 154, 332, 333

Kobau, R. 120

Kuhlmann, E. 74, 76

Kymlicka, W. 45

Kyoto Agreement 41, 42, 367

L

La Fontaine, J. 234

Labonte, R. 85

Labour Market Information 359

Lai, Y. M. 118, 120

laissez-faire approach 32, 57, 367

Lalonde Report (1974) 21, 22

Lambert, H. 154, 320, 321

Laverack, G. 77–8, 79

L-Dopa 16, 367

Le Fanu, J. 58

Learner Support Funds 351

learning disabilities
  and normalisation 112, 113

Ledger, W. 143, 331–2

Lee, S. H. 161

Leedy, P. D. 188

Leonard, L. 328

Lewis, J. and Ritchie, J. 253, 254

lewy body dementia (DLB) 167

liberal individualism/liberalism 13, 44–6,
    98, 153
  features of 44
  and health 45–6
  and liberty 44–5
  problems with 45

liberty 44–5
  negative and positive 45

life expectancy 87, 97, 110

lifestyle, rationing by 89, 91

Lincoln, Y. S. 222

Ling, R. 204, 213–14, 270, 313, 314, 318, 321

Liss, P. E. 104, 105, 106, 147

literature review 263–7, 296
  basic elements 266
  purpose and role of 263–5, 266–7
  skills involved in writing 265
  triangle 266–7, 267
  useful resources for writing 267

literature search 209–11, 263–5

Lloyd, L. 74

Locke, John 11, 44, 56, 93, 114

Loewy, E. H. 86

Lomborg, B. 41

Loughlin, M. 82

Lovelock, James 40

Lowe, C. R. 22, 66

lung cancer
  and smoking 49, 58, 229–30, 231

Lupton, D. 72–3

M

MacDonald, K. 295, 296

McKeith, I. 167, 168, 169, 177

McKeown, T. 22, 66

McKibben, B. 41

MacRae, H. 177, 180, 216–17, 220

managed care organisations (MCOs) 72

Mansfield, K. 17, 18

Manson, J. E. 199, 232–3

Marantz, P. 82

Marks, V. 26, 27

Marmot, M. 97, 98–9

Marx, Karl 31, 367

Marxism 47, 52, 71

Matthews, B. 222, 223–4, 234, 258, 259,
    260, 268, 295, 298, 303, 326, 329

Maynard, M. 50

means 202–3

medians 202

menopause 75

mental health/illness 25, 100

Changing Minds campaign 121
  need for increased public awareness of
    120–1
  and normalisation 112, 113
  and stigma 119–20, 121–2
Mental Health Foundation 171, 172
methodology 225
miasma theory 10
migration 83–4
Mill, John Stuart 55–6, 81, 93
Miller, W. L. 69, 263
Milne, A. 171, 172
mind-body dualism 93, 99–100, 170
Mini-Mental State Examination (MMSE)
    166
mixed method research 234, 261, 283,
    299–300, 367
  analalysing 331
modernism/modernity 38, 46–7, 49
  criticisms of 46
  and health 46–7
Montaño, D. E. 65
Moore, L. and Davis, B. 178
Moore, W.
  The Knife Man 39–40
morality 367
  and rights 116–17
morbidity rates 195
mortality
  and BMI (case study) 232–3
  and obesity 127
mortality rates 66, 96, 195
  age standardised 196
  infant 195–6
  and standardised mortality ratios 196–7
  world standardised 196
motherhood 143–4
Mulhall, A. 110, 111
Myers, D. G. 33, 35

N

Naidoo, J. 22
NAM 164
narrative analysis 328–9

National Child Measurement Programme
    (NCMP) 137
National Dementia Strategy 171, 176, 177,
    181
National Institute for Health and Clinical
    Excellence *see* NICE
National Institute for Health Research
    (NIHR) 189
National Institute for Mental Health in
    England (NIMHE) 121–2
National Service Framework (NSF) for
    Mental Health 121
National Skills Academy for Social Care
    (NSA) 345
natural capacity 103–4
Navarro, V. 33
Nazi Germany 45, 46, 83
needs (needs assessment) 98, 101–9, 113
  assessment of 106–8, 109
  autonomy as basic 102–3
  Bradshaw's taxonomy of 101–2, 111
  definition 101–2
  and fertility treatment 143, 147
  health 103–4
  healthcare 104, 106
  and life plans 102
  and notion of goal 104–5, 106, 108
  other concepts of 104–5
  physical survival/physical health as basic
    102
  population 108–9
  social 103
neo-classical economics 73, 367
networking 358
neural tube defects (NTD) 199, 200
neutrality
  and research 191, 367
Newcomb, P. A. 126
Newman, C. 157
Newman, J. 74, 75, 76
Newton, Sir Isaac 37–8
  Principia Mathematica 67
NHS (National Health Service) 87, 341–2
  career opportunities 343, 357

key dates of medical breakthroughs and policy changes 341–2
NHS Direct 76, 165
NICE (National Institute for Health and Clinical Excellence) 64, 88
report (2007) 59, 66
NIHR (National Institute for Health Research) 189
NIMHE (National Institute for Mental Health in England) 121–2
Noble, T. 228
non-governmental organisations (NGOs) 347
non-participant observation 319–20
non-probability sampling 279
Nordenfelt, L. 134
normal 109–10
normalisation 111
and health 112–13
normative 111, 118
norms 109–12, 113, 118
social 111–12
statistical 109–10
null hypothesis 231

O

Obama, Barack 53, 87
obesity 25, 42, 97, 124, 125–40, 137, 212
and Body Mass Index (BMI) 126, 134–5, 136
as child abuse 137
and children 126, 135–6
critique of as health concern 134–7
definition 126
and dieting 131
economic costs 126
feminist research into mothers of obese children 247
health problems linked with 127
and healthcare rationing 89, 137–8
measurement of 126, 135
medical treatment 133–4
and mortality 127
and physical activity 131–2

and population surveillance 137
prevalence and distribution 126–7, 134–6
reasons for 127–30, *128*
risk-factor questionnaire case study 287–8
and shifts in consumption habits 128–9
and shifts in energy expenditure 129–30
social constructions of 138–9
solutions to 130–4
stigma of 66
systematic review on older people and 291
waist measurement and waist to hip ratio 135
objectivity 191, 367–80
observation 313–23
case studies 315, 319–20, 322–3
covert 318
limitations 313–14
non-participant 319–20
participant 234, 236–7, 313, 320–3
qualitative 313, 316–18
structured 313, 314–16
O'Connor, D. 178
octuplets, birth of 146
odds ratios 200
Ogden, J. 50, 51, 66
Olapegba, P. O. 120, 121
Ollila, E. 85
'one-model fits all' approach 48
O'Neill, B. 42
ontology 221–3, 368
opportunity awareness 356
Orbach, S. 139
organ transplant 72
organisational change
and chaos/complexity theory 69
Ottawa Charter 78
ovarian hyperstimulation syndrome (OHSS) 142
ozone layer 41

P

Pain Assessment Checklist for Seniors with Limited Ability to Communicate (PACSLAC) 315–16

Palmlund, I. 75
Paoli, F. 154
paradigms 188, 368
    definition 221
    research 221–47
part-time work 364
participant observation 313, 320–3
    and ethnography 234, 236–7, 320
paternalism 58
patient choice 74, 75
patient, public involvement (PPI) 76
Paton, M. Q. 5
patriarchal/patriarchalism 44, 144, 368
Pawson, R. 114
Pennell, L. 33
person, definition 11
person-centred theory 177, 180
personhood
    and dementia 170, 177–8, 182, 183
Persson, A. 157
pesticides 40, 41
phenomenology 239–42, 297, 309
    case study 241–2
    challenging aspects and limitations
        240–1, 242
    key qualities of 240
Philippson, P. 50,51
Phillips, C. V. 51
physical activity
    and obesity 131–2
Pick's disease 168
Pickstone, J. V. 22
pilot research 282–3
Pitt, B. 74
placebo effect 199
planned behaviour, theory of (TPB) 61,
    287
plastic surgery 72–3
Plato 35
Plsek, P. E. 68, 69
pluralism 113
Popper, Karl 229, 230–1
population need 108–9
Porteous, M. 91, 137

Porter, R. 40
positivism/positivity 193, 222, 223, 225,
    227–33, 251–2, 284, 297, 334
    case study 232–3
    challenging aspects 229
    criticisms of 231–2
    and health-related research 229–31
    key qualities of research 228–9
    main principles of 228
post traumatic stress disorder 51
postal questionnaires 286, 305
postcode rationing 89–90, 91–2
postgraduate study 351, 364
postmodernism 39, 47–9, 113, 114
    criticisms of 48
    features of 47–8
    and health 48–9
poststructuralism 49–52
    criticisms of 50–1
    and health 51–2
poverty 10, 97
practitioner research 190, 368
pre-eclampsia 142, 368
pre-implantation genetic diagnosis (PGD)
    141, 145
prevalence data 196–7, 368
Prevention and Health (1977) 94
privatisation
    and healthcare 84–5
probability sampling 278–9
Prochaska, J. O. 62
professional bodies, joining 359
proportions 202–3, 368
prospective employers, researching
    356–7
Prospects website 358
public health 368–9
    documents 23–4
    policy 21–2
    and socialism 53
    see also health promotion
Public Service Agreements 98
Pulsford, D. 181–2
p-value 200–2

Q

qualifications (for working in healthcare)
    350–2
qualitative data analysis 325–9
  case studies 327, 330
  discourse analysis 329–30
  key resources 326
  narrative analysis 328–9
  qualities of 325–6
  thematic analysis 326–7
qualitative interviews 308–12
qualitative observations 313, 316–18
qualitative research 258–9, 282, 369
  credibility in 257–9
  features 282
  presenting and writing up of data 332–3
  and representativeness 257
  and research question 270–1
  and sampling 279
  trialling 283
  and validity 254–5
quality adjusted life years (QALYs),
    rationing by 90–1
quantitative data analysis 324–5
  descriptive statistics 325
  inferential statistics 325
  key qualities 324
  useful resources 325
quantitative research 282–3, 369
  features 282
  generalisations in 257
  piloting 282–3
  presenting and writing up of data
    331–2
  and sampling 278–9
questionnaires 284–8
  case study 287–8
  challenging elements and limitations
    285, 286, 287–8
  face-to-face 284–5, 286, 305
  key qualities of 286, 306
  online skills 355
  postal 286, 305
  purpose of 284
  useful resources 287
Quigley, R. 106

R

Radin, M. 71
random sampling 278–9
randomised control trials *see* RCTs
rapid appraisal
  and needs assessment 106, 107–8
rates 195–6
  standardisation of 196
rationalism 38
rationing of healthcare *see* healthcare
    rationing
RCTs (randomised control trials) 173, 193,
    197, 198–9, *198*, 288, 289, 292–4, 369
  case study 293–4
  and ethics 292–3
  limitations of 292–3, 294
  and systematic review 288, 289
reading 28–9
realism 224
reasoned action, theory of (TRA) 60, 61,
    111
reductionism/reductionist 67, 70, 99, 231,
    369
Redwood, H. 87, 89, 91–2
reflective activities, overview 5
reflective journal/diary 361–2, 363
reflective practice 361–2
reflexivity
  and research process 191–2, 215–16,
    218–19
Reid, John 143
relative risk 199–200, 203
relativism 11, 48, 50, 113–15
  criticisms of 114
  and health 114–15
reliability
  and research 251–2
representativeness 257, 296, 369
reproductive life cycle 44
research 185–335
  accessing the field process 280–1

core principles informing 220–81
credibility in qualitative 257–9
critical approaches to 225–6
and critical reasoning 189–90
data analysis 324–31
deductive and inductive reasoning 248–9
design of 259–63
and epidemiology study 194–204
ethics in 272–7
and evidence-based practice (EBP) 192–5
and generalisability 255–7
generating ideas 206
implications for practice/knowledge 334
interpretative 224, 225, 226–7, 260, 334
key characteristics of 189
limitations of your 333–4
and literature review 263–7, 296
meaning of 188–9
methods of 282–324
models of process of 204–5
motivation for 214–15
narrowing down 213–20
paradigms 221–47
and personal location 214–16
presenting and writing up of 331–5
purpose 214, 220
and reflexivity 191–2, 215–16, 218–19
and reliability 251–2
role of in healthcare 189
sampling in 257, 277–80
searching and reading around the topic 209–13
and self-reflection 215–16
source materials 210–11, 212
starting of 206–9
useful resources 187
and validity 252–5
and variables 250–1
research question 267–72, 278
responsibilities 33–4, 115–18
Rhodes, T. 156
Ridge, D. 151
rights 33–4, 37, 115–18

and autonomy 117
and fertility treatment 147
foundation of 116
and HIV/AIDS 162–3
and liberal individualism 44
limits of 118
moral context of 116–17
relationship between responsibilities and 116
social context of 116
rigour
and qualitative research 258
risk/risk ratios 199–200, 202, 203
Ritchie, C. 193
Robson, C. 251, 253, 313, 315, 328
Rogers, Anne Marie 90
Romanticism 38, 369
Rosenhan, D. L. 120
Ross, L. 222, 223–4, 234, 258, 259, 260, 268, 295, 298, 303, 326, 329
Rousseau, Jacques 38
Royal College of Psychiatrists 121
Ruger, J. P. 37
Ryan, T. J. 293

S
Sacks, Oliver 16, 17, 72
Sadiq-Sangster, A. 114
salutogenic health 15
same-sex parenting
and discourse analysis case study 330
sampling 257, 277–80, 369–70
issues to consider when selecting your sample 280
non-probability/purposive 279
probability/random 278–9
reasons for using 278
and target population 277–8
useful resources 280
Sanchez-Jankowski, M. 318
Sandelowski, M. 143, 145
Sarantakos, S. 191, 224, 234, 242–3, 276, 279, 280, 295
SARS 83

Sartorius, N. 121
Sartre, Jean-Paul 59, 81
Saving Lives – Our Healthier Nation (1999) 23
saviour babies 141, 145
Scambler, G. 154
schizophrenia 121
Scholes, S. 136
school meals, deregulation of 129
Schrecker, T. 85, 94
Schrimshaw, E. W. 161
sector skills councils (SSC) 359
Seedhouse, David 11, 14, 18–21, 28, 56, 57, 66, 71, 100, 104, 105, 147, 153, 170–1
    Health: The Foundations for Achievement 18–21
Siegal, K. 161
self-awareness 93, 354–5, 354, 361
self-efficacy 60, 61, 63–4, 65, 82
self-reflection
    and research process 215–16
semi-structured interviews 308–9, 311
Sen, Amartya 45
Sheaff, R. 103–4
Shefer, T. 154, 332–3
Sheon, N. 161
Sherr, L. 159, 161
Shircore, R. 42
Shiu, M. 82
Shoff, S. M. 126
short-term contracts 358
Silverman, D. 191, 272, 294, 296, 310
Sipos, A. 56, 57
skills development 353–64
    identifying your strengths and weaknesses through DOTS Model 254–9
    key transferable skills 353
Skills for Health 350, 359
slavery 83
Smajdor, A. 142, 145
small and medium-sized enterprises (SMEs) 357–8
SMART acronym 362–3

Smith, Adam 32
Smith, L. 293
smoking 68, 89, 105, 199
    ban on 45
    cost per QALY for cessation of 90
    and lung cancer 49, 58, 229–30, 231
    and Transtheoretical Model of Change 62
Snape, D. 191
Snow, John 194
'so what factor' 218, 260
social capital 97, 370
social care career/jobs 337, 341, 343, 345–6, 357–8
social class
    effect of on death and illness 96
Social Cognition Theory (SCT) 63
social construction/constructivism 6, 49–52, 54, 100, 143, 222, 223, 238–9, 370
    case study 238–9
    criticisms of 50–1
    and health 51–2
    of motherhood and fertility 143–4
    of obesity 138–9
social norms 111–12
social work careers 345
socialism 52–4
    criticisms of 53
    and health(care) 53–4
    principles of 52–3
SODT (self awareness, opportunity awareness, decision- making and transition learning) 354–7
Sonagachi STD/HIV Prevention Project (SHIP) 236–7
source materials
    and research 210–11, 212
Speedy, J. 238, 246
Spencer, L. 191
Spicker, S. F. 98
Spriggs, M. 144
standardised mortality ratios (SMRs) 196–7

STAR technique 360–1
statistical norms 109–10
statistics
    descriptive 325
    inferential 325
Steele, T. 73
Steptoe, Patrick 140
stigma 48, 118–23, 125
    definition 118–19
    and dementia 171–2, 180
    and HIV/AIDS 119, 120, 121, 122, 150,
        154, 159–60, 161, 162
    and mental health 119–20, 121–2
    and shame 119
    tackling of 120–3
Stilwell, Barbara 20–1
storytelling 328
Strawson, Peter 81
structuralism 49
structured interviews 305–7
studying health 26
Stylites, St Simeon 12
subjectivity 61, 94, 231, 236, 370
Sudnow, D. 182
suffrage movement 43
surveys 284, 287 *see also* questionnaires
Sutcliffe, A. 39
Swanson, V. 325, 334
Sweeting, H. 170, 180
Swindon Primary Care Trust 90
SWOT analysis 26, 339–40, *340*, 363
symbolic interactionism 171, 242–4, 332
    case study 243–4
    definition 242
    key qualities 243
    useful resources 243
Syrett, K. 86
systematic reviews 173, 192, 197, 288–91, 296
    case studies 290–1
    challenging aspects and limitations 289,
        290, 291
    key qualities 288–9
    purpose of 288
    useful resources 289

T
target population 277–8
Taylor, G. 201
Taylor, S. 51, 52
Tee, S. 79
ten Have, Henck 81
Terrence Higgins Trust 163, 164
text, engaging with 4
Thatcher, Margaret 73–4
thematic analysis 326–7
Theory of Planned Behaviour (TPB) 61
Theory of Reasoned Action (TRA) 60, 61,
    111
third sector organisations 357–8
Thirlaway, K. 61, 63, 66
Thomas, D. 112
Throsby, K. 146
Tipton, C. 295, 296
Tolson, D. 166, 181
Trade-Related Aspects of Intellectual
        Property Rights (TRIPS) 85
transferability
    and qualitative research 258
transferable skills 353
transition learning 357
transparency of research 258, 370
transplant treatment, and rationing 89
Transtheoretical Model of Change 60,
    61–3
trialling 283
triangulation/triangulated 234, 283, 370
Tudor, K. 113

U
United States 85
    healthcare system 53, 72, 87
    and HIV testing 161
unstructured interviews 309
Upton, D. 61, 63, 66

V
validity
    face and content 253–4
    internal and external 253

qualitative approaches to 254–5
and questionnaires 284, 285
values
and evidence 11–13
Van Balen, F. 143, 144, 146
variables
and research 250–1
vascular dementia 167–8
vertical banded gastroplasty 133
Vidler, E. 75
Virchow, Rudolf 98
Vitali, S. 193
voluntary organisations, working for 347–8
voluntary work 352, 358–9, 364
vulnerability issue
and research 275

W
waist to hip ratio (WHR) 135
wait measurement 135
Waller, B. N. 56, 81, 82
Walliman, N. 188–9, 206, 221, 251
Walton, D. 27
Wanless Report (2004) 23–4, 58
Warnock, Mary 34, 50, 59, 81, 114, 116, 117
Warnock Report 141
Waterman, H. 262
Weale, A. 87, 88
wealth gap
and health gap 97
web resources
and career development 358
weight
and health (case study) 232–3
monitoring of children's 137

obsession with 136
see also obesity
weight loss, RCT case study 293–4
well-being 12, 49, 370
Western/scientific theory of health see
biomedical model
White, K. 44, 71, 72
Whitehead, M. 95–6
Whiteside, A. 152
Who Cares? 168
Wilberforce, William 38
Wilkinson, S. 97, 171, 172, 174
Williams, R. 16, 17
Williams, S. J. 99, 100
Wills, J. 22
Wilton, T. 155
Wolitski, R. J. 160
Wollstonecraft, Mary 39, 43
women
and Enlightenment 39
see also feminism
Wood, M. J. and Kerr, J. C. 188
Woods, H. 112
work experience 343
World Health Organisation (WHO) 15–16,
126, 132, 164
World Psychiatric Association 121
Wright, C. 136
Wright, J. 138

Z
Zaccagnini, M. 122
Zarrilli, S. 84
Zwakhalen, S. M. G. 166, 176, 275, 283,
315, 331, 334

Lightning Source UK Ltd.
Milton Keynes UK
UKHW02f1349121117

312601UK00006B/417/P